Symptom Relief in Palliative Care

D1408840

Mervyn Dean
Palliative Care Physician
Western Memorial Hospital
Corner Brook, NL, Canada

Juan-Diego Harris
Director, Palliative Care Medicine
Roswell Park Cancer Institute
Buffalo, NY, USA

with

Claud Regnard
Consultant in Palliative Medicine
St Oswald's Hospice
Newcastle upon Tyne, UK

Jo Hockley
Clinical Nurse Specialist in Palliative Care
St Columba's Hospice
Edinburgh, UK

Radcliffe Publishing
Oxford • Seattle

Radcliffe Publishing Ltd
18 Marcham Road
Abingdon
Oxon OX14 1AA
United Kingdom

www.radcliffe-oxford.com
Electronic catalogue and worldwide online ordering facility.

British Library Cataloguing in Publication Data

A catalogue record for this book is available from the British Library.

ISBN 1 85775 629 0

Typeset by Anne Joshua & Associates, Oxford, UK
Printed and bound by TJ International Ltd, Padstow, Cornwall, UK

Contents

Foreword

In recent years, the need for expertise in palliative and end-of-life care has been increasingly recognized by health care providers, educators in health care disciplines, as well as by those who are affected by life-limiting illness.

One of the challenges in meeting this need for expertise is to increase the skill and confidence of practicing and training health care professionals in providing palliative care. Resources must be available reflecting the latest developments in symptom management, and addressing complex issues such as communication, decision making, and ethical dilemmas that arise. The majority of practicing clinicians have not had specific training in palliative and end-of-life care, and those currently in training have many competing demands for their time dedicated to learning.

Symptom Relief in Palliative Care very effectively fills an important role as an exceptional resource for health care professionals who wish to improve their knowledge of palliative and end-of-life care. It achieves what clinical reference texts strive towards, in successfully balancing a thorough, comprehensive content with a presentation that remains succinct, clinically relevant, and applicable to the common day-to-day challenges facing clinicians caring for the dying. The material is evidence based and remarkably thoroughly referenced, reflecting the high degree of academic rigueur that forms the foundation for the information presented.

The arrangement of topics and the consistent approach to the presentation of each chapter enables the reader to efficiently find relevant material. The content is very well organized and the information flows from the pages in an intuitive and accessible manner.

When clinicians are asked what their education needs are in palliative and end-of-life care, the response is often for information on pain management, communication issues, and ethical challenges. As is the case with the content throughout the text, these topics are very well addressed in *Symptom Relief in Palliative Care*.

The topic of pain management is covered comprehensively yet pragmatically, with information that can be readily applied to an immediate clinical situation. The importance of a detailed and knowledgeable assessment of pain is emphasized, and the reader is guided through the needed steps to evaluate and treat the various types of pain that can arise in palliative care.

The sections addressing communication issues will be a welcome resource to the health care team, for whom end-of-life discussions with patients and their families can seem daunting. Health care providers, as with society in general, often approach conversations on death and dying with trepidation. The guidance and advice in *Symptom Relief in Palliative Care* will be very helpful for clinicians, who often feel that neither clinical training nor life circumstances have provided adequate experience to feel confident in such situations.

Similarly, the material on decision making provides a framework for one of the most common tasks in palliative care yet one for which clinicians are generally ill-prepared: how to address the various choices that may arise for consideration, using an approach based on ethical principles through goal-oriented discussions with patients and families. When a palliative approach is chosen, the obligation to ensure ongoing provision of active and attentive care focused on comfort is emphasized.

The specific attention paid to the issues of competency as well as cardio-pulmonary resuscitation is particularly helpful. The highlighting of these topics reflects an awareness and recognition of the realities of clinical practice in palliative care. It is refreshing to see *Symptom Relief in Palliative Care* address such challenging issues with a practical approach that will guide clinicians in thoughtful and realistic discussions about care options.

The unique manner in which this text took shape – through presentation of chapters to peers on an international palliative care electronic mail discussion list – has contributed to a rich content, dense with useful information. The experience of the authors is evident in the style and overall feel of the material; one almost feels to be in the same room with them, receiving clinical pearls based on years of experience and a thorough knowledge of the literature.

Symptom Relief in Palliative Care is a comprehensive and practical resource, providing authoritative and accessible information for clinicians providing palliative and end-of-life care.

Mike Harlos MD, CCFP, FCFP
Professor, Faculty of Medicine, University of Manitoba
Medical Director, Palliative Care, Winnipeg Regional Health Authority
September 2005

Preface

This guide deals with the management of patients with advanced disease. Its foundation is a clinical decision approach based on what the patient has to tell us. It is our clear intention that the patient's information should guide the professional to appropriate management, rather than prescribe a specific approach. This provides a clearer framework and leaves the choice of route to the individual patient and professional. We are offering a map for guidance, not a route march! There is also no intention of providing a comprehensive palliative care text since there are many excellent examples available today. This guide is not written to be read cover-to-cover, but is intended as a bedside aid, to be consulted when you feel you need additional help and advice.

The practice of palliative care varies widely. Routes for administering medications as well as the variety of medications used may be significantly different when comparing a small rural hospice to a large urban hospice or to a university hospital-based palliative care unit. This book tries to provide information that is relevant to all practices but invariably some information may be omitted. Many people have helped us with this book, but any omissions are ours, not theirs. If you find an error, please let us know via the publisher.

We sincerely hope that it will guide professionals in a wide cross-section of caring environments involved in palliating advanced disease.

MD, Corner Brook, NL
JDH, Buffalo, NY
September 2005

Acknowledgments

Besides the continuing support of Claud Regnard, many people have helped with the editing of this Guide for the Canadian and US Health Systems. We especially wish to thank Karen Power, staff pharmacist at Western Memorial Regional Hospital (WMRH) Corner Brook, NL, for her invaluable, always cheerful, help with many questions about drugs in Canada. She became very used to the 'Monday morning questions'. Equally helpful was William Tompkins, RPH, from Pine Pharmacy in Niagara Falls, USA, who gave us his invaluable time and effort to provide information regarding medications that are only available in the US as compound formulations. Dr Robert Milch, medical director of the Center of Hospice and Palliative Care in Buffalo, NY, provided valuable information regarding specific details dealing with medications and routes of delivery in the US hospice setting. Carla Wells, also from WMRH, provided much useful information on wound dressing products, for which we are very grateful. Regarding ethical and legal issues, we wish to thank two members of the Canadian Medical Association (CMA): Dr Jeff Blackmer, Chair of the CMA Ethics Committee, and Judith Bedford-Jones of the CMA legal department. Both were very generous and thorough in responding to our queries. The ethical content pertaining to the US is a summation of the experience of one of us (JDH) at the Montefiore Medical Centre in the Bronx, especially the knowledge and advice imparted by Linda Farber Post JD, BSN, MA, bioethicist for the palliative care program. Dr Trish Feener, staff pediatrician at the WMRH also helped with some uncertainties about some aspects of Canadian pediatric practice as did Dr Hal Siden of Canuck Place, Vancouver. US pediatric content is a distillation from the experience of working at Memorial Sloan-Kettering, and Roswell Park Cancer Institute, and we would like to thank the staff at those institutes. Dr Mike Grabka in Corner Brook, NL provided advice, including a practical demonstration, on silicone materials for dressings.

We are indebted to the following colleagues who kept us on the right track and so kindly gave us their time and advice. We are particularly grateful to those colleagues who helped to co-write specific sections: Justin Amery, Susie Lapwood and Renee McCulloch for the sections relevant to children; Lynn Gibson and Dorothy Matthews for sections on issues around resuscitation and decisions around competency; Bryan Vernon for the section on making ethical choices; and Carmel Copeland for drug interactions in the drug information section. Thanks also go to Andrew Wilcock and Ben Zylicz who gave permission for the palliative medicine mailbase to be the site for the on-line writing of the Guide. We are also grateful to the following colleagues who gave us helpful advice and suggestions on the text: Chris Baxter, Doug Bridges, David Cameron, Sarah Charlesworth, Michael Cushen, Carol Davis, Frank Formby, Brother Francis, Margaret Gibbs, Mike Harlos, Andrew Hughes, Janet Jackson, Jeremy Keen, Marianne Klee, Andre Knols, Paul McIntyre, Kathryn Mannix, Stephen Mason, Sue Miller, Sandra Nesbitt, Tessa Nicoll, Doiminic Ö Branningaín, David Oliver, Christel Pakarinen, Eileen Palmer, Trevor Rimmer, Peter Robson, Claire Sinnott, Steve Tuplin, Martin Weber, Margaret Whipp and Roger Woodruff.

Finally, Gillian Nineham and Jamie Etherington of Radcliffe Publishing have also been encouraging, helpful and refrained from pressuring us to meet the deadlines we frequently revised. If we have left anyone out, we apologize. We are grateful to you all.

List of abbreviations

AB ratio	ankle/brachial ratio
ACE inhibitor	angiotensin-converting enzyme inhibitor
ACh_m	acetylcholine
ADH secretion	antidiuretic hormone secretion
AIDS	acquired immune deficiency syndrome
ALS	amyotrophic lateral sclerosis
AND	Allow a Natural Death
AV block	atrioventricular block
β blockers	beta blockers
BP	blood pressure
CADS	cancer-associated dyspepsia syndrome
CAT scan	computerized (axial) tomography
CBT	cognitive behavioural therapy
CCB	calcium channel blockers
CD	clinical decision
CETS	Containment, Exercise, Truncal massage, Skin care
Ch	chewable
CMV	cytomegalovirus
CNS	central nervous system
COPD	chronic obstructive pulmonary disease
CPDP	Care Pathway for the Dying Patient
CSCI	continuous subcutaneous infusion
CVA	cerebrovascular accident
D	dispersible
DIC	disseminated intravascular coagulation
DM	dextromethorphan
DNR	Do Not Resuscitate
DSM-IV	Diagnostic and Statistical Manual
eBNF	electronic British National Formulary
ECG	electrocardiogram
ENT	ear, nose and throat
EPA	(fatty acid) eicosapentaenoic acid
5HT	5-hydroxytryptamine
g/dl	grams/deciliter
g/l	grams/liter
GABA	gamma aminobutyric acid
GERD	gasto-esophageal reflux disease
GI	gastrointestinal
Gy	gray (SI unit)
HAD scale	Hospital Anxiety and Depression scale
Hb	haemoglobin
IADH	inappropriate anti-diuretic hormone
IC pressure	intracranial pressure
IgM	immunoglobulin A
IM	intramuscular
Inj	injection
INR	international normalized ratio
IPP	intermittent positive pressure

ir	immediate release
IU	international unit
IV	intravenous
IVC	inferior vena cava
IVCO	inferior vena caval obstruction
K+	potassium ions
LA	local anesthetic
LAMS	Lambert–Eaton myesthenic syndrome
mcg	microgram
ME	medical examiner
mg	milligram
Mg++	magnesium ions
mm/hg	millimeter mercury (pressure)
mmol/l	millimoles per liter (concentration)
MND	motor neuron disease
mr	modified release
MRI	magnetic resonance imaging
MST	(slow release) morphine sulphate
N_2O	nitrous oxide
NG tube	nasogastric tube
NIV	non-invasive ventilation
NSAIDs	non-steroidal anti-inflammatory drugs
O_2	oxygen
OPT	oral to pharyngeal transit time
P	powder
PCA	patient controlled analgesia
PD	peritoneal dialysis
PEG	percutaneous gastrostomy
pH	degrees of acidity/alkalinity
PPI	proton pump inhibitor
PQRST	Precipitating factors; Quality; Radiation; Site and severity; Timing
PRN	breakthrough dose
qid	four times daily
S_aO_2	oxygen saturation
SC	subcutaneous injection
SIADH	syndrome of inappropriate antidiuretic hormone
SL	sublingual
SNRI	serotonin and norepinephrine reuptake inhibitors
soln	solution
sr	sustained release
SSRIs	selective serotonin reuptake inhibitors
supps	suppositories
susp	suspension
SVC	superior vena cava
SVCO	superior vena caval obstruction
T	tablet
TB	tuberculosis
TC	tricyclic
TD	transdermal
TENS	transcutaneous electrical nerve stimulation
U	units
UTI	urinary tract infection
Uv	ultraviolet
ViPoma	(tumor secreting) vasoactive intestinal peptide
WPC	Warn Pause Check approach

Introduction

The consequences of advanced disease

Life-threatening, progressing disease is a creeping crisis that affects patients, partners and carers alike. The time of diagnosis is a bereavement that faces them with multiple losses. Although some people will grow from the experience, it remains distressing for all.

The distress of the patient

Patients already have to face the loss of their future life and to this has to be added any loss of function as they become more ill. Everyday activities can become a source of distress and irritation. This may require so much effort that sleep, appetite and concentration are affected, leaving the individual physically and emotionally drained. Activities which once gave life meaning and purpose are curtailed, reduced or abandoned. Suffering alters social interactions, reducing an individual's ability or desire to communicate with others, causing that individual to become dissociated from life around them. Valued relationships suffer and may be lost. One woman explained:[1]

> 'I've come to hate the way I am towards my grandchildren. I love them to bits, I love to see them, but then I just couldn't be bothered with them. I'd get tired easily because of the pain and I didn't have the energy or patience left for them, and I'd be short. I'd never been like that. Their mother stopped bringing them to the house. Now when they visit they treat me like a stranger. It saddens me to think how they will remember me.'

These losses make patients question their situation:

- Why has this happened to me?
- What is it all about?
- What next?

How a person copes, and is helped to cope, with these big questions will have an impact on their distress, whatever its cause.

The distress of the partners and family

Carers also suffer losses. They try to be understanding, but often feel 'shut out' by the patient. Used to facing difficulties together, carers find it difficult to reach the patient, producing a feeling of powerlessness. Guilt and anger and a sense of injustice are particularly common in parents and siblings confronted with the reality of outliving a dying child or young adult.

Unprepared for their new role, carers learn by trial and error. Not surprisingly, they question their skills and may even question whether they were responsible for the patient's present suffering. They have little time for relaxation, reflection or for thinking about the future. In long-term illnesses such as slowly progressive degenerative neurological disease carers have the additional burden of managing even the most basic daily needs over many months or years:

> 'I used to love the evenings together when the house would be locked up, and we would curl up to watch a film. We can't really do that now, it's difficult to relax, it's always on our mind that they'll be coming to get him ready and put him to bed.'[1]

The distress of the professional carers

The sense of isolation in patients and carers is reflected in professionals. They are faced with multiple physical, psychological, spiritual and social issues and yet often have had little or no training in managing these problems. This sense of loss can cloud judgement so that sensible, caring professionals can make illogical and inappropriate decisions. The consequence is unrelieved distress. Unrelieved pain persists and surveys have shown that severe pain remains unrelieved in over half of cancer patients,[2] and over 60% of AIDS patients.[3,4]

Is there a solution?

Such distress seems insurmountable. But palliative care is now well established as an effective means of managing such distress. It cannot remove all distress, but people can be helped to shift their focus of hope and cope with their losses. It provides a path through the distress and confusion that helps the patient (adult or child), partner, family and professional achieve a worthwhile quality of life.

Sharing the consequences of advanced disease

Pain and other symptoms often cause psychological distress. Initially, anxiety or a low mood results, but these usually settle rapidly if the symptom is relieved. If, however, the symptom persists or there are fears and unresolved issues concerning the disease, relationships, beliefs, money or the home, then the psychological distress will continue and is likely to delay attempts to manage the symptom. Indeed, it is unusual for a symptom to exist as the only cause of distress, and the phrase 'total pain' was coined by Dame Cicely Saunders to stress the broad nature of such distress in advanced disease.[5] Three essential human needs risk becoming blocked: *choice* (to choose or be chosen), *understanding* (to understand or be understood), and *love* (to love or be loved).[6,7] Symptoms such as pain can block choice by limiting actions and plans. Understanding can become blocked if information is not forthcoming or the nature and extent of the symptom are not believed. Love can become blocked by the effect of anger, irritability or low mood on close relationships. The result of blocking choice is frustration, anger and bitterness; the result of blocking understanding is fear and anxiety; while blocking love causes isolation and loneliness. If any of the feelings persist, depression is often the result. Sometimes patients develop behaviors that further complicate treatment and recovery.

Issues around these needs must be addressed.[8] The support and co-operation of the interprofessional team (nurses, doctors, specialists, social worker, physiotherapist, occupational therapist, pharmacist and chaplain) are necessary to achieve success. Help starts with assessment and supportive communication. Anxiety, anger and depression in particular need to be managed. The full range of additional treatments possible is wide and depends on the enthusiasm of the team, but includes touch,[9] hypnosis,[10,11] art therapy,[12] music therapy,[13] imagery,[14] aromatherapy and other complementary therapies.[15] When the psychological distress is severe, expert help will be required. The skills needed may be those of cognitive therapy, psychiatry or family therapy, although the choice sometimes depends on availability of personnel rather than suitability of the approach. Palliative care is a speciality[16] whose trained professionals are essential in complex or severe situations.

WHO characteristics of palliative care[17]
- Provides relief from pain and other distressing symptoms.
- Affirms life and regards dying as a normal process.
- Intends neither to hasten nor to postpone death.
- Integrates the psychological and spiritual aspects of patient care.
- Offers a support system to help patients live as actively as possible until death.
- Offers a support system to help the family cope during the patient's illness and in their own bereavement.
- Uses a team approach to address the needs of patients and their families, including bereavement counseling, if indicated.
- Will enhance quality of life, and may also positively influence the course of illness.
- Is applicable early in the course of illness, in conjunction with other therapies that are intended to prolong life, such as chemotherapy or radiation therapy, and includes those investigations needed to better understand and manage distressing clinical complications.

Mary, a 34-year-old woman with two young children, developed a recurrence of breast carcinoma with bone metastases. She became increasingly troubled with bone pain and was admitted to hospital and seen by the palliative care team. Her codeine was changed to oral morphine and the dose titrated so that she was sufficiently comfortable to return home. The community palliative care team continued her care, supporting her during the process of explaining her illness to her children.

Freddie was 22 months with infantile Battens disease causing neurological degeneration resulting in troublesome insomnia. In the children's hospice monitoring showed his sleep patterns were due to cerebral irritability, multi-focal seizures and hallucinations. This allowed assessment of new treatment strategies and suggestions for ongoing medical management. Freddie's exhausted parents benefited from the respite care provided, and were able to learn massage techniques to use on Freddie.

David had rapidly progressing dementia related to Down's syndrome. Communication was very poor. He became increasingly distressed but the cause was unclear. The palliative care specialist noticed the distress was occurring every few minutes, suggesting colic. An injection of hyoscine butylbromide (Buscopan)* stopped the distress, confirming the diagnosis. He was started on a gentle laxative with no further distress.

---

* Hyoscine butylbromide is not available in the US and hyoscyamine would be used instead.

Principles of symptom relief in palliative care

- **Effective supportive care is the right of every patient and partner, and the duty of every professional.**

  Access to training, updating, and to specialist palliative care services should be widely available.

- **Ensure adequate team skills, knowledge, attitudes and communication.**

  Individuals and teams need basic skills in communication and diagnosis, together with the knowledge of symptoms in advanced disease, their effects and management.

- **Create a 'safe place to suffer'.**

  This is not a building, but the *relationship* between patient and carer (lay and professional), one that enables the patient and family to feel safe to express their distress. Not all distress can be removed, but the expression of that distress is therapeutic.[18]

- **Establish a relationship with the patient, the partner and family.**

  The flow of information and treatment decisions should be controlled by the patient and negotiated with the partner and family.

- **Do not wait for a patient to complain – ask and observe.**

  Patients with persistent distress do not always look distressed. They may be withdrawn, with poor sleep or mobility, and the effects of the pain may have spread to the partner or relative. Assessing these factors is more important than estimating severity that is open to bias and often unhelpful in deciding treatment. The comments of the partner, parents or other relatives and carers are often helpful.

- **Accurately diagnose the cause of the problem.**

  A successful treatment is dependent on a clear diagnosis, together with the willingness to modify the choice depending on the response. This tailors the treatment to the individual person.

- **Patients often have multiple problems.**

  Problems are often multiple and mixed. In advanced cancer, for example, 85% of patients have more than one site of pain, and 40% have four or more pains.[19]

- **Do not delay starting treatment.**

  Symptoms should be treated promptly since they become more difficult to treat the longer they are left. This is partly because their persistence makes it increasingly difficult for the patient to cope. Treatment must start as soon as the diagnosis is made.

- **Administer drugs regularly in doses titrated to each individual, that ensure the symptom does not return.**

   If a drug gives effective relief for 4 hours, then prescribe it 4-hourly. 'As required' or 'PRN' administration on its own will not control continuous symptoms.
- **Set realistic goals.**

   Accept the patient's goals. If these seem overly optimistic, negotiate some additional *shorter*-term goals. If the patient's goals seem overly pessimistic then negotiate some additional *longer*-term goals. A clear plan of action based on negotiated goals helps the patient, partner and family see a way out of their distress.
- **Reassess repeatedly and regularly.**

   Accurate titration of medication demands reassessment.
- **Treat concurrent symptoms.**

   Patients with other symptoms such as nausea and breathlessness experience more pain than those without these symptoms.[20]
- **Empathy, understanding, diversion and elevation of mood are essential adjuncts.**

   Drugs are only part of overall management. What matters most is the relationship between the carer and patient, partner and family.

References

B = book; C = comment; Ch = chapter; CS-n = case study-number of cases; CT = controlled trial; E = editorial; GC = group consensus; I = interviews; LS = laboratory study; MC = multi-center; OS = open study; R = review; RCT = randomized controlled trial; RS = retrospective survey; SA = systematic or meta analysis.

1 McKeever M, Regnard C (1997) Qualitative interviews. In: *Palliative Crisis Response Service (PCRS) Needs Assessment. Final Report: February 1997*. St Oswald's Hospice, Newcastle. (RCT)

2 Addington-Hall J, McCarthy M (1995) Dying from cancer: results of a national population based investigation. *Palliative Medicine*. **9**: 295–305. (MC, OS, I)

3 Breitbart W (1997) Pain in AIDS. In: TS Jensen, JA Turner, Z Wiesenfield-Hallin (eds) *Proceedings of the 8th World Congress on Pain. Progress in Pain Research and Management Vol 8*. IASP Press, Seattle. pp. 63–100. (Ch)

4 Larue F, Fontaine A, Colleau SM (1997) Underestimation and undertreatment of pain in HIV disease: multicentre study. *BMJ*. **314**: 23–8. (MC, OS)

5 Saunders CM (1967) In: *The Management of Terminal Illness*. Hospital Medicine Publications, London. (Ch)

6 Heron J (1977) In: *Catharsis in Human Development*. British Postgraduate Medical Federation (University of London), London. (Ch)

7 Liossi C, Mystakidou K (1997) Heron's theory of human needs in palliative care. *European Journal of Palliative Care*. **4**: 32–5. (C)

8 Gamlin R, Leyland M, Regnard C (1997) Unit 3: Meeting the psychological needs of patients. In: *CLIP Open Learning Series*. Hochland and Hochland, Manchester. (Ch)

9 Sims S (1988) The significance of touch in palliative care. *Palliative Medicine*. **2**: 58–61. (R)

10 Spiegel D (1985) The use of hypnosis in controlling cancer pain. *CA*. **35**: 221–31. (R)

11 Hilgard ER, Hilgard JR (1975) *Hypnosis in the Relief of Pain*. William Kaufman Inc, California. (Ch)

12 Connell C (1992) Art therapy as part of a palliative care programme. *Palliative Medicine*. **6**: 18–25. (R)

13 Mandel SE (1992) Music therapy in the hospice: 'Musicalive'. *Palliative Medicine*. **5**: 155–60. (R)

14 Kearney M (1996) In: *Mortally Wounded: Stories of soul pain: death and healing*. Mercier, Dublin. (B)

15 Tavares M (2003) *National Guidelines for the Use of Complementary Therapies in Supportive and Palliative Care*. Prince of Wales Foundation for Integrated Health and the National Council for Hospice and Specialist Palliative Care Services, London.

16 Doyle D (2003) Editorial. *Palliative Medicine*. **17**(1): 9–10. (E)

17 World Health Organization (2002) *National Cancer Control Programmes, Policies and Managerial Guidelines* (2e). World Health Organization, Geneva. 1–4.

18 Stedeford A (1987) A safe place to suffer. *Palliative Medicine*. **1**: 73–4. (C)

19 Twycross RG, Harcourt J, Bergl S (1996) A survey of pain in patients with advanced cancer. *Journal of Pain and Symptom Management*. **12**: 273–82. (OS)

20 Desbiens NA, Mueller-Rizner N, Commors AF, Wenger NS (1997) The relationship of nausea and dyspnoea to pain in seriously ill patients. *Pain*. **71**: 149–56. (MC, OS)

Getting started

- Setting the scene and starting the interview
- Helping the person to share their problems
- Answering difficult questions
- Breaking difficult news
- Helping the person with the effects of difficult news
- Identifying distress in the person with severe communication difficulty

Advice on children written by Susie Lapwood, Justin Amery
and Renee McCulloch

Setting the scene and starting the interview

Clinical decision and action checklist

1 Are you unfamiliar with the patient's details?
2 Is the location for the interview unsuitable?
3 Greet the person, introduce yourself.
4 Is the person accompanied?
5 Is only a short time available for the interview?
6 Does the person object to your roles and objectives?
7 Does the person object to the time available?
8 Does the person object to you taking notes?
9 Does the person object to you sharing information with the team?
10 Is the patient's competency uncertain?

Key points

- Spending time on 'setting the scene' enables the person to share their concerns.
- This part of the interview is usually brief (a few minutes at most).
- Seeing the patient alone increases disclosure, but this does not have to be at the first meeting.
- Only a few major problems can be discussed in under 30 minutes.
- Taking notes shows the person you value their comments.
- Sharing information within the team is essential for effective care.
- In the case of children it is imperative to seek input from the parents and carers, as well as the child.

Introduction

In most situations, care starts with talking to the patient, their partner or relative. Spending a little time in setting the scene for this discussion can make the experience more helpful for both the professional and the person in the discussion.

Setting the scene

Introducing yourself is surprisingly easy to forget, especially if you are on familiar territory such as a hospital. An introduction helps to explain your role and the reason for seeing them.

Seeing the person alone will result in more disclosure of the person's concerns.[1] This needs to be balanced against the important need to include partners and relatives in the care, if the patient wishes this. It is common practice in palliative care to see patients and partners together on the first meeting, and then to see individuals on their own at a later stage. Similarly, when looking after children and young people with life-limiting illness, it is usual to meet first with the family and child together, taking account of the child's age and competence. It is important to be vigilant for the undisclosed needs of the child and family members, and separate interviews can be planned with the child or young person alone, and with the parent(s) alone.

Time available for discussion: It is not possible to elicit the problems of a patient with advanced disease in less than 30 minutes. Less time than this only allows for a few major issues to be elicited. Nevertheless, it is important to make the time available clear to the person. People disclose their problems more quickly knowing how much time is available.

Taking notes: It is essential to make notes of important cues and issues because it shows the person that you are taking their problems seriously, it does not hinder disclosure and gives you a record for the future. However, taking notes should not absorb you so much that there is prolonged loss of eye contact and empathy is lost.

Sharing information: This is essential to team working and makes best use of the team's pooled expertise. It also reduces the risk of over-dependency on the professional, or unrealistic expectations.[1] Holding 'secrets' for patients is unhelpful for patients and potentially harmful to professionals. The only exceptions are priests in a confessorial role or professionals who receive individualized professional support to fulfil their work.

A note about children: With dying children and their families there can be powerful dynamics of fear, guilt, protection and counter-protection that can prevent good communication within the family. These can manifest verbally or non-verbally. They often cannot be dealt with immediately but need discussion with the care team. To protect their parents, dying children will often explore concerns and fears with those outside the main healthcare team such as siblings, other child patients or junior staff members. This is poignantly demonstrated by the way some children, on being told difficult news, apologize to their parents. It is important to anticipate, support and manage such situations.

Clinical decision	If YES ⇒ Action
1 **Are you unfamiliar with the patient's details?**	• Read the chart before seeing the patient, partner or relative.
2 **Is the location for the interview unsuitable?**	• Find somewhere that is quiet and private enough to allow the person to feel safe enough to share their problems. • When interviewing children and their families, choose a child-friendly environment and ensure that you have sufficient helpers and toys around to enable each person's needs to be disclosed, understood and addressed. • If possible, switch off beepers and cell phones, and disconnect telephones.
3 **Greet the person and introduce yourself by name – explain your role.**	
4 **Is the person accompanied?**	• Ask the patient if they want the other person to come in with them. – *If person agrees:* ask who the other person is and see them both together. Arrange a time later to see the patient alone. – *If person disagrees:* ask whether they would like to include the other person later in the interview or on another occasion. • With dying children and their families, consider who should most helpfully and appropriately be present at each stage of the interview.
5 **Is only a short time available for the interview?**	• *If less than 30 minutes available or patient too unwell for full interview:* focus on recent changes or major problems only.
Explain your role and objectives.	
6 **Does the person object to these?**	• Explore the reasons and renegotiate the objectives, e.g. concentrate on main problem only.
Mention the time available.	
7 **Does the person object to the time available?**	• **If time is too short:** explore the reasons and try to negotiate follow-up interviews. – *If person objects to negotiation:* acknowledge this and end interview. – *If person agrees to negotiation:* arrange longer interview for later. • **If time is too long:** explore reasons and negotiate more limited objectives, e.g. main problem only.
Mention that you would like to take notes during the interview.	
8 **Does the person object to you taking notes?**	• Explore the reasons: – *If person objects to negotiation:* agree not to take notes. – *If person agrees to negotiation:* take notes of what has been agreed (person may ask for some information to be left unrecorded).
Mention that you are part of a team and need to share what is discussed with colleagues.	
9 **Does the person object to you sharing information with team?**	e.g. person insists that some or all information is kept secret. • Advise person that you cannot agree to secrecy. – *If person objects:* offer to refer to a professionally supported counselor. – *If person agrees:* go on to elicit the current problems.
10 **Is the patient's competency uncertain?**	• Competency needs to be established early on, especially in children. *see* Decisions around competency (p. 189).

Adapted from Maguire, Faulkner and Regnard[1]

Helping the person to share their problems

Clinical decision and action checklist

1 Greet the person and introduce yourself.
2 Do you find it difficult to let the person do the talking?
3 Does the person have an obvious, overriding problem?
4 Is the person unable to prioritize?
5 Ask the person to list the most troublesome problems.
6 Clarify and specify each problem in turn.
7 Is the person obviously distressed?
8 Have the main problems been disclosed?
9 Is the agreed time for the interview almost at an end?

Key points

- Encouraging the person to tell their own story encourages them to share their problems and is itself therapeutic.[2]
- Avoid closed questions, focusing on physical problems or switching the subject.
- Withhold giving advice until the full story has unfolded.
- Avoid false reassurance.

Introduction

Advanced disease can create multiple problems for patients, partners and families.[3,4] Despite this, nurses and doctors have difficulty enabling people to disclose their concerns.[4,5] Doctors and nurses commonly use behaviors that discourage a person from sharing their concerns, especially emotional issues.[5-7] Patients are *less* likely to disclose problems if the professional uses closed or leading questions, focuses on physical aspects, switches the subject to avoid a difficult question, or moves rapidly to give advice or reassurance.[6]

Eliciting the problems

Overriding problem: A person may be obviously in severe pain, vomiting or frightened. This needs to be addressed before any interview can continue.

Ask the person to list the problems: This is essential, as professionals fail to pick up more than half of patients' concerns.[5]

Check each problem: Use short and precise questions to detail the problems. Summarize your understanding with the person to make sure you have understood the issues correctly.

Distress: People who are distressed would like this acknowledged, together with help to understand why they are feeling this way. Professionals often feel anxious when this distress is openly expressed, fearing that they have 'upset' the person or caused psychological damage. In reality, it shows that the person feels safe enough to show distress.

Summarize and explain: This is the time to discuss the plan for help and treatment, and to set realistic goals.

Concluding the interview: This is as important as starting the interview. If the professional does not finish within the agreed time, the person may think they have unlimited time and demand more time, which prevents the professional spending time with other patients.

Factors making disclosure *more* likely

People are more likely to share their problems if:
- The professional is *actively listening* by:
  - enabling the person to tell the story their way with a minimum of interruptions
  - asking open questions, e.g. 'Can you tell me about any difficulties you're having?' rather than 'Is the pain better?'
  - using questions about emotions early in the interview, e.g. 'How has this affected you emotionally?' This should be in the first 10 minutes of the interview[6]
  - not avoiding a difficult question (*see* Answering difficult questions, p. 21).
- Reassurance is used wisely: it must never be false reassurance; the facts must be clear; it must not be used to avoid a difficult situation or question.
- Further training: attending interactive workshops and sessions on communication improves communication skills.[8,9]

Children: Young children may not understand the abstract concepts of death and dying, but this does not mean that they have no understanding of what they are facing. These understandings can be elicited, especially if the skills and tools of the whole team are used to enable the child to communicate through word, storytelling, art or music. Children will test adults carefully before opening up. This may take the form of casual questions dropped into conversations in inappropriate places. The answers must be appropriate to the child (*see* Answering difficult questions (p. 21)).

Clinical decision	If YES ⇒ Action
1 Greet person and introduce yourself by name and position.	
2 **Do you find it difficult to let the person do the talking?**	If you prevent the person saying things in their own way at the beginning of the interview, they are much less likely to tell you their problems. • Ask the person to tell their story, e.g. 'I've read your chart but I would like you to tell me what has happened since.' • Keep interruptions to a minimum. • Avoid early or false reassurance. • Ask about feelings early on in the interview (in the first 10 minutes). • Avoid explanations about disease process and treatment until the patient has presented all their current issues. • Be aware of your own embarrassment or awkwardness in some areas such as sexual issues. If this is difficult, arrange for training or for someone else to ask on your behalf. NB: Allowing the patient to talk in this way does not lengthen the interview.
3 **Is there an obvious, overriding problem?** e.g. severe pain	• Agree this is a priority, e.g. 'It seems to me that your main problem is . . .' • Check if they want help with the problem now, e.g. 'Do you want me to give you something now for the pain?' • See appropriate clinical decision table for guidance to management. • Return later to complete the interview.
4 **Is the person unable to prioritize?**	• Focus on the most obvious problem or the first problem chosen or mentioned.
5 Ask the person to list the most troublesome problems.	
6 Check each problem using short and precise questions:	• **clarify** its precise nature • **specify** when it started, its severity, duration and pattern • **briefly** summarize your understanding of the problem.
7 **Is the person obviously distressed?**	• Acknowledge the distress, e.g. 'You seem anxious, do you want to talk about it?' *If person can bear to talk about it:* • Identify, clarify and specify each emotion. *If person cannot bear to talk about it:* • Agree that the person can discuss this later if they feel the need.
8 **Have the main problems been disclosed?**	• Explain to the patient what you think is the cause of each problem. • Give an overview of your short- and long-term plans. • Explain what the patient can do. • Provide a realistic goal for treatment. • Agree on future plans.
9 **Is the agreed time for the interview almost at an end?**	• Explain that time is nearly up. • Summarize issues, e.g. 'So the main problems are . . .' • Check if there is anything the person wants to add. • Make concluding statement, e.g. 'I'd like to arrange the next appointment . . .' • Arrange next interview.

Adapted from Maguire, Faulkner and Regnard.[1]

Answering difficult questions

Clinical decision and action checklist

1 Acknowledge the importance of the question.
2 Is the setting inappropriate?
3 Check why the question is being asked.
4 Is the person reluctant to pursue the question?
5 Is a clear answer difficult?
6 Is a clear answer impossible?
7 Is the answer bad news?

Key points

- Difficult questions arise out of a person's uncertainty.
- Acknowledging the question is key.
- Answers may be unclear or impossible.
- Being honest about not knowing improves rather than hinders relationships.
- Some answers mean more bad news.

Introduction

People take time to adjust to the shock of advanced disease. During this time they will often seek clarification and information from health professionals. While some questions will be straightforward, other questions are more difficult to answer, e.g. 'Why has this happened to me?'

Why are questions difficult?

Many factors can make some questions difficult.[10,11]

For the patient and partner there is a need for information to make rational choices, but this may conflict with the fears of advancing illness (treatment, symptoms, emotions, dying, relationships and finances) and the need to maintain hope in the face of uncertainty. These factors inevitably generate difficult questions.

For the professional there are fears of being blamed, of eliciting an emotional reaction, of admitting ignorance, of expressing emotions, of medical hierarchy and of doing something for which they have received little or no training.[11] These factors make the questions from a patient or partner more difficult to answer.

Cultural issues

Different cultures have different views about what information should be exchanged, based on differing views of individualism.[12,13] This needs to be taken into account since open disclosure is a Western belief that is not shared universally.

The first steps

Acknowledge the importance of the question: Acknowledging a person's concern is a recurring key action. It emphasizes that you have listened and are taking the issue seriously.

The setting: While a quiet, private setting seems ideal, difficult questions are often asked at the foot of the stairs or on busy wards. Remember that the person may be asking in that setting because they feel safe to do so.

Check the question: It is important to ensure that you are both on the same wavelength. This is the opportunity to check through any problems with the person's understanding or any difficulties the professional is having with the question.

Finding an appropriate response

Difficult answers: These are difficult because the answers are unclear, not known, or may make the person or professional distressed. If there is no clear answer, then being honest about not knowing is respected and often enhances rather than diminishes the relationship.

Impossible answers: Professionals may find a question impossible to answer. If this is because of a lack of knowledge or experience then the person should be referred to someone who has the knowledge, or has the experience in answering such questions.

Children: A common error is to give an adult understanding to a child's question. For example, in answering a child's question 'Where will I go when I die?', an adult may launch into images of heaven, terrifying the child with images of a disconnected and faraway place full of walking dead people. In reality, motivated by his fear of closed spaces and the dark, the child may be asking if he will be buried like his grandmother. Therefore, checking why the child is asking that question is very important.

Bad news: If the answer is likely to be bad news then the decisions on Breaking difficult news (*see* p. 25) can be used. Avoiding the truth is unhelpful: 'The truth may hurt, but deceit hurts more.'[14]

Clinical decision	If YES ⇒ Action
1 **Acknowledge the importance of the question**, e.g. 'That's an important question'.	
2 **Is the setting inappropriate?**	• Difficult questions are often asked in inappropriate places and dropped nonchalantly into conversations. Children are particularly likely to do this when checking out an adult before opening up. • Offer to move somewhere quieter or more private. *If the person seems frightened or reluctant to go elsewhere:* • Accept the setting the person has chosen and continue with the conversation.
3 **Check why the question is being asked**, e.g. 'What makes you ask that?'	
4 **Is the person reluctant to pursue the question?**	• Acknowledge the ambivalence and check if they want to continue, e.g. 'You seem uncertain whether you want to discuss this, do you want to continue?' *If they misunderstood:* • Check for deafness, drowsiness or confusion. • Ask again in a different way. *Were **you** unprepared for the question?* • Apologize for the inattention. • Show that you are listening by acknowledging the importance of the question. • Check if they want to continue. *Are **you** uncomfortable with the question?* • Be prepared to describe your feelings, e.g. 'I don't know what to say.' *If the person is clear about stopping the interview:* • Acknowledge the refusal and inform them that they can speak again to you or another team member in the future.
5 **Is a clear answer difficult?**	• Acknowledge the uncertainty faced by the person, e.g. 'I can see this uncertainty is not easy for you.' • Explore whether the patient can accept small chunks of certainty such as asking the patient how quickly or slowly they feel their condition is changing. *If the person needs to make realistic plans:* • Give a 'best guess' response, but make it clear this is based on knowledge and experience, not certainty.
6 **Is a clear answer impossible?**	*If this is because you do not have the knowledge or experience:* • Acknowledge this, e.g. 'I don't have the answer.' • Offer to refer person to someone who may be able to help.
7 **Is the answer bad news?**	• Go to Breaking difficult news (*see* p. 25).

Adapted from Faulkner, Regnard[10]

Breaking difficult news

Clinical decision and action checklist

- Is the setting appropriate?
- 3 things to check:
  1. Is the person unable to understand?
  2. What does the person know?
  3. Does the person want to know more?
- 3 steps to breaking the news (WPC):
  1. Warn
  2. Pause
  3. Check
- 3 reactions a person could have:
  1. Does the person want to continue?
  2. Does the person want to stop the discussion?
  3. Is the person uncertain?

Key points

- Difficult news cannot be made easier, but telling it badly creates new difficulties.
- It is the patient who decides how much they should be told, not the professional.
- Breaking difficult news is done in stages, at the person's pace.
- Denial often helps people to cope more effectively. Denial is not a knowledge gap, but a coping gap.
- An unwillingness to openly discuss difficult news is not usually a barrier to informed consent.

Introduction

Difficult news is any news that is unexpected and may cause distress. It is usually 'bad' news, but this label is one decided by care professionals. There are occasions when apparently 'good' news causes as much distress as 'bad' news. For example, the news that radiotherapy for a frontal lobe brain tumour has resulted in a long remission may seem good news from a professional's view, but could be devastating to a relative who has now to cope with months or years of someone with an altered personality. In contrast the diagnosis of a cancer may be a relief to someone whose symptoms have been a puzzle for many months.

Three steps of three

Three things to check

1 *The person's understanding:* This involves making sure that the person can hear and is capable of understanding. Confusion, anxiety and depression can all reduce concentration.
2 *The person's knowledge:* This is crucial. It is unhelpful to guess what a person knows.
3 *The person's desire to know more:* This is not so difficult as it sounds: e.g. 'Do you want me to explain the results of the tests?'

Three steps to breaking the news (WPC)

Most people are already worried that something might be seriously wrong. Even so, they still need to be warned that this is the case.

1 *Warn:* Carer – 'I'm afraid the results were more serious than we thought.'
2 *Pause:* wait for a response: Person – 'What do you mean more serious?'
3 *Check:* Carer – 'We found some abnormal cells, do you want me to explain what these were?'

It is important to check that the person has understood the news. This WPC approach is repeated until the person has all the information they want at that time. It is equally important that the person knows that 'the door is open' to return for further information or clarification. It is good practice to offer a follow-up interview.

Three reactions a person could have

1 More information is requested, e.g. 'I think it's better that I know.'
2 No more information is wanted, e.g. 'Oh, I'll leave all that to you.'
3 Uncertainty about how much information is wanted, e.g. 'I'm not sure.'

Many patients are clear that they want to hear all the information, and they only need one or two sets of 'Warn, Pause, Check'. If the person is uncertain, the carer might ask some further questions, e.g. 'Are you the sort of person who likes to know everything that is happening to them?'

If the uncertainty persists this is best acknowledged and left open. The carer might say, 'I can see you're not sure. That's not a problem, you can ask me sometime in the future.'

This does not prevent the discussion of treatment. This may seem strange, but remember this is not usually a lack of knowledge, but a struggle to cope with the knowledge they do have. Discussing treatment is a way of dealing with this knowledge.

Clinical decision	If YES ⇒ Action
Is the setting appropriate?	• Find somewhere confidential and, if possible, quiet, comfortable and free from interruptions. • Ask if the person would like someone else to be present.

3 things to check:

1 Is the person unable to understand?	• *If this is reversible* (e.g. deafness responding to a hearing aid): treat the cause. • *If this is irreversible:* unless patient has previously objected, consider breaking difficult news to the relative or partner using these clinical decisions.
2 Does the person know all the facts? e.g. try asking, 'What have you understood about the tests?'	• Go to Helping the person with the effects of difficult news (*see* p. 29).
3 Does the person want to know more? e.g. try asking 'Do you want me to explain the results of the tests?'	• Follow the 3 steps to breaking difficult news (WPC) below.

3 steps to breaking the news (WPC):

1 **Warn:** give 'warning shot' (e.g. try saying 'The test results are more serious than we thought').
2 **Pause:** to give the person time to react and analyze what has been said. This often needs no more than a few seconds.
3 **Check:** if the person wants to continue (e.g. try asking 'Do you want me to explain further?') and if they have understood the information so far.

3 reactions a person could have:

1 Does the person want to continue?	• Continue repeating the WPC process above until the person has as much information as they want:
	  – answer invitation for more information (e.g. try saying 'We found some abnormal cells')
	  – ensure person understands this information
	  – keep giving information as long as person continues to request information.
	• Consider audio-taping the conversation for the person or providing written material.

2 Does the person want to stop the discussion?	• Acknowledge the refusal. • Offer the opportunity to discuss this further in the future if the person wishes. NB: Denial is not usually a lack of knowledge, but a way of coping with difficult news.
3 Is the person uncertain about knowing more?	• Acknowledge the uncertainty. • Offer the opportunity to discuss this further in the future if the person wishes. NB: Uncertainty is not usually a lack of knowledge, but a struggle to openly face difficult news. It is often accompanied by anxiety.

Adapted from Faulkner, Maguire, Regnard[15]

Helping the person with the effects of difficult news

Clinical decision and action checklist

1 Pause to check the person's reactions.
2 Acknowledge any distress.
3 Is the person accepting the difficult news?
4 Is the person overwhelmingly distressed?
5 Is the person denying, or holding on to unrealistic expectations?
6 Is the person ambivalent?
7 Is the patient colluding?
8 Is the relative or partner colluding?

Key points

- Bad news will result in emotions being expressed. Fear of such emotions being expressed prevents professionals from allowing them to occur. Expression of emotions is a helpful part of adjustment.
- Denial may be an effective coping mechanism for some people.
- Collusion between patients, partners and relatives is common and is usually driven by a wish to protect the other person.

Introduction

Although bad news cannot be made less bad, it can be broken badly. When a person perceives they have too much (or too little) information, their concerns are kept hidden and unresolved. This increases the risk of clinical anxiety and/or depression.[16] Faced with difficult news most people respond with some acceptance or denial. Some will be firm in this reaction while many will fluctuate between the two. A few people will be ambivalent about whether they want to know more or not.

29

Possible reactions

Distress: This indicates that the difficult news has been heard. There will be a wide range of possible reactions to difficult news such as anger, bitterness, sadness and fear. Sometimes this is expressed openly at the time; sometimes it appears later. Professionals are often fearful of this reaction and worry that they have 'upset' the person or caused psychological damage. This is often a reason for not exploring emotional issues.[5,7] As long as the disclosure has been at the person's pace with them in control, no damage will be caused. Open expression can be helpful to the individual and allows the professional to explore feelings further. The fact that a person has become distressed usually shows that the professional has made the person feel safe enough to express their distress.

Coping with denial or unrealistic expectations: These reactions are important and powerful protective mechanisms for anyone facing difficult news. The key is deciding whether their presence is helping the individual cope. If the person is coping then no action need be taken – thoughtless intervention in such a patient shows little regard for the patient, partner and family.[17] Obviously, if these reactions are failing to protect the individual, then gently challenging the presence of denial or unrealistic expectations may enable the person to express their distress more clearly. This expression is in itself therapeutic and may lead to some resolution of that distress.

Collusion: This is usually between the patient and the partner or relative. Collusion is another reaction that is seen as abnormal by professionals, and yet it is often an act of love, protecting someone they love and know well. This reaction is understandable and like denial can be left if it is working for those involved. However, collusion can cause difficulties if it is damaging the relationship through a 'conspiracy of silence', in which case this cost will need to be explored and gently challenged.

Children: Parents often wish to protect their dying child ('He's such a happy child . . .'), while the child may try to protect the parents ('I don't want to make her cry'). While this can work for some families, in many it hampers communication at a time when mutual trust, support and sharing are so important. Parents are often surprised to hear that the child knows more about the situation than they admitted to the parent. Children are often relieved to hear that it is not them but the situation that is making their parents unhappy, and that crying is not always a bad thing. Carers can be in an important position to encourage such communication within the family. Since different family members may open up to different carers, team communication and support are vital.

Clinical decision	If YES ⇒ Action
1 Pause to check the person's reactions.	
2 Acknowledge any distress.	
3 Is the person accepting the difficult news?	• Acknowledge and explore any feelings and concerns. • Monitor regularly for feelings of defeat, spiritual anguish, anger and withdrawal (*see* Anger (p. 161) and Withdrawal and depression (p. 177)).
4 Is the person overwhelmingly distressed?	• Acknowledge the distress, e.g. 'I can see that's distressing news.' NB: although this seems a trite and obvious response from the professional, it shows the person that you have noticed. A 'poker' face gives the person the impression of not caring or not wishing to deal with feelings. • Explore the individual concerns to work out why the reaction has been so disturbing.
5 Is the person denying, or holding on to unrealistic expectations?	*If the person is coping well with these feelings:* • Do not persist in challenging denial or unrealistic expectations (after all, they *are* coping!). *If the person is **not** coping with these feelings:* • Acknowledge the denial or unrealistic expectations. • Check for a window on the denial (e.g. 'Are there times, even for a second, when you're less sure that everything is all right?'). • Gently challenge inconsistencies (e.g. 'You say everything is fine, but you're worried about the weight loss.'). • Avoid being defensive about unrealistic expectations.
6 Is the person ambivalent?	• Acknowledge the uncertainty (e.g. 'It seems that you're uncertain about this.'). • Offer time for help (e.g. 'When you need more information, please ask.').
7 Is the patient colluding?	i.e. wanting to withhold information from the partner or relative. • Recognize that this is often due to a wish to protect the partner. • Accept that the patient does know the partner or relative better than any professional. • Explore the reasons for the collusion and check the cost of that collusion. • Ask for permission to speak to the partner or relative to find out what they think about the situation.
8 Is the relative or partner colluding?	i.e. wanting to withhold information from the patient. • Accept that the carer does know the patient better than any professional. • Explore reasons for collusion (remember that the carer is doing what they think best at the time). • Ask for permission to find out from the patient what they think of the situation. • Check the cost of collusion on the patient–carer relationship.

Adapted from Faulkner, Maguire, Regnard[15]

Identifying distress in the person with severe communication difficulty

Clinical decision and action checklist

1 Observe and document distress signs or behavior (or ask carers).
2 Document the context.
3 Compare the new sign or behavior with:
   - previous episodes of distress
   - signs and behaviors when content
   - any long-term behaviors.
4 Check through possible causes.

Key points

- Even comatose patients can show signs or behaviors of distress.
- Relatives can provide valuable information and, especially in children, their perspective is essential.
- Professional carers have the skills to pick up distress, but often do so intuitively and do not have confidence in their observations.
- Distress signs and behaviors should be documented and compared with signs and behaviors in other situations.

Introduction

In some situations and conditions the ability of a patient to express his or her distress clearly can be severely affected. This includes adults or children with severe learning disability, people with dementia, severe dysphasia (stroke, cerebral tumor), severe depression or psychosis, and people in a comatose or semi-comatose state. There has been little research on distress in people with profound communication problems.[18,19] Carers have found it difficult to articulate their intuitive sense that the individual has an unmet need. The difficulty in identifying distress is magnified when people move between care environments or come into contact with new carers. The concept of identifying distress, rather than pain, is an essential component of achieving comfort in people with severe communication difficulties. The key is to document the carers' existing skills in identifying distress, take note of the context and then apply clinical decisions to identify the cause.

What are the behaviors and signs of distress?

Even in the absence of speech or the presence of severe intellectual impairment, distress can still be observed through the following:[20]

- *Verbal:* This may be simple descriptions, e.g. 'I'm not right' or using sounds (crying, screaming, sighing, moaning, grunting).
- *Facial:* These may be simple expressions (grimacing, clenched teeth, shut eyes, wide open eyes, frowning, biting lower lip) or more complex.
- *Adaptive:* Rubbing or holding an area, keeping an area still, breath holding, hypersensitivity to stimuli, approaching staff, avoiding stimulation, reduced or absent function (reduced movement, lying or sitting).
- *Distractive:* Rocking (or other rhythmic movements), pacing, biting their hand or lip, gesturing, clenched fists.
- *Postural:* Increased muscle tension (extension or flexion), altered posture, flinching, head in hands, limping, pulling cover or clothes over their head, knees drawn up.
- *Autonomic:* This may be either sympathetic (the flight or fright response with ↑pulse rate, ↑BP, wide pupils, pallor and sweating) or parasympathetic (in response to nausea or visceral pain with ↓BP and ↓pulse rate).

In 80% or more of distress episodes there may be changes in facial appearance, verbal expression, posture, mannerisms or the appearance of the eyes, as well as autonomic skin changes.[21] These changes may be a new sign or behavior, or the absence of signs and behavior seen during content times.

Picking up distress

Relatives and parents have often learnt the signs and behaviors of distress and can provide valuable information. Professional carers have the skills to observe the same signs and behaviors of distress, but often do not have the confidence in their observations. Daily observation increases the number of distress signs and behaviors that are picked up and teams pick up more signs and behaviors than individuals.[21] Documenting the observations of all new signs and behaviors is a key step.[20]

Making sense of distress signs and behaviors

Common mistakes are to misinterpret distress as a behavior that needs treating, or to assume that distress indicates pain.[20] There is no evidence that any single cause of distress produces distinct signs or behaviors.[20] In contrast, individuals tend to use the same signs and behaviors for different types of distress.[21] The context in which the new sign or behavior occurs is important. For example, a distress sign or behavior on moving an arm suggests arm pain, while the same behavior in a frightening situation (e.g. hospital visit) suggests fear. However, it is necessary to work through the checklist opposite to ensure that the most likely causes have been considered.

Clinical decision	If YES ⇒ Action
1 Observe and document signs or behavior (or ask carers).	• See notes opposite for examples of distress signs and behaviors. • Establish baselines during episodes of known contentment.
2 Document the context in which a new sign or behavior is occurring.	
3 Compare the new sign or behavior of distress with: • previous episodes of distress • signs and behaviors when content • any long-term behaviors.	

4 Is the new sign or behavior of distress:

• repeated rapidly?	*Consider these causes:* • pleuritic pain (in time with breathing): *see* cd-3d in Diagnosing and treating pain (p. 41) • colic (comes and goes every few minutes): *see* cd-4 in Diagnosing and treating pain (p. 42) • repetitive behavior due to boredom or fear: *see* Anxiety (p. 165), Anger (p. 161) or Withdrawal and depression (p. 177).
• associated with breathing?	*Consider these causes:* • pleuritic pain due to infection; fractured rib(s): *see* cd-3d in Diagnosing and treating pain (p. 41) • breathlessness due to COPD, pleural effusion, tumor, mucus plugging, aspiration, bronchospasm: *see* Respiratory problems (p. 131).
• worsened or precipitated by movement?	*Consider:* movement-related pains: *see* cd-3 in Diagnosing and treating pain (p. 41).
• related to eating?	*Consider these causes:* • food refusal through illness, fear, depression, or due to swallowing problems: *see* Nutrition and hydration problems (p. 119) and Dysphagia (p. 91) • oral problems: dental problems, mucosal infection, oromotor dysfunction: *see* Oral problems (p. 125) • upper GI problems (oral hygiene, peptic ulcer, esophageal reflux, dyspepsia) or abdominal problems: *see* cd-7 in Diagnosing and treating pain (p. 42).
• related to a specific situation?	*Consider these causes:* • frightening, unfamiliar or painful situations: e.g. hospital visit, unfamiliar person. • painful procedures: *see* cd-5 in Diagnosing and treating pain (p. 42).
• associated with vomiting?	*Consider causes of nausea and vomiting: see* Nausea and vomiting (p. 113) and Dyspepsia (p. 85)
• associated with elimination (urine or fecal)?	*Consider these causes:* • urinary problems (infection, retention): *see* Urinary and sexual problems (p. 151) • GI problems (diarrhea, constipation): *see* Diarrhea (p. 81), or Constipation (p. 75).
• present in a normally comfortable position or situation?	*Consider these causes:* • pains at rest (*see* Diagnosing and treating pain (p. 39)) • nausea (*see* Nausea and vomiting (p. 113)) • infection: check urine and chest for signs of infection • anxiety, anger or depression: *see* Anxiety (p. 165), Anger (p. 161) or Withdrawal and depression (p. 177).

cd = clinical decision

Distress may be hidden, but it is never silent.

References

B = book;   C = comment;   Ch = chapter;   CS-n = case study-number of cases;   CT = controlled trial; E = editorial; GC = group consensus; I = interviews; LS = laboratory study; MC = multi-center; OS = open study; PhD = PhD thesis; R = review; RCT = randomized controlled trial; RS = retrospective survey; SA = systematic or meta analysis.

1 Maguire P, Faulkner A, Regnard C (1995) Eliciting the current problems. In: *Flow Diagrams in Advanced Cancer and Other Diseases*. Edward Arnold, London. pp. 1–4. (Ch)

2 Price J, Leaver L (2002) ABC of psychological medicine: beginning treatment. *BMJ*. **325**: 33–5.

3 Maguire P, Walsh S, Jeacock J, Kingston R (1999) Physical and psychological needs of patients dying from colo-rectal cancer. *Palliative Medicine*. **13**: 45–50. (OS, I)

4 Maguire P, Parkes CM (1998) Surgery and loss of body parts. *BMJ*. **316**: 1086–8. (R)

5 Heaven CM, Maguire P (1996) Training hospice nurses to elicit patient concerns. *Journal of Advanced Nursing*. **23**: 280–6. (RCT)

6 Maguire P, Faulkner A, Booth K, Elliott C, Hillier V (1996) Helping cancer patients disclose their concerns. *European Journal of Cancer*. **32A**: 78–81. (OS)

7 Maguire P (1985) Barriers to psychological care of the dying. *British Medical Journal Clinical Research Ed*. **291**: 1711–13. (R)

8 Maguire P (1999) Improving communication with cancer patients. *European Journal of Cancer*. **35**: 2058–65. (R)

9 Maguire P (1999) Improving communication with cancer patients. *European Journal of Cancer*. **35**: 1415–22. (R)

10 Faulkner A, Regnard C (1995) Handling difficult questions. In: *Flow Diagrams in Advanced Cancer and Other Diseases*. Edward Arnold, London. pp. 92–5. (Ch)

11 Buckman R (1997) Communication in palliative care: a practical guide. In: D Doyle, GWC Hanks, N MacDonald (eds) *The Oxford Textbook of Palliative Medicine* (2e). Oxford Medical Publications, Oxford. pp. 141–56. (Ch)

12 Dein S, Thomas K (2002) To tell or not to tell. *European Journal of Palliative Care*. **9**(5): 209–12. (R, 30 refs)

13 Fainsinger RL, Núñez-Olarte JM, Demoissac DM (2003) The cultural differences in perceived value of disclosure and cognition: Spain and Canada. *Journal of Pain and Symptom Management*. **19**(1): 43–8. (I-200)

14 Fallowfield LJ, Jenkins VA, Beveridge HA (2002) Truth may hurt but deceit hurts more: communication in palliative care. *Palliative Medicine*. **16**: 297–303.

15 Faulkner A, Maguire P, Regnard C (1995) Breaking bad news. In: *Flow Diagrams in Advanced Cancer and Other Diseases*. Edward Arnold, London. pp. 86–91. (Ch)

16 Maguire P (1998) Breaking bad news. *European Journal of Surgical Oncology*. **24**: 188–91. (R)

17 Vachon MLS (1997) The emotional problems of the patient. In: D Doyle, GWC Hanks, N MacDonald (eds) *The Oxford Textbook of Palliative Medicine* (2e). Oxford Medical Publications, Oxford. pp. 883–907. (Ch)

18 Hunt A (2001) Towards an understanding of pain in the child with severe neurological impairment. Development of a behaviour rating scale for assessing pain. PhD thesis. University of Manchester. (PhD)

19 Tuffrey-Wijne I (2003) The palliative care needs of people with intellectual disabilities: a literature review. *Palliative Medicine*. **17**: 55–62. (R)

20 Regnard C, Matthews D, Gibson L, Clarke C (2003) Difficulties in identifying distress in people with severe communication problems. *International Journal of Palliative Nursing*. **9**(3): 173–6. (R)

21 Regnard C, Matthews D, Gibson L, Clarke C, Watson B, Reynolds J (2003) *Developing and Validating a Clinical Tool to Assess Distress in People with Severe Communication Problems*. Poster, 3rd Congress of the European Association of Palliative Care, The Hague.

Managing pain

- Diagnosing and treating pain
- Choosing an analgesic
- Using opioids
- Managing the adverse effects of analgesics

Advice on children written by Susie Lapwood and Renee McCulloch

Diagnosing and treating pain

Clinical decision and action checklist

Are the pain descriptions, behaviors or signs:
1   Severe or overwhelming?
2   Breakthrough pain?
3   Related to movement?
4   Periodic?
5   Related to a procedure?
6   Due to visceral pain?
7   Related to eating?
8   Made worse by passing urine or stool?
9   Associated with skin changes?
10 Worsened by touch or described as an unpleasant sensory change at rest?
11 In an area supplied by a peripheral nerve?
12 Persisting despite treatment?

Key points

- Pain treatment cannot start until an assessment has been made of the likely cause of pain.
- Work through these 12 pain clinical decisions in order – they cover most of the pains seen in advanced disease.
- Use the information provided to help you decide which pain is present.
- Finally, follow the suggestions in the tables for managing the pain.

Assessing pain

Most adults and older children can clearly describe pain and its nature, and will be able to describe the PQRST features of pain (Precipitating factors; Quality; Radiation; Site and severity; Timing). In addition, it is important to ask how the pain has affected feelings, daily activities and relationships, and to ascertain the patient's expectations. Information from parents and carers can be invaluable, but the basic rule is that 'pain is what the patient says hurts'.[1] A clinical examination is essential. Assessment or scoring tools specific to pain can be used in adult palliative care, but are more often used in monitoring children in pain and can help communicating children express their pain in their own way.[2–4]

Understanding pain: In both adults and children, cognitive, behavioral, emotional, cultural and family issues affect the experience and understanding of pain.[5] Children beyond infancy, and adults with moderate learning disability, can accurately point to the body area or mark the site of the pain on a drawing, but may need to use their own words for pain such as 'hurt', or 'feeling bad'.[6,7]

Is it pain? Pain is a distressing experience.[8,9] Making clear that the distress is due to pain can be difficult or impossible for a pre-verbal child, or anyone with severe anxiety, depression, confusion or neurological impairment. It is tempting to assume that a distressed person with advanced disease has pain since the solution of giving analgesia seems simple. There is no evidence that pain tools are of value in differentiating pain from other causes of distress, but identifying the cause of distress is still possible.[10] *See* Identifying distress in the person with severe communication difficulty (p. 33).

Checklist for pain

1 Severe or overwhelming pain

Pain of this severity needs urgent treatment (*see* cd-5 in Emergencies (p. 207)).

2 Breakthrough pain

Despite good pain relief with regular analgesia, a brief worsening of pain can 'break through' the analgesia.[11] This will need a boost of analgesia. The causes can be:

- related to movement or a procedure (incident pain)[12]
- inadequate regular analgesia
- an unpredictable worsening of the pain, e.g. pathological fracture
- episodic pain caused by a pain less responsive to the current analgesia, e.g. colic, neuropathic pain.

3 Pain related to movement

Fracture: Movement of the affected part by the examiner will usually result in severe pain on the slightest movement. Pathological fractures (e.g. bone metastases) are not always painful when they occur, but pain is usually a feature within minutes. Follow the advice for severe pain in cd-5 in Emergencies (p. 207).

Bone metastases or infection: Local tenderness over a bone suggests a local weakness. Severe skeletal instability can cause pain on minimal movement such as coughing. In immunocompromised patients infection should be excluded, especially mycobacteria. Bone metastases are best picked up on bone scan, except for myeloma and renal carcinoma, which may show up better on X-rays or MRI scan. Weak or strong opioids are first line treatment, but such pains may be less opioid-responsive.[13] Radiotherapy produces complete relief after one month in 25% and partial relief in a further 40%.[14] If skeletal instability is severe, operative fixation can be used followed by radiotherapy.[15] The pain of *multiple* metastases requires systemic treatments. There is no evidence to support the routine, first-line use of NSAIDs in bone pain,[16] but they can be useful second- or third-line treatment in some patients. A proven treatment is an intravenous infusion of pamidronate or zoledronic acid,[17–22,156] used when analgesics and/or radiotherapy have failed.[23] Pain relief can be seen within 6 days.[24] When used regularly bisphosphonates have the added advantage of reducing skeletal complications.[18,19,156,157] For persistent pain from vertebral metastases, vertebroplasty (injection of cement) can be effective.[25]

Joint pains: These are common in immobile patients due to muscle atrophy, weakness and poor positioning. Spasticity due to neurological impairment can be exacerbated by contractures that can be severe enough to cause subluxation or dislocation of joints.

Myofascial pain: This is common in advanced disease. The pain is distributed in a myotomal pattern and charts showing the typical distribution of all the main muscles are available.[26,27] A trigger point is usually present in the affected muscle and consists of a single spot which reproduces the pain when pressed, accompanied by a palpable band of muscle in spasm beneath the trigger point.

Skeletal muscle strain: This occurs suddenly during exertion. Although a cold compress is said to be effective, the evidence base is poor.[28] Local warmth is more pleasant for the patient.

Spasticity and dystonia: Infection or tumor involving muscle will cause that muscle to go into painful spasm. Infection must be excluded and treated if present. The pain of tumor infiltration can be helped with dexamethasone, possibly with a local nerve or spinal block. Spasticity is also seen in several neurological conditions (upper motor neurone disease, cerebral palsy, multiple sclerosis, spinal cord injury).[43] Spasticity is a motor disorder characterized by an increase in muscle tone in response to a cerebral or spinal insult, which includes the upper motor neurones of the corticospinal tracts. Dystonia is recognized as a state of sustained muscle contraction producing involuntary fluctuating movements and postures, without pyramidal deficit. Spasticity caused by cerebral palsy is associated with other problems such as reduced movement control, weakness and fatigue, abnormal tone and posture, muscle contractures leading to bone and joint deformity, and abnormal rate of bone growth relative to muscle growth

Clinical decision	If YES ⇒ Action
1 Is the pain severe or overwhelming?	*See* cd-5 in Emergencies (p. 207).
2 Is this breakthrough pain? (i.e. pain occurring despite regular analgesia)	NB: All breakthrough doses may need to be adjusted up or down for the individual patient. • *If already on a non-opioid analgesic:* give one dose of the regular analgesic, e.g. 1 g acetaminophen. • *If already on a regular oral opioid:* give 50% of the q4h dose q1h (q2–4h in children), e.g. 60 mg/day (10 mg q4h = breakthrough dose of 5 mg). • *If on a transdermal opioid patch*: Fentanyl: give 1-hourly dose, e.g. 25 microgram/hour patch = 25 microgram dose SC or sublingual or for every 25 microgram/hour give equivalent of morphine 10 mg PO. Buprenorphine: give 6-hourly dose of buprenorphine (available in the US as a transdermal gel which can be made by a compounding pharmacist). • *If on continuous SC infusion of opioid*: Hydromorphone: give 50% of q4h dose, e.g. 30 mg/24 hours (5 mg q4h) = 2.5 mg dose SC. Fentanyl: give 1-hourly dose, e.g. 500 microgram/24 hours ≈ 20 microgram dose SC. *If there is a response to the breakthrough dose:* • Consider increasing the regular analgesic dose if the breakthrough pain tends to occur before the next regular dose, and/or three or more breakthrough doses are required per 24 hours. *If there is no response:* • *After one breakthrough dose:* for a non-opioid, repeat in 4 hours. For an opioid, repeat after one hour with the same dose. If there is still no response, consider changing from a non-opioid to a weak opioid, or from a weak opioid to a strong opioid. • *If there is still no response after three breakthrough doses:* reconsider the cause of pain using the following cd-3–12 below.
3 Is the pain related to movement? (i.e. worsened or precipitated by movement)	**(a) Worsened by the slightest passive movement** • *Fracture* (deformity may be present): immobilize. *See* cd-5 in Emergencies (p. 207). Metastasis: consider elective orthopedic surgery and radiotherapy. Osteoporosis: consider bisphosphonate and calcium treatment. • *Severe soft tissue inflammation:* usually due to infection: *see* cd-9 (p. 43). If the infection is deeper, movement pain may be the only sign. • *Joint problems* (common in immobile and neurologically impaired patients): Exclude infection, subluxation, dislocation, metastases or a fracture involving the joint. For inflammatory arthropathies: ask a rheumatologist for advice. Ask the physiotherapist and occupational therapist for advice on positioning, and modifying mobility and function. Consider: NSAIDs or strong opioids. May need specialist pain or palliative care help. • *Inflammation or irritation of muscle* (affected muscle in spasm): *see* cd-3c below. • *Nerve compression: see* cd-11 (p. 43). **(b) Worsened by straining bone during examination (e.g. percussing spine, pressing rib)** • Consider nerve compression (*see* cd-11 (p. 43)) or bone infection. • *Bone metastases* (may need to be confirmed on bone or MRI scan): If in pain at rest, start a strong opioid. If no improvement after three dose increases, add an NSAID (e.g. diclofenac) for one week's trial. For pain at a single site, arrange radiotherapy. If pain is in multiple sites, or pain is persisting (and patient is not hypocalcemic) use pamidronate 60–90 mg IV infusion over 2 hours. If this makes no difference after 1 week, try zoledronic acid 4 mg IV infusion over 15–30 minutes. Effects can last 1–2 months. **(c) Worsened by active movement (i.e. movement against resistance)** • *Skeletal instability:* pain on minimal active movement such as coughing or standing suggests there is a risk of bone fracture or collapse. Treat bone metastases as in cd-3a above. Arrange for an urgent X-ray and consider referral for orthopedic and radiotherapy opinion. • *Myofascial pain* (myotomal distribution, trigger point in muscle which reproduces pain when pressed): inject the trigger point with 0.25% bupivacaine,[29] or use low frequency TENS over the trigger point.[30,31] • *Skeletal muscle strain* (history of sudden onset during exertion): TENS, local warmth/cold. • *Spasticity:* start with baclofen 10 mg q8h and titrate dose. Alternatives include dantrolene or gabapentin,[32–34] botulinum toxin,[35] intrathecal baclofen,[36] neurolytic blocks,[37] surgery,[38] and the help of physical therapists.[39] Diazepam can be used as a single bedtime dose, but adverse effects are common.[40,41] **(d) Worsened by inspiration (or breathing is more shallow)** • *Rib metastases/fracture* (local tenderness is present): refer for intercostal nerve block. For multiple sites *see* cd-3b above. • *Pleuritic pain* (local rub may be present): consider a pulmonary embolus. Treat infection if present. Consider an NSAID ± intercostal block. • *Peritoneal pain due to local metastases*: start an NSAID, e.g. diclofenac 50 mg q8h. If the pain is localized to one or two dermatomes, try an intercostal block.

cd = clinical decision

Table continued overleaf

(e) Consider also:
- *Joint pain:* treat local infection if this is present. Start an NSAID, e.g. diclofenac 50 mg q8h. Check for dislocation or subluxation. Ask the physiotherapist for advice.
- *Gastric distension due to gastric stasis* (fullness, early satiation, hiccups, heartburn): metoclopramide or domperidone (obtained in the US from a Compounding Pharmacy – 10 mg, 20 mg).
- *Local distension due to hemorrhage:* exclude bleeding disorder. Consider opioid or ketamine.
- *Local distension due to tumor:* strong opioid ± high dose dexamethasone (10–16 mg daily). A local block or spinal analgesia is sometimes needed.
- *Local inflammation due to tumor, infection or trauma:* exclude and treat infection. Consider using topical morphine[60–62] or radiotherapy if this is due to tumor.
- *Trauma:* do a 'first aid' examination (head, neck, shoulders, limbs, back, chest, abdomen).
- *Gastro-esophageal reflux: see* cd-4 in Dyspepsia (p. 85).

4 Is the pain periodic? (i.e. comes and goes regularly)	**(a) Occurring regularly every few seconds:** • Consider rib metastases or pleuritic pain (*see* cd-3d (p. 41)). • Consider severe skeletal instability (*see* cd-3c (p. 41)). **(b) Occurring regularly every few minutes: this is likely to be smooth muscle colic** • *Abdominal pain:* probably bowel colic due to constipation, bowel obstruction or bowel irritation (drugs, radiotherapy, chemotherapy, infection). Treat the cause, but for relief use hyoscine butylbromide (Canada only) 10–20 mg SC as required. Can be used as continuous SC infusion (30–180 mg per 24 hrs). In the US use hyoscyamine (Levsin) 0.125–0.25 mg PO/SL tid-qid PRN. • *Suprapubic pain with urinary frequency or urgency:* this may be bladder colic due to infection, outflow obstruction, unstable bladder, or irritation by tumor. Treat the cause, but for relief use hyoscine butylbromide (Canada) or hyoscyamine (US) as for bowel colic above. *See* Urinary and sexual problems (p. 151). • *If the pain is in the groin:* this may be ureteric colic due to irritation or obstruction. Treat the cause, but for relief use hyoscine butylbromide (Canada) or hyoscyamine (US) as for bowel colic above, or ketorolac 30–60 mg IV or SC. Consider starting a strong opioid (or giving a breakthrough dose of an existing opioid). An NSAID can be tried if renal function is good. For obstruction due to tumor, try dexamethasone 6 mg once daily.
5 Is the pain related to a procedure? (e.g. a dressing change)	• Change the technique (e.g. different dressings or use a topical opioid).[60–62] Gabapentin may have a role.[55] Local anesthetic cream can help.[46] • If available, try Entonox (50% O_2, 50% N_2O) just before and during procedure. Do not use in the presence of pneumothorax or distended bowel. • Try a 4-hourly dose of usual analgesic given PO or SC (*see* p. 52 for opioid equivalents). • Consider asking for advice from palliative care specialist. Options are ketamine 2.5–5 mg SC or buccal, fentanyl or sufentanil SL[158] or reducing fear with midazolam 1–5 mg titrated IV or buccal.[56] • *For children:* distraction and cuddling is almost always helpful.
6 Is this visceral pain?	• *Cardiac pain persisting despite adequate anti-anginal management:* start regular strong opioid. Consider referral for spinal analgesia. • *Liver capsule distension:* start dexamethasone 6 mg PO daily, reducing to lowest dose that controls symptoms. Consider an opioid (*see* Choosing an analgesic (p. 45)). • *Celiac plexus pain:* start gabapentin (± opioid and/or steroid) 100 mg q8h and titrate (up to 800 mg q8h may be needed).[57] Consider referral for spinal analgesia or celiac plexus block. • *Related to bowels or bladder:* see cd-4b above and cd-8 below.
7 Is the pain related to eating?	• *Pain in the mouth: see* cd-4 in Oral problems (p. 127). • *Pain on swallowing: see* cd-6 in Dysphagia (p. 93). • *Dyspepsia causing abdominal pain:* see Dyspepsia (p. 85). • *Gastritis:* treat cause. Consider ranitidine or lansoprazole (omeprazole in children). For NSAID gastritis: use lansoprazole or omeprazole.[58,59] If bleeding is present add sucralfate suspension 10 ml q6h as a hemostatic agent. • *Duodenitis:* start ranitidine, lansoprazole or omeprazole. • *Gastric stasis causing heartburn:* metoclopramide or domperidone (obtained in the US from a Compounding Pharmacy – 10 mg, 20 mg). • *Gastro-esophageal reflux: see* cd-4 in Dyspepsia (p. 87).
8 Is the pain made worse by passing urine or stool?	• *Pain on micturition: see* cd-3 in Urinary and sexual problems (p. 151). • *Pain on passing stool:* Consider these causes: hard stool (*see* Constipation (p. 75)), anal fissure (use nitroglycerin (NTG) ointment), hemorrhoids (use topical soothing cream), infection (treat). • *Rectal pain (proctalgia) or strong sensation of evacuation (tenesmus):* – exclude rectal impaction with stool. – if due to tumor, dexamethasone 6 mg PO once daily may help. – if due to inflammation of rectal mucosa (tumor, infection, radiotherapy), try rectal steroid (as retention enema (Entocort, Cortenema) or foam enema (Cortifoam)) every 1–2 days. The following are available in the US: Cortenema (Hydrocortisone rectal 100/60 ml), Entocort EC, Cortifoam, Anusol HC 1%, 2.5% (hemorrhoid cream containing hydrocortisone). Additional corticosteroid preparations can be obtained at Compounding Pharmacies, e.g. dexamethasone via suppository.

cd = clinical decision

9 Are there associated skin changes in the area of the pain?	• *Skin ulcers: see* Skin problems (p. 139) and Malignant ulcers and fistulae (p. 109). Consider using topical morphine,[60–62] e.g. 10 mg preservative-free morphine injection solution in 5 ml water-soluble gel or local anesthetic gel. • *Red/hot skin:* Exclude eczema or dermatitis. If cellulitis is suspected, start antibiotic (amoxicillin or erythromycin in lymphedematous limb, otherwise use flucloxacillin). In the US, cephalexin (Keflex) is generally used. Consider whether this pain is a sympathetic hypoactivity pain (*see* cd-10c below). • *Pale/cold or black skin:* Arterial insufficiency (pale or black skin): contact a vascular surgeon for advice. An opioid is only partly effective, and alternatives are ketamine as a continuous SC infusion (50–300 mg in 24 hours), a local nerve block or spinal analgesia. Sympathetic hyperactivity pain (pale, cold skin): *see* cd-10c below. • *For other skin disease:* treat the cause.
10 Is this an unpleasant sensory change at rest, or does touch make the pain worse?	**(a) Pain in a dermatome** (i.e. in the distribution of a spinal nerve root) = deafferentation pain: • Start low dose amitriptyline (10–25 mg once at night) and titrate. If this helps but adverse effects are troublesome, try imipramine (10–25 mg at night and titrate). If the pain is no better, add gabapentin 100 mg q8h and titrate (up to 800 mg q8h may be needed). • *If the pain persists:* contact a pain or palliative care specialist. Possibilities include ketamine, nerve blocks or spinal analgesia. **(b) Pain in area supplied by peripheral nerve** = neuropathy or neuralgia: • Exclude reversible causes (e.g. B12 deficiency). Treat as for deafferentation pain. **(c) Pain in a sympathetic distribution** (i.e. the same distribution as the arterial supply, since sympathetic nerves run along arteries) = sympathetically maintained pain. • Start treating in the same way as deafferentation pain. If the skin is cold and pale, this is hyperactive sympathetic activity and a pain specialist may advise a chemical sympathectomy. If skin is warm and red or dusky, this is hypoactive sympathetic activity and this can sometimes be helped by placing TENS electrodes over the main artery supplying the area (do not use this over the carotid arteries). **(d) Hemibody pain:** this may be due to destructive brain lesions (metastases, CVA). It can also occur in neurologically impaired children with complex seizures. Anticonvulsants such as gabapentin may help.[72–75]
11 Is the pain in an area supplied by a peripheral nerve? (e.g. sciatica)	• If this is an unpleasant sensory change at rest: *see* cd-10 above. • *Nerve compression:* Start an opioid. Exclude (with X-rays ± bone scan) nerve compression by skeletal instability (a CAT or MRI scan may be necessary). Exclude or treat bone infection. For tumors or metastases consider dexamethasone (6 mg once daily) or radiotherapy. A TENS may help. Occasionally a nerve block or spinal analgesia is needed.
12 Is the pain persisting?	• *Consider these as causes:* Total pain: unresolved fear, anger or depression (*see* Anxiety (p. 165), Anger (p. 161), Withdrawal and depression (p. 177)). Poor compliance – fear, misunderstanding of instructions or an unacceptable form of medication. Inappropriate analgesic dose or timing. Onset of a new pain (go through previous pain clinical decisions).

Adapted from Thompson and Regnard[42]
cd = clinical decision

in children. Pain is a common feature which may occur during movement and as a result of muscle spasm. Pain is often severe and can be the cause of general distress and agitation in the child. It may fluctuate in severity or be constant. Pain due to muscle spasm may well precipitate seizures in those with a predisposition. Relieving pain can help to stop the cycle of spasm and seizure. The advice of the physiotherapist and occupational therapist is important since correct positioning and seating can reduce the pain of the spasticity. Simple measures may alleviate spasticity such as repositioning the person or gentle stretching of the muscles involved. Aromatherapy may have a role in muscle relaxation. Unfortunately, no well-designed studies have compared the effects and side effects of the available oral medications on spasticity. In general these drugs are mildly effective orally, are more effective in younger children and

are often limited by unacceptable side effects. These include weakness, sedation and increased secretions. If the spasticity does not respond to simple drug treatment, advice from a neurorehabilitation specialist is invaluable as multiple options are available[44] but there is no clear evidence base to choose one treatment over another.[45]

Severe soft tissue inflammation: This is usually due to an acute infection. Overlying skin is usually red and swollen, and antibiotics are indicated (*see* cd-9 above). Deeper infections or those in AIDS patients may have few signs and may be an abscess that needs draining and IV antibiotics. In head and neck cancer, the rapid onset of severe pain may be the only symptom, but responds rapidly to flucloxacillin (in the US, cephalexin (Keflex) is generally used) and metronidazole.

Pleuritic pain: This is due to local inflammation and persistent pain can be eased with an NSAID or an intercostal block of the affected area.

Other causes: Structures that are inflamed, infected or distended may cause pain on movement. Recent trauma needs to be excluded, especially in frail or elderly patients.

4 Periodic pain

Smooth muscle spasm causes regular episodes of pain lasting a few minutes. This periodic feature is characteristic of colic, although occasionally colic is continuous. Bowel is the commonest source, followed by bladder and ureter. Bile duct is an unusual source. Opioids are ineffective and may worsen the pain. A smooth muscle relaxant (antispasmodic) is the treatment of choice. Hyoscine butylbromide (Buscopan) (Canada only) is preferred since it has fewer central effects than hyoscine hydrobromide (known as scopolamine in the US) or glycopyrrolate. In the US use hyoscyamine (Levsin) 0.125–0.25 mg PO/SL tid-qid prn.

5 Pain related to a procedure

Procedures that are painful produce increasing fear and pain with further procedures. Adequate analgesia prevents this build-up of anxiety. Nitrous oxide is a quick, effective analgesia for procedure-related pain in adults and children.[47–51] However, it is less effective than sedation and may not control more severe pain.[52,53] It should not be used in the presence of abnormal air cavities, e.g. pneumothorax, or bowel distension due to obstruction.[51]

6 Visceral pain

This is caused by disorders of the internal organs due to tumor, ischemia, or inflammation.[54] Cardiac pain and bowel distension are examples. Liver metastases can cause pain, but only if the liver capsule is stretched or inflamed. Damage to the celiac plexus or the lumbosacral plexus by tumor or fibrosis can cause a visceral neuropathic pain. It can be difficult to separate visceral neuropathic pain (gabapentin ± opioid) from compression of the celiac plexus (which might benefit from opioids + steroids) or a soft tissue pain due to retroperitoneal disease.

7 Pain related to eating

Pain will be caused by anything that causes inflammation of the mucosa of the mouth, pharynx, esophagus or stomach. Related structures must also be considered, such as teeth.

8 Associated with elimination

Problems such as constipation or a urine infection can cause pain. This may be periodic (colic), due to mucosal irritation (e.g. dysuria), pressure from local tumor causing a persistent sensation of wanting to defecate (tenesmus) or rectal tumor or inflammation causing rectal pain (proctalgia).

9 Associated skin changes

The most painful part of an ulcer is usually the damaged skin edge. Topical morphine may be helpful.[60–62] When pain is due to damage to deeper structures, systemic opioids or local nerve or spinal block may be needed.

10 Unpleasant sensory changes at rest

Neuropathic pain is due to persistent changes in the spinal cord in receptor and neurotransmitter functioning.[63] The term covers deafferentation pain (due to altered sensory processing following previous nerve damage causing pain in a dermatomal distribution), sympathetically maintained pain (pain in an autonomic nerve distribution), painful peripheral neuropathies, and peripheral neuralgias. Features are shown in the box below:

Clinical features of neuropathic pain[64]

> Spontaneous symptoms:
> - superficial burning pain
> - deep pain
> - paresthesia, e.g. tingling
> - dysesthesia, e.g. stabbing, stinging
> - paroxysms, i.e. severe episodes.
>
> On examination:
> - reduced temperature sensation (cool vs warm)
> - reduced light touch
> - pain on touching (allodynia)
> - increased sensitivity to touch
> - reduced vibration sensation.

No single test can confirm the presence of neuropathic pain, so it is diagnosed on the patient descriptions, together with the signs elicited on examination.[64]

Treatment can be complex,[65] and the advice of a pain or palliative care specialist should be sought. In cancer, pains often have multiple causes and opioids may be helpful, but neuropathic pain is often only partly responsive to opioids. Secondary analgesics (e.g. low dose amitriptyline or gabapentin) are often needed.[66–69] Amitriptyline has the best evidence for efficacy in neuropathic pain, but also has the most adverse effects.[67] Carbamazepine is usually seen as second choice, but has many potential interactions with drugs used in palliative care (*see* Drug information (p. 234)). The evidence for the efficacy of gabapentin is growing and it has fewer interactions or adverse effects.[69]

11 Nerve compression

If the cause is a tumor, the aim is to shrink the tumor (e.g. radiotherapy) or reduce the edema around the tumor with dexamethasone.[70] A local nerve block or spinal analgesia may be needed.

12 Persistent pain

If pain persists despite going through these clinical decisions, then a complete reassessment is necessary. A new pain or poor compliance are common reasons for persistent pain. It is also important to exclude unresolved psychological and spiritual issues, since these reduce the ability to cope with pain. These will need to be addressed by an interdisciplinary team, including a chaplain/spiritual advisor and a psychologist. Involving the adult or child in the management of their pain increases self-esteem and reduces pain perception.[71]

Choosing an analgesic

Clinical decision and action checklist

1 Check through 'Diagnosing and treating pain – clinical decisions' on pp. 41–3.
2 Is a rapid control of the pain needed?
3 Is the patient vomiting or unable to swallow?
4 Which opioid preparation is preferred?
5 Is there a medical precaution or contraindication?
6 Are adverse effects troubling the patient?
7 Is a combination of analgesics indicated?

Key points

Choice of analgesic depends on:

• the cause of the pain
• the route of administration
• patient preference for a preparation
• coexisting conditions
• adverse effects
• the need for combination analgesia.

Introduction

There are many analgesic types and preparations to suit most patients. However, comparative trials are few. For example, there is no evidence that any one strong opioid is better than any other.[76] An analgesic must be chosen on the basis of the cause of the pain, its pharmacokinetics, route of administration and convenience for the patient.

Choice based on the cause of pain

Pains vary in their sensitivity to opioids and some pains will only respond to other drugs (adjuvant analgesics, e.g. hyoscine butyl-bromide (Canada) or hyoscyamine (US) for colic) or approaches (e.g. pressure relieving devices for skin pressure pain).[77–80] Use the 12 clinical decisions in Diagnosing and treating pain (pp. 41–3) to decide what drugs or approaches are needed.

Choice based on analgesic staircase

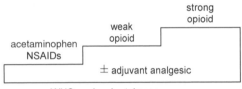

WHO analgesic staircase

This analgesic staircase uses the key principle of broad spectrum analgesia with non-opioids, opioids and adjuvant analgesics.[1] Weak opioids remain a key middle step,[76,81] while morphine remains the strong opioid of choice.[82] However, it is necessary to individualize the staircase to each patient. For example, the staircase for a patient with neuropathic pain would look very different:

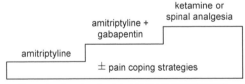

Example of analgesic staircase for neuropathic pain

Choice based on the patient

The cause of the pain will often suggest the type of analgesic needed. Choosing a specific analgesic depends on:

- *Speed of response:* There is a time delay before the affects of an analgesic can be assessed. This delay is shorter for some routes (e.g. intravenous) than others (e.g. oral). Using a route that allows a rapid assessment may be preferred in severe pain.
- *Ability to take oral medication:* If a patient is vomiting or unable to swallow, non-oral routes are necessary. These are usually subcutaneous or rectal.
- *Patient choice:* Patients may prefer tablets, solutions or transdermal patches. Controlled-release preparations are necessary for optimal pain management.[82,83]
- *Medical precautions and contraindications:* Analgesic choice can be influenced by coexisting illness (e.g. renal failure) or a history of previous illness (e.g. history of peptic ulceration). Also beware of drug interactions (*see* p. 223).
- *Adverse effects:* A change to a similar analgesic may reduce or stop drug adverse effects (e.g. diclofenac to ibuprofen, morphine to hydromorphone).
- *Need for combination analgesia:* Some conditions (e.g. pelvic tumors) can produce complex pains with multiple causes that need combinations of non-opioid, opioids and adjuvant analgesics.

Clinical decision	If YES ⇒ Action
1 Check through clinical decisions 1–12 in Diagnosing and treating pain, pp. 41–3.	
2 Is a rapid control of the pain needed?	Use analgesic routes with a rapid action. If pain relief is needed in: • less than 2 minutes: use the intravenous route • 15 minutes: use the intramuscular (deltoid muscle), buccal, intranasal or rectal route* • 30 minutes: use the subcutaneous route • 60 minutes: use an oral instant release preparation. * Rectal route: for a rapid response an instant release preparation must be used.

3 Is the patient vomiting or unable to swallow?	• For opioids, use subcutaneous hydromorphone or morphine (continuous infusion or bolus).
	• Alternatives for regular analgesic administration:
	  – rectal: non-opioid (acetaminophen), opioid (hydromorphone, morphine, or oxycodone), NSAID (naproxen). NB: The rectal route for controlled release morphine has been reported,[84–87] and may be an alternative at home for short-term use when pumps or parenteral drugs are temporarily unavailable.
	  – transdermal: (this route is only suitable for patients with stable pain) fentanyl or buprenorphine. (Buprenorphine is not available in Canada. In the US, a compounding pharmacy can provide a transdermal gel preparation of buprenorphine but a patch is not available).
	  – buccal (transmucosal): fentanyl (injection liquid in Canada and US; fentanyl lozenge (Actiq) in US or sufentanil) (this produces brief pain relief of up to 2 hours).[82,88,89]
	NB The IV, IM and buccal routes are not suitable for regular, bolus doses of analgesia.[82,90] The intravenous route can be used for titration or continuous administration.[91]

4 Does the patient have a preference for an opioid preparation?	• *Controlled-release opioid preparations:*
	  – oral capsules, e.g. morphine (MOS SR, MS-Contin, Oramorph SR), oxycodone (OxyContin)
	  – capsules, e.g. hydromorphone (Hydromorph Contin), morphine (M-Eslon)
	  – transdermal, e.g. fentanyl (Duragesic).
	• *Instant release opioid preparations:*
	  – oral tablets, e.g. morphine (MOS, MS-IR, Statex)
	  – buccal/sublingual preparations, e.g. fentanyl or sufentanil injection solution (or fentanyl lozenge (Actiq) in US). Sublingual buprenorphine is available in US (but not in Canada) as Subutex but has restricted access and is little used in palliative care.
	  – liquids, e.g. morphine (Morphitec, Statex, MOS)
	  – capsules, e.g. hydromorphone (Dilaudid), oxycodone (Oxy-IR)
	  – suppositories, e.g. morphine (MOS, MS-IR, Statex), hydromorphone (Dilaudid, PMS-Hydromorphone), Oxycodone (Supeudol).

Table continued overleaf

5 Is there a medical precaution or contraindication?	• *Renal impairment:*
	  – use NSAIDs with care (may cause further renal impairment).
	  – use acetaminophen with care.
	  – use morphine, hydromorphone or oxycodone with care.[92–97] Hydromorphone may be safe for mild-moderate impairment.[98,99] Fentanyl may be safe in severe impairment, but caution is still required.[100]
	• *Hepatic impairment:*
	  – use NSAIDs and acetaminophen with care.
	  – use all opioids with care.[101–103] Morphine may be the preferred choice, but if hepatic encephalopathy is present, *any* opioid can precipitate coma.
	• *Peptic ulceration:*
	  – previous history: cover NSAIDs with proton pump inhibitor (e.g. omeprazole),[104] cover corticosteroids with H_2 blocker (e.g. ranitidine) or proton pump inhibitor.[105,106]
	  – current ulceration: avoid NSAIDs or corticosteroids. Consider switching to a selective COX2 inhibitor (but only reduces risk by half and may be less effective analgesic than standard NSAIDs).[107]
	• Infants < 1 year are very sensitive to opioids. *See* Drugs in palliative care for children: starting doses (p. 253).
	• *Drug interactions: see* pp. 225–8 for interactions of analgesics with drugs used in palliative care.

6 Are adverse effects troubling the patient?	Switch to alternative analgesic, for example: • diclofenac to ibuprofen • morphine to hydromorphone, oxycodone or fentanyl (*see* Using opioids (p. 49)) • amitriptyline or carbamazepine to gabapentin.
7 Is a combination of analgesics indicated?	• Review clinical decisions 1–12 in Diagnosing and treating pain (pp. 41–3) and list possible pain mechanisms to decide the combination of non-opioid, opioid and adjuvant analgesic needed.

cd = clinical decision

Using opioids

1 Check Diagnosing and treating pain (pp. 41–3) to ensure that an opioid is needed.
2 Check Choosing an analgesic (pp. 45–8) to decide the starting opioid and route.
3 Are you uncertain about starting dose, frequency or titration rate?
4 If changing between opioids, check correct conversions.

Key points

- The starting dose and titration rate are tailored to the individual.
- The frequency of doses depends on the preparation used.
- Conversion ratios between opioids are guides only and dose adjustments may be needed.
- Final dose requirements cannot be predicted.
- Breakthrough doses may also need to be titrated to the individual.

Starting dose

Because dose requirements cannot be predicted, starting doses should be low, especially in infants under one year, or in frail or elderly adults. Starting with high doses produces adverse effects and increases the chance of the patient rejecting the analgesic. Starting doses for a frail, elderly adult previously on a non-opioid may be as low as codeine 10 mg q4h, while younger adults may cope with higher doses such as codeine 30 mg q4h. Starting doses in children depend in part on their age (*see* p. 253). Patients on non-opioids should not be started on potent strong opioids such as transdermal fentanyl. Patients already on higher doses of a regular weak opioid can start a strong opioid equivalent to their current dose.

Frequency of dose

This will depend on:

1   the duration of action of a controlled-release preparation
2   the half-life of the opioid.

Oral morphine is normally given q4h for an instant-release preparation, but infants and children may need it every 2–3 hours. A double dose at bedtime does not reduce the need for a night-time dose.[108] Morphine can be given once or twice daily depending on which controlled-release preparation is used. Controlled-release morphine is well tolerated by children,[109] but some may need to take it three times daily. Remember that patients using transdermal fentanyl still need breakthrough medication prescribed (usually morphine or hydromorphone).

Conversions

The table on p. 52 is a guide to conversions. However, conversion values are approximations and caution is needed.[82,110–113] Convert to the equivalent dose of the current opioid, and then reduce that dose by 25%.[111] Monitor the patient and in particular, look out for opioid toxicity and opioid withdrawal.

Rules of opioid conversion:

1   Know your opioid.
2   Use a conversion factor with which you are familiar.
3   Be prepared to retitrate the dose.
4   If in doubt, ask.

More potent opioids or routes DO NOT provide greater efficacy, e.g. a pain that is not responsive to oral morphine will not respond to injectable hydromorphone either, even though this drug by this route is about 10 times as potent. However, an alternative route may be needed to ensure adequate absorption.

Example of conversion: Oral morphine to hydromorphone infusion

- Conversion factor is ÷ 10.
- So 60 mg/24 hours oral morphine ≡ 6 mg/24 hours SC hydromorphone.

Fentanyl

- Check the manufacturer's conversion tables.
- Quick conversion: oral morphine in mg/24 hr ÷ 3 = TD fentanyl in microgram/hr (e.g. 75 mg oral morphine/day ≈ 25 microgram/hour TD fentanyl).
- Transdermal fentanyl is less flexible than other opioid preparations and should be reserved for patients with stable pain.[82] It can be used in children.[114]

Titration, laxatives and 'PRN' analgesia

Opioids should not be increased by more than 50%. For children some use smaller routine increases of 25%.[115] Increases are usually every third day, but faster titration (e.g. twice daily) can be done under supervision. Faster titration is useful if urgency is an issue, but it also increases the likelihood of adverse effects. For 'PRN' or breakthrough doses, *see* cd-2 in Diagnosing and treating pain (p. 41).

Concurrent laxatives are essential in 90% of patients. Breakthrough medication must also be prescribed.

Use of opioids in children

There are important differences in using opioids in children with respect to starting doses, dosing frequency, adverse effects and useful routes. For more details, *see* Drugs in palliative care for children: starting doses (p. 253).

Clinical decision	If YES ⇒ Action
1 Check through clinical decisions 1–12 in Diagnosing and treating pain (pp. 41–3).	
2 Check Choosing an analgesic (p. 45) to decide the starting opioid and route.	
3 Are you uncertain about starting dose, frequency or titration rate?	*Starting dose:* • For breakthrough pain: *see* cd-2 in Diagnosing and treating pain (p. 41). • If previously on non-opioid: start a weak opioid (e.g. codeine 30 mg q4h for adults). If ineffective, titrate the weak opioid. *See* p. 253 for doses in children. • If previously on a weak opioid, start with the equivalent dose of a strong opioid (*see* conversion chart overleaf) and then titrate to the individual's requirements. *Frequency of doses for regular analgesia:* • Instant release: oral or SC morphine, hydromorphone or oxycodone = q4h (may need 2–3 hourly in children). • Controlled release = q12h (may need q8h in children) (M-Eslon, Oramorph SR, MOS-SR) or once daily (Kadian). • Transdermal = change patch every third day (Duragesic). *Titration, laxatives and 'PRN' (breakthrough) medication:* • Increase opioid by 25–50%, usually every third day, but can be faster under supervision. • Prescribe laxative and breakthrough medication (*see* p. 41 for breakthrough doses).
4 If changing between opioids, check conversion according to table on p. 52.	
cd = clinical decision	

3 step conversion

1   Find the current opioid and route at the **top** of the table.
2   Find the new opioid and route you are changing to on the **right** of the table.

3   Where the lines cross, read the conversion factor.
× Multiply current opioid by this factor
÷ Divide current opioid by this factor
ask Ask for advice

Current opioid and route ▶	PO codeine	PO morphine	PO oxycodone	SC morphine	PO hydromorphone	SC hydromorphone	TD or SC fentanyl	New opioid and route ▼
		× 10	× 15	× 20	ask	ask	ask	PO codeine
	÷ 10		× 1.5	× 2	× 5	× 10	ask	PO morphine
	÷ 15	÷ 1.5		× 1.3	× 3	× 6	ask	PO oxycodone
	÷ 20	÷ 2	÷ 1.3		× 2.5	× 5	ask	SC morphine
	ask	÷ 5	÷ 3	÷ 2.5		× 2	ask	PO hydromorphone
	ask	÷ 10	÷ 6	÷ 5	÷ 2		ask	SC hydromorphone
	ask	ask	ask	ask	ask	ask		TD or SC fentanyl

Managing the adverse effects of analgesics

Clinical decision and action checklist

1   Is coma or respiratory depression present?
2   Is there nausea and vomiting?
3   Has stool consistency changed?
4   Is there drowsiness, confusion, nightmares or hallucinations?
5   Are there antimuscarinic symptoms?
6   Is movement affected?
7   Is the patient fearful of the opioid?
8   Is there evidence of recent liver or renal problems?
9   Has blood pressure changed?
10 Is this a drug interaction?

Key points

- NSAID adverse effects are common.
- Tolerance develops to some opioid effects (e.g. nausea) but not others (e.g. constipation).
- Co-analgesics are often forgotten as a cause of troublesome adverse effects.

Introduction

Although there is no evidence that death is a consequence of the correct use of oral morphine in palliative care,[1,116–118] analgesics are not free of adverse effects and minimizing their impact on patients is part of effective symptom control.

Non-opioid analgesics

Acetaminophen: This is usually well tolerated in doses of 1 g q4h,[119] but hepatotoxicity can occur,[120] and nausea and vomiting are early symptoms.[121]

Non-steroidal anti-inflammatory drugs (NSAIDs): These can be effective in some cancer pains,[122] but adverse effects are common.[123] Gastrointestinal mucosal damage is the commonest, risking dyspepsia, ulceration and bleeding.[124,125] Renal impairment is a risk, especially with longer acting NSAIDs (e.g. piroxicam).[126] COX2 specific NSAIDs can be an alternative, but recent cardiovascular concerns and severe skin reactions have led to the withdrawal from the market of rofecoxib and valdecoxib respectively (only celecoxib is presently available in North America):

1 they only reduce peptic ulceration by half[127]
2 bleeding from the gut can still occur[125,128,129]
3 the risk of renal impairment may be no different[130]
4 they may be less effective than a dual COX1/COX2 inhibitor (such as diclofenac)[107]
5 Health Canada advises that patients with cardiac risk factors for heart attack or stroke should not use celecoxib.[160]

Proton pump inhibitors (e.g. lansoprazole) and misoprostol can help protect against NSAID-induced ulceration.[58] H_2-antagonists should not be used as they are less effective in protecting the stomach from NSAID damage.[123,131]

Opioid analgesics

Tolerance: Opioids show 'selective tolerance'[132] so that tolerance to euphoria takes 1–2 days, to drowsiness 5–7 days, while no tolerance develops to constipation. Tolerance to analgesia is not a clinical problem.[133]

Respiratory depression is rarely a problem in patients on long-term morphine.[134] The only exception is when pain (a stimulus to respiration) is suddenly relieved without prior dose reduction, e.g. after a nerve block.

Addiction (a pleasurable craving for a chemical or situation)[159] is rare in patients with advanced disease taking opioids for pain.[135,136] Physical dependence does occur but withdrawal symptoms are unusual (usually colic, diarrhea) and do not prevent gradual reductions over 5 days.[137]

Drowsiness: This usually wears off over a few days, but persistent drowsiness may necessitate a switch to a different opioid. If this is not possible, an alternative is to use a psychostimulant such as methylphenidate.[138]

Other: Constipation occurs in 90% of patients and concurrent laxatives are essential.[139] Dry mouth occurs in up to 40% of patients.[140] Myoclonus is seen with morphine,[141] but has also been reported with hydromorphone,[141] methadone[142] and fentanyl.[143,144] Opioids are an unusual cause of hallucinations and other causes should be considered.[145]

Children: The frequency of adverse effects from opioids and NSAIDs is similar in neonates, children and adults.[146–148]

Adjuvant analgesics

These drugs have a wide range of adverse effects and the drug monographs should be consulted.

Antidepressants: Amitriptyline still has the best evidence base for neuropathic pain,[149] but it causes many antimuscarinic effects at higher doses (dry mouth, constipation, blurred vision, hypotension, movement disorders, drowsiness, confusion).

Anticonvulsants: Carbamazepine has a high rate of adverse effects and interactions, and gabapentin is a safer alternative in advanced disease.[149,150]

Corticosteroids: These can cause many adverse effects including diabetes, edema, proximal weakness (due to a myopathy) and osteoporosis.[151]

Antispasmodics: Hyoscine butylbromide (Buscopan) (Canada only) usually has few adverse effects, but hyoscine hydrobromide (known as scopolamine in the US) can cause marked central antimuscarinic effects. In the US use hyoscyamine (Levsin) 0.125–0.25 mg PO/SL tid-qid PRN.

Antispastics: These can cause a wide range of effects from confusion to weakness.

Clinical decision	If YES ⇒ Action
1 Is coma or respiratory depression present?	• *See* cd-3b in Emergencies (p. 205).
2 Is there nausea and/ or vomiting?	• *Gastric irritation (NSAID any type, corticosteroids):* start a proton pump inhibitor (PPI), e.g. lansoprazole 30 mg daily (omeprazole in children) (a PPI is preferable to misoprostol).[59] If vomit or stool are positive for blood, stop the NSAID. • *Central effects (opioid, carbamazepine, dantrolene):* when the pattern is mixed nausea and vomiting start haloperidol 1.5–3 mg once at night. Consider switching to a different opioid.[113] If constipation is present: *see* Constipation (p. 75). • *Gastric stasis (opioid, amitriptyline):* If large volume vomiting is the main problem this suggests gastric stasis. *See* cd-2a in Nausea and vomiting (p. 115).
3 Has stool consistency changed?	• Consider these drugs as causes: amitriptyline, carbamazepine, dantrolene, NSAIDs, opioids. • *See* Constipation (p. 75), Diarrhea (p. 81).
4 Are drowsiness, confusion, nightmares or hallucinations present?	• Consider these drugs as causes: amitriptyline, carbamazepine, dantrolene, baclofen, gabapentin, ketamine, NSAIDs, opioids. Reduce the dose or change to an alternative drug. *See* Confusional states (delirium and dementia) (p. 171). • *If drowsiness persists:* check for other causes (*see* Fatigue, drowsiness, lethargy and weakness (p. 101)). Consider using methylphenidate 2.5–5 mg in the morning, increasing if necessary to 10–15 mg. A second dose can be given, but no later than lunchtime to avoid insomnia.
5 Are antimuscarinic symptoms present? (i.e. blurred vision, drowsiness, dry mouth, hypotension, urinary retention)	• Consider these drugs as causes: amitriptyline, hyoscine hydrobromide (known as scopolamine in the US), opioids. Reduce dose or change to an alternative analgesic.
6 Is movement affected?	• *Myoclonus (opioids):* change opioid.[152] Alternatively, try dantrolene[153] or SC midazolam.[154] • *Dyskinesia, Parkinson's:* consider amitriptyline, carbamazepine, haloperidol, phenothiazine or gabapentin as causes. Reduce the dose or change to a different drug, or give benztropine 1–2 mg od or bid (or procyclidine 2.5 mg q8h and titrate). • *Muscle weakness* (baclofen, corticosteroids): reduce the dose.
7 Is the patient fearful of the opioid?	Usually this is due to a fear of opioid adverse effects. • Explain the facts about opioids (*see* opposite). Offer written information.[155]
8 Is there evidence of recent liver or renal impairment?	*Liver impairment:* consider carbamazepine, gabapentin, NSAIDs, acetaminophen as causes. Change to alternative. *Renal impairment:* consider carbamazepine or NSAIDs as causes. Change to alternative.
9 Is there a recent change in blood pressure?	*Increased:* consider dantrolene, dexamethasone, ketamine, prednisolone or tramadol (not currently available in Canada) as causes. Reduce dose or change to alternative. *Decreased:* consider amitriptyline, baclofen, dantrolene or tramadol as causes. Reduce dose or change to alternative.
10 Is the problem due to a drug interaction?	• Check interactions of analgesic drugs with other drugs used in palliative care (pp, 225–8).

cd = clinical decision

References

B = book; C = comment; Ch = chapter; CS-n = case study-number of cases; CT = controlled trial; E = editorial; GC = group consensus; I = interviews; Let = letter; LS = laboratory study; MC = multi-center; OS-n = open study-number of cases; R = review; RCT-n = randomized controlled trial-number of cases; RS = retrospective survey; SA = systematic or meta analysis.

1 Twycross R, Wilcock A (2001) Pain relief. In: *Symptom Management in Advanced Cancer*. Radcliffe Medical Press, Oxford. (Ch)

2 Baker CM, Wong DL (1987) Q.U.E.S.T.: a process of pain assessment in children. *Orthopedic Nursing*. **6**(1): 11–21.

3 Gauvain-Piquard A, Rodary C, Rezvani A, Serbouti S (1999) The development of the DEGR(R): a scale to assess pain in young children with cancer. *European Journal of Pain*. **3**(2): 165–76.

4 Hain RDW (1997) Pain scales in children: a review. *Palliative Medicine*. **11**: 341–50. (R)

5 McGrath PA (1998) Pain control in paediatric palliative care. In: D Doyle, GWC Hanks, N MacDonald (eds) *The Oxford Textbook of Palliative Medicine* (2e). Oxford Medical Press, Oxford. (Ch)

6 Eland JM (1985) Paediatrics. In: *Pain*. Springhouse Corporation, Springhouse (PA). (Ch)

7 McGrath PJ, McAlpine L (1993) Psychologic aspects on paediatric pain. *Journal of Paediatrics*. **5**(2): S2–8.

8 Craig KD (1994) Emotional aspects of pain. In: PD Wall, R Melzack (eds) *Textbook of Pain on CD-ROM* (3e). Churchill Livingstone, Edinburgh.

9 International Association for the Study of Pain (IASP) (1979) Pain terms: a list of definitions and notes on usage recommended by the IASP Subcommittee on Taxonomy. *Pain*. **6**: 249–52. (GC)

10 Regnard C, Matthews D, Gibson L, Clarke C. Distressed people with severe communication difficulties: is it pain? *International Journal of Palliative Nursing*. In press.

11 Portenoy RK, Payne D, Jacobsen P (1999) Breakthrough pain: characteristics and impact in patients with cancer pain. *Pain*. **81**(1–2): 129–34. (OS-164)

12 Swanwick M, Haworth M, Lennard RF (2001) The prevalence of episodic pain in cancer: a survey of hospice patients on admission. *Palliative Medicine*. **15**(1): 9–18. (OS-245)

13 Luger NM, Sabino MAC, Schwei MJ, Mach DB, Pomonis JD, Keyser CP, Rathbun M, Clohisy DR, Honore P, Yaksh TL, Mantyh PW (2002) Efficacy of systemic morphine suggests a fundamental difference in the mechanisms that generate bone cancer vs inflammatory pain. *Pain*. **99**: 397–406. (LS)

14 McQuay HJ, Collins SL, Caroll D, Moore RA (1995) Radiotherapy for the palliation of painful bone metastases (Cochrane Review). In: *The Cochrane Library, Issue 4, 2002*. Oxford Update Software, Oxford. www.cochrane.org (SA)

15 Townsend PW, Smalley SR, Cozad SC, Rosenthal HG, Hassanein RE (1995) Role of postoperative radiation therapy after stabilization of fractures caused by metastatic disease. *International Journal of Radiation Oncology, Biology, Physics*. **31**: 43–9. (OS-60)

16 Eisenberg E, Berkey CS, Carr DB, Mosteller F, Chalmers TC (1994) Efficacy and safety of non-steroidal antiinflammatory drugs for cancer pain: a meta-analysis. *Journal of Clinical Oncology*. **12**(12): 2756–65. (SA)

17 Berenson JR (2001) Zoledronic acid in cancer patients with bone metastases: results of Phase I and II trials. *Seminars in Oncology*. **28**(Suppl 6): 25–34. (R, 33 refs)

18 Coleman RE, Seaman JJ (2001) The role of zoledronic acid in cancer: clinical studies in the treatment and prevention of bone metastases. *Seminars in Oncology*. **28** (Suppl 6): 11–16. (R, 36 refs)

19 Berenson JR, Rosen LS, Howell A, Porter L, Coleman RE, Morley W, Dreicer R, Kuross SA, Lipton A, Seaman JJ (2001) Zoledronic acid reduces skeletal-related events in patients with osteolytic metastasis. *Cancer*. **91**: 1191–200. (MC, RCT-280)

20 Hortobagyi GN, Theriault RL, Porter L, Blayney D, Lipton A, Sinoff C, Wheeler H, Simeone JF, Seaman J, Knight RD (1996) Efficacy of pamidronate in reducing skeletal complications in patients with breast cancer and lytic bone metastases. *New England Journal of Medicine*. **335**: 1785–91. (MC, RCT-382)

21 Berenson JR, Lichtenstein A, Porter L, Dimopoulos MA, Bordoni R, George S, Lipton A, Keller A, Ballester O, Kovacs MJ, Blacklock HA, Bell R, Simeone J, Reitsma DJ, Heffernan M, Seaman J, Knight RD (1996) Efficacy of pamidronate in reducing skeletal events in patients with advanced multiple myeloma. *New England Journal of Medicine*. **334**: 488–93. (RCT-392)

22 Mannix K, Ahmedzai SH, Anderson H, Bennett M, Lloyd-Williams M, Wilcock A (2000) Using bis-phosphonates to control the pain of bone metastases: evidence-based guidelines for palliative care. *Palliative Medicine*. **14**(6): 455–61. (SA, 32 refs)

23 Wong R, Wiffen PJ (2002) Bisphosphonates for the relief of pain secondary to bone metastases (Cochrane Review). In: *The Cochrane Library, Issue 4, 2002*. Oxford Update Software, Oxford. (www.cochrane.org) (SA)

24 Petcu EB, Schug SA, Smith RH. Clinical evaluation of onset of analgesia using intravenous pamidronate in metastatic bone pain. *Journal of Pain and Symptom Management*. **24**(3): 281–4. (Let, OS-10)

25 Predey TA, Sewall LE, Smith SJ (2002) Percutaneous vertebroplasty: new treatment for vertebral compression fractures. *American Family Physician*. **66**(4): 611–15. (R, 19 refs)

26 Borg-Stein J, Simons DG (2002) Focused review: myofascial pain. *Archives of Physical Medicine & Rehabilitation*. **83**(Suppl 2): S40–7. (R, 99 refs)

27 Travell JG, Simons DG (1989) Myofascial pain. In: PD Wall, R Melzack (eds) *Textbook of Pain* (2e). Churchill Livingstone, Edinburgh. (Ch)

28 Sauls J (1999) Efficacy of cold for pain: fact or fallacy? *Online Journal of Knowledge Synthesis for Nursing*. **6**(8).

29 Iwama H, Ohmori S, Kaneko T, Watanabe K (2001) Water-diluted local anesthetic for trigger-point injection in chronic myofascial pain syndrome: evaluation of types of local anesthetic and concentrations in water. *Regional Anesthesia & Pain Medicine*. **26**(4): 333–6. (OS-40)

30 Offenbacher M, Stucki G (2000) Physical therapy in the treatment of fibromyalgia. *Scandinavian Journal of Rheumatology Supplement*. **113**: 78–85. (R, 58 refs)

31 Graff-Radford SB, Reeves JL, Baker RL, Chiu D (1989) Effects of transcutaneous electrical nerve stimulation on myofascial pain and trigger point sensitivity. *Pain*. **37**(1): 1–5. (CT-60)

32 Francisco GE, Kothari S, Huls C (2001) GABA agonists and gabapentin for spastic hypertonia. *Physical Medicine & Rehabilitation Clinics of North America*. **12**(4): 875–88. (R, 84)

33 Elovic E (2001) Principles of pharmaceutical management of spastic hypertonia. *Physical Medicine & Rehabilitation Clinics of North America*. **12**(4): 793–816. (R, 180 refs)

34 Ward AB, Ko CK (2001) Pharmacological management of spasticity. In: MP Barnes, RJ Garth (eds) *Upper Motor Neurone Syndrome and Spasticity: clinical management and neurophysiology*. Cambridge University Press, Cambridge. (Ch)

35 Yablon SA (2001) Botulinum neurotoxin intramuscular chemodenervation. Role in the management of spastic hypertonia and related motor disorders. *Physical Medicine & Rehabilitation Clinics of North America*. **12**(4): 833–74. (R, 84 refs)

36 Ivanhoe CB, Tilton AH, Francisco GE (2001) Intrathecal baclofen therapy for spastic hypertonia. *Physical Medicine & Rehabilitation Clinics of North America*. **12**(4): 923–38. (R, 57 refs)

37 Zafonte RD, Munin MC (2001) Phenol and alcohol blocks for the treatment of spasticity. *Physical Medicine & Rehabilitation Clinics of North America*. **12**(4): 817–32. (R, 53 refs)

38 Grabb PA, Doyle JS (2001) The contemporary surgical management of spasticity in children. *Physical Medicine & Rehabilitation Clinics of North America*. **12**(4): 907–22. (R, 53 refs)

39 Gracies JM (2001) Physical modalities other than stretch in spastic hypertonia. *Physical Medicine & Rehabilitation Clinics of North America*. **12**(4): 769–92. (R, 222 refs)

40 Abbruzzese G (2002) The medical management of spasticity. *European Journal of Neurology*. **9**(Suppl 1): 30–4; discussion 53–61. (R, 27 refs)

41 Wagstaff AJ, Bryson HM (1997) Tizanidine. A review of its pharmacology, clinical efficacy and tolerability in the management of spasticity associated with cerebral and spinal disorders. *Drugs*. **53**(3): 435–52. (R, 112 refs)

42 Thompson JW, Regnard C (1995) Pain. In: *Flow Diagrams in Advanced Cancer and Other Diseases*. Edward Arnold, London. pp. 5–10. (Ch)

43 Barnes M (2001) An overview of the clinical management of spasticity. In: MP Barnes, RJ Garth (eds) *Upper Motor Neurone Syndrome and Spasticity: clinical management and neurophysiology*. Cambridge University Press, Cambridge. (Ch)

44 Burchiel KJ, Hsu FP (2001) Pain and spasticity after spinal cord injury: mechanisms and treatment. *Spine*. **26**(24 Suppl): S146–60. (R, 176 refs)

45 Shakespeare DT, Young CA, Boggild M (2000) Anti-spasticity agents for multiple sclerosis. *Cochrane Database Syst Rev*. (**4**): CD001332. (SA, 172 refs)

46 Briggs M, Nelson EA (2003) Topical agents or dressings for pain in venous leg ulcers (Cochrane Review). In: *The Cochrane Library*, Issue 2. Update Software, Oxford. www.cochrane.org

47 Masood J, Shah N, Lane T, Andrews H, Simpson P, Barua JM (2002) Nitrous oxide (Entonox) inhalation and tolerance of transrectal ultrasound guided prostate biopsy: a double-blind randomized controlled study. *Journal of Urology*. **168**(1): 116–20. (RCT-110)

48 Cleary AG, Ramanan AV, Baildam E, Birch A, Sills JA, Davidson JE (2002) Nitrous oxide analgesia during intra-articular injection for juvenile idiopathic arthritis. *Archives of Disease in Childhood*. **86**(6): 416–18. (OS-55)

49 Rosen MA (2002) Nitrous oxide for relief of labor pain: a systematic review. *American Journal of Obstetrics & Gynecology*. **186**(5 Suppl Nature): S110–26. (R, 69 refs)

50 Gerhardt RT, King KM, Wiegert RS (2001) Inhaled nitrous oxide versus placebo as an analgesic and anxiolytic adjunct to peripheral intravenous cannulation. *American Journal of Emergency Medicine*. **19**(6): 492–4. (RCT-11)

51 Sealey L (2002) Nurse administration of Entonox to manage pain in ward settings. *Nursing Times*. **98**(46): 28–9. (R, 9 refs)

52 Forbes GM, Collins BJ (2000) Nitrous oxide for colonoscopy: a randomized controlled study. *Gastrointestinal Endoscopy*. **51**(3): 271–7. (RCT-102)

53 Enting RH, Oldenmenger WH, van der Rijt CCD, Koper P, Smith PAE (2002) Nitrous oxide is not beneficial for breakthrough cancer pain. *Palliative Medicine*. **16**: 257–9. (CS-2)

54 Al-Chaer ED, Traub RJ (2002) Biological basis of visceral pain: recent developments. *Pain*. **96**: 221–5. (R, 39 refs)

55 Devulder J, Lambert J, Naeyaert JM (2001) Gabapentin for pain control in cancer patients' wound dressing care. *Journal of Pain and Symptom Management*. **22**(1): 622–6. (CS-1)

56 Camfield PR (1999) Buccal midazolam and rectal diazepam for treatment of prolonged seizures in childhood and adolescence: a randomised trial. *Journal of Pediatrics*. **135**(3): 398–9. (RCT)

57 Pelham A, Lee MA, Regnard CBF (2002) Gabapentin for coeliac plexus pain. *Palliative Medicine*. **16**: 355–6 (CS-3)

58 Graham DY, Agrawal NM, Campbell DR, Haber MM, Collis C, Lukasik NL, Huang B (2002) NSAID-Associated Gastric Ulcer Prevention Study Group. Ulcer prevention in long-term users of nonsteroidal anti-inflammatory drugs: results of a double-blind, randomized, multicenter, active- and placebo-controlled study of misoprostol vs lansoprazole. *Archives of Internal Medicine*. **162**(2): 169–75. (GC)

59 Yeomans N, Wilson I, Langstrom G, Hawkey C, Naesdal J, Walan A, Wiklund I (2001) Quality of life in chronic NSAID users: a comparison of the effect

of omeprazole and misoprostol. *Scandinavian Journal of Rheumatology.* **30**(6): 328–34. (OS-610)

60 Back IN, Finlay I (1995) Analgesic effect of topical opioids on painful skin ulcers. *Journal of Pain and Symptom Management.* **10**: 493. (Let)

61 Krajnik M, Zylicz Z (1997) Topical morphine for cutaneous cancer pain. *Palliative Medicine.* **11**: 325–6. (CS-6)

62 Twillman RK, Long TD, Cathers TA, Mueller DW (1999) Treatment of painful skin ulcers with topical opioids. *Journal of Pain and Symptom Management.* **17**(4): 288–92. (CS-9)

63 Portenoy RK (1992) Cancer pain: pathophysiology and syndromes. *Lancet.* **339**: 1026–31. (R, 34 refs)

64 Jensen TS, Baron R (2003) Translation of symptoms and signs into mechanisms in neuropathic pain. *Pain.* **102**: 1–8. (R, 40 refs)

65 Hanks GW, Justins DM (1992) Cancer pain: management. *Lancet.* **339**: 1031–6. (R, 34 refs)

66 Jensen TS (2002) Anticonvulsants in neuropathic pain: rationale and clinical evidence. *European Journal of Pain.* **Suppl A**: 61–8. (R, 31 refs)

67 McQuay HJ (2002) Neuropathic pain: evidence matters. *European Journal of Pain.* **Suppl A**: 11–18. (SA, 30 refs)

68 Koltzenburg M, Scadding J (2001) Neuropathic pain. *Current Opinion in Neurology.* **14**(5): 641–7. (R, 65 refs)

69 Serpell MG (2002) Neuropathic Pain Study Group. Gabapentin in neuropathic pain syndromes: a randomised, double-blind, placebo-controlled trial. *Pain.* **99**: 557–66. (RCT-305)

70 Twycross R (1994) The risks and benefits of corticosteroids in advanced cancer. *Drug Safety.* **11**(3): 163–78. (R)

71 Twycross A *et al.* (1998) *Paediatric Pain Management: a multidisciplinary approach.* Radcliffe Medical Press, Oxford. (B)

72 Holtom N (2000) Gabapentin for treatment of thalamic pain syndrome. *Palliative Medicine.* **14**(2): 167. (Let, CS-1)

73 Kaplan KM, Barron TF, Jones BV (1998) Thalamic pain in a child with acute disseminated encephalomyelitis. *Clinical Pediatrics.* **37**(7): 441–3. (CS-1)

74 Nasreddine ZS, Saver JL (1997) Pain after thalamic stroke: right diencephalic predominance and clinical features in 180 patients. *Neurology.* **48**(5): 1196–9. (SA)

75 Segatore M (1996) Understanding central post-stroke pain. *Journal of Neuroscience Nursing.* **28**(1): 28–35. (R, 74 refs)

76 Mercadante S, Salvaggio L, Dardanoni G, Agnello A, Garofalo S (1998) Dextropropoxyphene versus morphine in opioid-naïve cancer patients with pain. *Journal of Pain and Symptom Management.* **15**: 78–81. (RCT-32)

77 Hanks GW, Forbes K (1997) Opioid responsiveness. *Acta Anaesthesiologica Scandinavica.* **41**(1 Pt 2): 154–8. (R)

78 Mercadante S, Portenoy RK (2001) Opioid poorly-responsive cancer pain. Part 3. Clinical strategies to improve opioid responsiveness. *Journal of Pain and Symptom Management.* **21**(4): 338–54. (R, 189 refs)

79 Mercadante S, Portenoy RK (2001) Opioid poorly-responsive cancer pain. Part 2: basic mechanisms that could shift dose response for analgesia. *Journal of Pain and Symptom Management.* **21**(3): 255–64. (R, 86 refs)

80 Mercadante S, Portenoy RK (2001) Opioid poorly-responsive cancer pain. Part 1: clinical considerations. *Journal of Pain and Symptom Management.* **21**(2): 144–50. (R, 56 refs)

81 Mercadante S (2001) Is morphine the drug of choice in cancer pain? *Progress in Palliative Care.* **5**: 190–3. (R)

82 Hanks GW, Conno F, Cherny N, Hanna M, Kalso E, McQuay HJ, Mercadante S, Meynadier J, Poulain P, Ripamonti C, Radbruch L, Casas JR, Sawe J, Twycross RG, Ventafridda V (2001) Expert Working Group of the Research Network of the European Association for Palliative Care. Morphine and alternative opioids in cancer pain: the EAPC recommendations. *British Journal of Cancer.* **84**(5): 587–93. (GC)

83 Davis M, Wilcock A (2001) Modified-release opioids. *European Journal of Palliative Care.* **8**: 142–6. (R)

84 Kaiko RF, Fitzmartin RD, Thomas GB, Goldenheim PD (1992) The bioavailability of morphine in controlled-release 30-mg tablets per rectum compared with immediate-release 30-mg rectal suppositories and controlled-release 30-mg oral tablets. *Pharmacotherapy.* **12**: 107–13. (RCT-14)

85 Wilkinson TJ, Robinson BA, Begg EJ, Duffull SB, Ravenscroft PJ (1992) Pharmacokinetics and efficacy of rectal versus oral sustained-release morphine in cancer patients. *Cancer Chemotherapy and Pharmacology.* **31**: 251–4. (RCT-10)

86 Campbell WI (1996) Rectal controlled-release morphine: plasma levels of morphine and its metabolites following the rectal administration of MST Continus 100 mg. *Journal of Clinical Pharmacology and Therapeutics.* **21**: 65–71. (OS-8)

87 Maloney CM, Kesner RK, Klein G, Bockenstette J (1989). The rectal administration of MS Contin®: clinical implications of use in end stage cancer. *American Journal of Hospice Care.* **6**: 34–5. (OS-39)

88 Christie JM, Simmonds M, Patt R, Coluzzi P, Busch MA, Nordbrock E, Portenoy RK (1998) Dose-titration, multicenter study of oral transmucosal fentanyl citrate for the treatment of breakthrough pain in cancer patients using transdermal fentanyl for persistent pain. *Journal of Clinical Oncology.* **16**(10): 3238–45. (RCT-62)

89 Fallon M (2001) Oral transmucosal fentanyl citrate – the UK experience. *European Journal of Palliative Care.* **8**: 7–8. (R)

90 Hanks GW, Thomas EA (1985) Intravenous opioids in chronic cancer pain. *British Medical Journal Clinical Research Ed.* **291**(6502): 1124–5. (C)

91 Radbruch L, Loick G, Schulzeck S, Beyer A, Lynch J, Stemmler M, Lindena G, Lehmann KA (1999) Intravenous titration with morphine for severe cancer pain: report of 28 cases. *Clinical Journal of Pain.* **15**(3): 173–8. (MC, OS-28)

92 Portenoy RK, Thaler HT, Inturrisi CE, Friedlander-Klar H, Foley KM (1992) The metabolite morphine-6-glucuronide contributes to the analgesia produced by morphine infusion in patients with pain and normal renal function. *Clinical Pharmacology and Therapeutics.* **51**: 422–31. (OS-14)

93 Faura CC, Moore A, Horga JF, Hand CW, McQuay HJ

(1996) Morphine and morphine-6-glucuronide plasma concentrations and effect in cancer pain. *Journal of Pain and Symptom Management.* **11**: 95–102. (OS-39)

94 Mazoit JX, Sardouk P, Zetlaoui P, Scherrmann JM (1987) Pharmacokinetics of unchanged morphine in normal and cirrhotic patients. *Anaesthesia and Analgesia.* **66**: 293–8. (CT-14)

95 Portenoy RK, Foley KM, Stulman J *et al.* (1991) Plasma morphine and morphine-6-glucuronide during chronic morphine therapy for cancer pain: plasma profiles, steady state concentrations and the consequences of renal failure. *Pain.* **47**: 13–19. (CS-2)

96 Ashby M, Fleming B, Wood M, Somogyi A (1997) Plasma morphine and glucuronide (M3G and M6G) concentrations in hospice patients. *Journal of Pain and Symptom Management.* **14**: 157–67. (OS-36)

97 Kirvela M, Lindgren L, Seppala T, Olkkola KT (1996) The pharmacokinetics of oxycodone in uremic patients undergoing renal transplantation. *Journal of Clinical Anesthesia.* **8**(1): 13–18. (CT-20)

98 Lee MA, Leng ME, Tiernan EJ (2001) Retrospective study of the use of hydromorphone in palliative care patients with normal and abnormal urea and creatinine. *Palliative Medicine.* **15**(1): 26–34. (RS-55)

99 Babul N, Darke AC, Hagen N (1995) Hydromorphone metabolite accumulation in renal failure. *Journal of Pain and Symptom Management.* **10**(3): 184–6. (C)

100 Davies G, Kingswood C, Street M (1996) Pharmacokinetics of opioids in renal dysfunction. *Clinical Pharmacokinetics.* **31**(6): 410–22. (R, 93 refs)

101 Tegeder I, Lotsch J, Geisslinger G (1999) Pharmacokinetics of opioids in liver disease. *Clinical Pharmacokinetics.* **37**(1): 17–40. (R, 257 refs)

102 Labroo RB, Paine MF, Thummel KE, Kharasch ED (1997) Fentanyl metabolism by human hepatic and intestinal cytochrome P450 3A4: implications for interindividual variability in disposition, efficacy, and drug interactions. *Drug Metabolism & Disposition.* **25**(9): 1072–80. (LS)

103 Tallgren M, Olkkola KT, Seppala T, Hockerstedt K, Lindgren L (1997) Pharmacokinetics and ventilatory effects of oxycodone before and after liver transplantation. *Clinical Pharmacology & Therapeutics.* **61**(6): 655–61. (CS-6)

104 Seager JM, Hawkey CJ (2001) ABC of the upper gastrointestinal tract: Indigestion and non-steroidal anti-inflammatory drugs. *BMJ.* **323**(7323): 1236–9. (R)

105 Pecora PG, Kaplan B (1996) Corticosteroids and ulcers: is there an association? *Annals of Pharmacotherapy.* **30**(7–8): 870–2. (R)

106 Ellershaw JE, Kelly MJ (1994) Corticosteroids and peptic ulceration. *Palliative Medicine.* **8**(4): 313–19. (R)

107 McCormack K, Twycross R (2002) Cox-2 selective inhibitors and analgesia. *Pain Clinical Updates.* **10**: 1–4. (R)

108 Todd J, Rees E, Gwilliam B, Davies A (2002) An assessment of the efficacy and tolerability of a 'double dose' of normal-release morphine sulphate at bedtime. *Palliative Medicine.* **16**(6): 507–12. (RCT-20)

109 Zernikow B, Lindena G (2001) Long-acting morphine for pain control in paediatric oncology. *Medical & Pediatric Oncology.* **36**(4): 451–8. (RS-95)

110 Barnett M (2001) Alternative opioids to morphine in palliative care: a review of current practice and evidence. *Postgraduate Medical Journal.* **77**(908): 371–8. (R, 35 refs)

111 Pereira J, Lawlor P, Vigano A, Dorgan M, Bruera E (2001) Equianalgesic dose ratios for opioids: a critical review and proposals for long-term dosing. *Journal of Pain and Symptom Management.* **22**: 672–87. (R, 46 refs)

112 Anderson R, Saiers JH, Abram S, Schlicht C (2001) Accuracy in equianalgesic dosing: conversion dilemmas. *Journal of Pain and Symptom Management.* **21**: 397–406. (R, 55 refs)

113 Cherny N, Ripamonti C, Pereira J, Davis C, Fallon M, McQuay H, Mercadante S, Pasternak G, Ventafridda V (2001) Expert Working Group of the European Association of Palliative Care Network. Strategies to manage the adverse effects of oral morphine: an evidence-based report. *Journal of Clinical Oncology.* **19**(9): 2542–54. (R, 72 refs)

114 Hunt A, Goldman A, Devine T, Phillips M (2001) FEN-GBR-14 Study Group. Transdermal fentanyl for pain relief in a paediatric palliative care population. *Palliative Medicine.* **15**(5): 405–12. (OS-41)

115 World Health Organization (1998) *Cancer Pain Relief and Palliative Care in Children.* WHO, Geneva. (B)

116 Regnard C, Badger C (1987) Opioids, sleep and the time of death. *Palliative Medicine.* **1**(2): 107–10. (RS)

117 Cools HJ, Berkhout AM, De Bock GH (1996) Subcutaneous morphine infusion by syringe driver for terminally ill patients. *Age & Ageing.* **25**(3): 206–8. (RS)

118 Morita T, Tsunoda J, Inoue S, Chihara S (2001) Effects of high dose opioids and sedatives on survival in terminally ill cancer patients. *Journal of Pain and Symptom Management.* **21**(4): 282–9. (OS-209)

119 Clissold SP (1986) Paracetamol and phenacetin. *Drugs.* **32** Suppl 4: 46–59. (R, 58 refs)

120 Twycross RG *et al.* (2000) Paracetamol. *Progress in Palliative Care.* **8**: 198–202. (R)

121 Meredith TJ, Vale JA, Proudfoot AT (1995) Poisoning caused by analgesic drugs. In: DJ Weatherall, JGG Leadingham, DA Warrell (eds) *The Oxford Textbook of Medicine* (3e). Oxford University Press, Oxford. (Ch)

122 Mercadante S (2001) The use of anti-inflammatory drugs in cancer pain. *Cancer Treatment Reviews.* **27**(1): 51–61. (R, 100 refs)

123 Hawkins C, Hanks GW (2000) The gastroduodenal toxicity of nonsteroidal anti-inflammatory drugs: a review of the literature. *Journal of Pain and Symptom Management.* **20**(2): 140–51. (R)

124 Griffin MR (1998) Epidemiology of nonsteroidal anti-inflammatory drug-associated gastrointestinal injury. *American Journal of Medicine.* **104**(3A): 23S–29S. (R, 92 refs)

125 Laine L (2003) Gastrointestinal effects of NSAIDs and coxibs. *Journal of Pain and Symptom Management.* **25**(2S): S32–40. (R, 43 refs)

126 Sturmer T, Erb A, Keller F, Gunther KP, Brenner H (2001) Determinants of impaired renal function with use of nonsteroidal anti-inflammatory drugs: the

importance of half-life and other medications. *American Journal of Medicine.* **111**(7): 521–7. (MC, OS-802)

127 Laine L (2002) Gastrointestinal safety of coxibs and outcomes studies: what's the verdict? *Journal of Pain and Symptom Management.* **23**(Suppl): S11–13. (R, 13 refs)

128 Foral PA, Wilson AF, Nystrom KK (2002) Gastrointestinal bleeds associated with rofecoxib. *Pharmacotherapy.* **22**(3): 384–6. (R)

129 Bjorkman DJ (2002) Commentary: gastrointestinal safety of coxibs and outcomes studies: what's the verdict? *Journal of Pain and Symptom Management.* **23**(Suppl): S5–10. (C)

130 Brater DC (2002) Renal effects of cyclooxygenase-2 selective inhibitors. Commentary: gastrointestinal safety of coxibs and outcomes studies: what's the verdict? *Journal of Pain and Symptom Management.* **23**(Suppl): S15–20. (C)

131 British National Formulary (2003) NSAID-associated ulcers. In: *BNF 45.* Pharmaceutical Press and BMJ Books, London. (Ch)

132 Taub A (1982) Opioid analgesics in the treatment of chronic intractable pain of non-neoplastic origin. In: LM Kitahata, JG Collins (eds) *Narcotic Analgesics in Anaesthesiology.* Williams and Wilkins, Baltimore. pp. 199–208. (Ch)

133 Collin E, Poulain P, Gauvain-Piquard A, Petit G, Pichard-Leandri E (1993) Is disease progression the major factor in morphine 'tolerance' in cancer pain treatment? *Pain.* **55**(3): 319–26. (OS-29)

134 Borgbjerg FM, Nielsen K, Franks J (1996) Experimental pain stimulates respiration and attenuates morphine-induced respiratory depression: a controlled study in human volunteers. *Pain.* **64**(1): 123–8. (CT)

135 Passik S, Portenoy R (1998) Substance abuse issues in palliative care. In: A Berger (ed) *Principles and Practice of Supportive Oncology.* Lippincott-Raven, Philadelphia. (Ch)

136 Joranson DE, Ryan KM, Gilson AM, Dahl JL (2000) Trends in medical use and abuse of opioid analgesics. *JAMA.* **283**(13): 1710–14. (RS)

137 Twycross RG, Wald SJ (1976) Longterm use of diamorphine in advanced cancer. In: JJ Bonica (ed) *Advances in Pain Research and Therapy, Vol 1.* Raven Press, New York. (Ch)

138 Wilwerding MB, Loprinzi CL, Mailliard JA, O'Fallon JR, Miser AW, van Haelst C, Barton DL, Foley JF, Athmann LM (1995) A randomized, crossover evaluation of methylphenidate in cancer patients receiving strong narcotics. *Supportive Care in Cancer.* **3**(2): 135–8. (RCT)

139 Sykes N (1998) The relationship between opioid use and laxative use in terminally ill patients. *Palliative Medicine.* **12**: 375–82. (RS)

140 White ID, Hoskin PJ, Hanks GW, Bliss JM (1989) Morphine and dryness of the mouth. *BMJ.* **298**(6682): 1222–3. (OS)

141 Smith MT (2000) Neuroexcitatory effects of morphine and hydromorphone: evidence implicating the 3-glucuronide metabolites. *Clinical & Experimental Pharmacology & Physiology.* **27**(7): 524–8. (R, 30 refs)

142 Sarhill N, Davis MP, Walsh D, Nouneh C (2001) Methadone-induced myoclonus in advanced cancer. *American Journal of Hospice & Palliative Care.* **18**(1): 51–3. (CS-1)

143 Stuerenburg HJ, Claassen J, Eggers C, Hansen HC (2000) Acute adverse reaction to fentanyl in a 55 year old man. *Journal of Neurology, Neurosurgery & Psychiatry.* **69**(2): 281–2. (Let, CS-1)

144 Adair JC, el-Nachef A, Cutler P (1996) Fentanyl neurotoxicity. *Annals of Emergency Medicine.* **27**(6): 791–2. (Let, CS-1)

145 Fountain A (2002) Before you blame the morphine: visual hallucinations in palliative care. *CME Cancer Medicine.* **1**(1): 23–6. (R, 78 refs)

146 Kart T, Christrup LL, Rasmussen M (1997) Recommended use of morphine in neonates, infants and children based on a literature review: Part 2–Clinical use. *Paediatric Anaesthesia.* **7**(2): 93–101. (R, 82 refs)

147 Litalien C, Jacqz-Aigrain E (2001) Risks and benefits of nonsteroidal anti-inflammatory drugs in children: a comparison with paracetamol. *Paediatric Drugs.* **3**(11): 817–58. (R, 325 refs)

148 Cuzzolin L, Dal Cere M, Fanos V (2001) NSAID-induced nephrotoxicity from the fetus to the child. *Drug Safety.* **24**(1): 9–18. (R, 98)

149 Collins SL, Moore RA, McQuay HJ, Wiffen P (2000) Antidepressants and anticonvulsants for diabetic neuropathy and postherpetic neuralgia: a quantitative systematic review. *Journal of Pain and Symptom Management.* **20**(6): 449–58. (SA)

150 Jensen TS (2002) Anticonvulsants in neuropathic pain: rationale and clinical evidence. *European Journal of Pain: Ejp.* **6** Suppl A: 61–8. (R, 31 refs)

151 Twycross R (1994) The risks and benefits of corticosteroids in advanced cancer. *Drug Safety.* **11**(3): 163–78. (R)

152 Ashby MA, Martin P, Jackson KA (1999) Opioid substitution to reduce adverse effects in cancer pain management. *Med J Aust.* **170**: 68–71. (OS-49)

153 Mercadante S (1995) Dantrolene treatment of opioid-induced myoclonus. *Anesthesia & Analgesia.* **81**(6): 1307–8. (R)

154 Holdsworth MT, Adams VR, Chavez CM, Vaughan LJ, Duncan MH (1995) Continuous midazolam infusion for the management of morphine-induced myoclonus. *Annals of Pharmacotherapy.* **29**(1): 25–9. (CS-1)

155 Twycross RG (1999) *Morphine and the Relief of Cancer Pain. Information for patients, families and friends.* Beaconsfield Publishers, Beaconsfield. (B)

156 Neville-Webbe HL, Coleman RE (2003) The use of zolendronic acid in the management of metastatic bone disease and hypercalcemia. *Palliative Medicine.* **17**: 539–53. (R, 61 refs)

157 Ross JR, Saunders Y, Edmonds PM, Patel S, Broadley KE, Johnston RD (2003) Systematic review of role of bisphosphonates on skeletal morbidity in metastatic cancer. *BMJ.* **327**: 469–72. (SA–30, 21 refs)

158 Gardner-Nix J (2001) Oral transmucosal fentanyl and sufentanil for incident pain (letter). *Journal of Pain and Symptom Management.* **2**: 627–30.

159 Goodman A (1990) Addiction: definition and implications. *British Journal of Addiction.* **85**(11): 1403–80.

160 *Pharmacist's Letter* (2005) **21**(5): 25–6.

Other physical symptoms

- Ascites

- Bleeding

- Bowel obstruction

- Constipation

- Diarrhea

- Dyspepsia

- Dysphagia

- Edema and lymphedema

- Fatigue, drowsiness, lethargy and weakness

- Malignant ulcers and fistulae

- Nausea and vomiting

- Nutrition and hydration problems

- Oral problems

- Respiratory problems

- Skin problems

- Terminal phase (the last hours and days)

- Urinary and sexual problems

Ascites

1 Is there doubt that this is ascites?
2 Is the prognosis short?
3 Is the condition causing distress?
4 Can the patient tolerate diuretics?
5 Is the ascites persisting?

Key points

- Paracentesis offers immediate relief but poor long-term control.
- Combination diuretics offer useful long-term control in some patients.

Introduction

Ascites in cancer or liver disease usually carries a poor prognosis.[1] The commonest causes for malignant ascites are primary tumors of breast, ovary, colon, stomach, pancreas and bronchus. Symptoms of ascites include nausea, vomiting, abdominal distension or pain, edema (legs, perineum or lower trunk) and breathlessness due to diaphragmatic splinting.[2]

Types of ascites

Four types can be identified.[3]

- *Raised hydrostatic pressure:* caused by cirrhosis, congestive heart failure, inferior vena caval obstruction and hepatic vein occlusion.
- *Decreased osmotic pressure:* caused by protein depletion (nephrotic syndrome, protein-losing enteropathy), reduced protein intake (malnutrition) or reduced protein production (cirrhosis).
- *Fluid production exceeding resorptive capacity:* caused by infection or neoplasms.
- *Chylous:* due to obstruction and leakage of the lymphatics draining the gut.

Treatment

Diuretics and paracentesis are still the mainstay of treatment.[4,5]

Diuretics

Patients with liver metastases (and resulting portal hypertension) are most likely to respond to diuretics,[6] and a serum-ascites albumin gradient > 11 g/l is a simple way of selecting such patients.[7] The use of spironolactone and furosemide in combination is well established.[7–10] However, diuretics can cause electrolyte disturbances and hypotension. They also need to be used with caution in patients with poor renal or hepatic function.

Paracentesis

Insertion methods vary from using a peritoneal dialysis (PD) catheter attached to a standard PD collection bag, to using a large bore IV cannula or a suprapubic trochar and catheter. The use of 0.5% bupivacaine as local anesthetic (LA) for the puncture site allows pain-free drainage for up to 8 hours if necessary. Puncture sites should be away from scars, tumor masses, distended bowel, bladder, liver or the inferior epigastric arteries that run 5 cm either side of the anterior midline. The best sites are in the left iliac fossa (at least 10 cm from the midline) and in the midline suprapubically (the bladder must be empty). A lateral approach is advisable in patients with distended bowel – marked distension is a contraindication to paracentesis. As a precaution, the LA needle can be used to check if ascitic fluid is present before inserting the drainage tube. Ultrasound evaluation is only required when the diagnosis is uncertain or if it is suspected that the ascites is loculated.[5] In malignant ascites it is safe and effective to drain up to 5 liters over a few hours without intravenous fluid replacement, even in children.[4,11,12] Most symptoms can be relieved after only 2 hours' drainage, although it may take 72 hours after drainage has stopped before breathlessness improves.[13] Many patients can have their paracentesis done at home or as an outpatient.[14] Patients with other causes of ascites can have much larger volumes drained but this needs to be done over several days,[15] and may need an infusion of Dextran.[8] After removal of the catheter any leakage of ascites from the puncture site can be collected with a colostomy bag. Leakage usually stops after 2–3 days and so the patient is spared a suture.

Catheters and shunts

Peritoneal catheters can be inserted and left for periods of up to a month,[16] but are limited by complications.[6] Shunts can be inserted percutaneously,[17,18] but the long-term use of shunts results in troublesome complications in both cirrhosis and cancer-related ascites.[19,20] Using a shunt to drain ascites does not give a better quality of life than using regular paracentesis.[6] A disadvantage of repeated paracentesis is the steady loss of albumin.[21] This will result in a low serum albumin and increasing peripheral edema.

Other treatments

In malignancy, systemic or intraperitoneal chemotherapy has been used,[22] but no large studies have shown a benefit, especially in advanced disease.[4] Intraperitoneal triamcinalone may have a role.[23] Octreotide has been reported to reduce ascites in cancer.[24] In mucinous ascites that is too viscous for tube drainage, an artificial fistula can be formed to drain the ascites.

Clinical decision	If YES ⇒ Action
1 **Is there doubt that this is ascites?**	Signs of ascites: flank dullness, shifting dullness, fluid thrill. • Exclude: other causes of abdominal distension such as bowel obstruction, abdominal tumor or hepatomegaly. • If still uncertain, consider an abdominal ultrasound examination.
2 **Is the prognosis short?** (day by day deterioration)	• *If free of symptoms:* no further action is required. • *If symptoms are troublesome:* Nausea and vomiting: *see* Nausea and vomiting (p. 113). Abdominal stretch pain: – consider a brief paracentesis of 2 liters to reduce discomfort. – acetaminophen or diclofenac may help discomfort. Consider TENS. Peripheral edema: *see* cd-6 in Edema and lymphedema (p. 99).
3 **Is the distension causing distress?**	• *If dehydrated, hypotensive or the ascites is due to cirrhosis:* start IV infusion of Dextran 70. • *In the **absence** of gross bowel distension or abdominal tumor:* Carry out therapeutic paracentesis (see opposite for details): – drain 2 liters over 1 hour, then drain up to a further 3 liters over 3–4 hours (larger volumes will need drainage over 24 hours or more). (There are anecdotal reports of suction drainage of up to 5 litres in under an hour with no adverse sequelae.) – remove tube and place ostomy bag over puncture site. – if hypotension develops start IV infusion of Dextran. • *If no fluid is obtained:* the ascites may be loculated. Arrange for drainage under ultrasound control. • *If ascites is too viscous to drain (e.g. ovarian carcinoma):* Consider paracentesis with suction. Alternatively, ask a surgeon to form an artificial fistula (*see* notes opposite).
4 **Can the patient tolerate diuretics?**	• *For patients able to take oral medication and with good renal function:* Measure abdominal girth at a marked site each week. Start spironolactone 100 mg with furosemide 40 mg PO once daily. Increase doses up to 300 mg spironolactone and 80 mg furosemide to achieve a weight loss of 0.5–1 kg/day.[25] Patients with peripheral edema may tolerate doses up to furosemide 160 mg + spironolactone 400 mg daily for a limited period.[9,26,27] NB: Spironolactone takes up to two weeks to reach a steady plasma level.[28] • *For patients with poor renal function:* Avoid diuretics. Use paracentesis to drain sufficient for comfort. • *If hypotension develops:* Start IV infusion of Dextran and reduce diuretic dose. • Check serum electrolytes weekly. Continue diuretics at lowest dose that will control symptoms.
5 **Is the ascites persisting?**	• Consider systemic octreotide or intraperitoneal triamcinalone. • Discuss options with oncologist, e.g. systemic chemotherapy, immunotherapy. • Discuss options with gastroenterologist, e.g. peritoneovenous shunt.

Adapted from Regnard and Mannix[29]
cd = clinical decision

References

B = book; C = comment; Ch = chapter; CS-n = case study-number of cases; CT-n = controlled trial-number of cases; E = editorial; GC = group consensus; I = interviews; Let = letter; LS = laboratory study; MC = multi-center; OS-n = open study-number of cases; R = review; RCT-n = randomized controlled trial-number of cases; RS-n = retrospective survey-number of cases; SA = systematic or meta analysis.

1 Bieligk SC, Calvo BF, Coit DG (2001) Peritoneovenous shunting for nongynecologic malignant ascites. *Cancer.* **91**(7): 1247–55. (RS-55)

2 Keen J, Fallon M (2002) Malignant ascites. In: C Ripamonti, E Bruera *Gastrointestinal Symptoms in Advanced Cancer Patients.* Oxford University Press, Oxford. pp. 279–90. (Ch)

3 Parsons SL, Watson SA, Steele RJC (1996) Malignant ascites. *British Journal of Surgery.* **83**: 6–14. (R, 92 refs)

4 Aslam N, Marino CR (2001) Malignant ascites: new concepts in pathophysiology, diagnosis, and management. *Archives of Internal Medicine.* **161**(22): 2733–7. (R, 28 refs)

5 Stephenson J, Gilbert J (2002) The development of clinical guidelines on paracentesis for ascites related to malignancy. *Palliative Medicine.* **16**(3): 213–18. (R)

6 Parsons SL, Lang MW, Steele RJ (1996) Malignant ascites: a 2-year review from a teaching hospital. *European Journal of Surgical Oncology.* **22**: 237–9. (RS-164)

7 Runyon BA (1994) Current concepts: care of patients with ascites. *New England Journal of Medicine.* **330**: 337–42. (R)

8 Jelan R, Hayes PC (1997) Hepatic encephalopathy and ascites. *Lancet.* **350**: 1309–14. (R, 62 refs)

9 Greenway B, Johnson PJ, Williams R (1982) Control of malignant ascites with spironolactone. *British Journal of Surgery.* **69**: 441–2. (OS-15)

10 Fogel MR, Sawhney VK, Neal EA, Miller RG, Knauer CM, Gregory PB (1981) Diuresis in the ascitic patient: a randomised controlled trial of three regimens. *Journal of Clinical Gastroenterology.* **3**(Suppl 1): 73–80. (RCT-90)

11 Forouzandeh B, Konicek F, Sheagren JN (1996) Large-volume paracentesis in the treatment of cirrhotic patients with refractory ascites. The role of post-paracentesis plasma volume expansion. *Journal of Clinical Gastroenterology.* **22**(3): 207–10. (R, 51 refs)

12 Kramer RE, Sokol RJ, Yerushalmi B, Liu E, MacKenzie T, Hoffenberg EJ, Narkewicz MR (2001) Large-volume paracentesis in the management of ascites in children. *Journal of Pediatric Gastroenterology & Nutrition.* **33**(3): 245–9. (RS-21)

13 McNamara P (2000) Paracentesis – an effective method of symptom control in the palliative care setting? *Palliative Medicine.* **14**(1): 62–4. (OS)

14 Moorsom D (2001) Paracentesis in a home care setting. *Palliative Medicine.* **5**(2): 169–70. (Let)

15 Smith GS, Barnard GF (1997) Massive volume paracentesis (up to 41 liters) for the outpatient management of ascites. *Journal of Clinical Gastroenterology.* **25**(1): 402–3. (CS-1)

16 Lee A, Lau TN, Yeong KY (2000) Indwelling catheters for the management of malignant ascites. *Supportive Care in Cancer.* **8**(6): 493–9. (RS-38)

17 Orsi F, Grasso F, Bonomo G, Monti C, Marinucci I, Bellomi M (2002) Percutaneous peritoneovenous shunt positioning: technique and preliminary results. *European Radiology.* **12**(5): 1188–92. (CS-9)

18 Barnett TD, Rubins J (2002) Placement of a permanent tunneled peritoneal drainage catheter for palliation of malignant ascites: a simplified percutaneous approach. *Journal of Vascular & Interventional Radiology.* **13**(4): 379–83. (RS-29)

19 Zervos EE, McCormick J, Goode SE, Rosemurgy AS (1997) Peritoneovenous shunts in patients with intractable ascites: palliation at what price? *American Surgeon.* **63**(2): 157–62. (OS-48)

20 Schumacher DL, Saclarides TJ, Staren ED (1994) Peritoneovenous shunts for palliation of the patient with malignant ascites. *Annals of Surgical Oncology.* **1**: 378–81. (OS-89)

21 Schiano TD, Black M, Hills C, Ter H, Bellary S, Miller LS (2000) Correlation between increased colloid osmotic pressure and the resolution of refractory ascites after transjugular intrahepatic portosystemic shunt. *Southern Medical Journal.* **93**(3): 305–9. (OS-23)

22 Malik I, Abubakar S, Rizwana I, Alam F, Rizvi J, Khan A (1991) Clinical features and management of malignant ascites. *JPMA – Journal of the Pakistan Medical Association.* **41**(2): 38–40. (RS-45)

23 Mackey JR, Wood L, Nabholtz J, Jensen J, Venner P (2000) A phase II trial of triamcinolone hexacetanide for symptomatic recurrent malignant ascites. *Journal of Pain and Symptom Management.* **19**(3): 193–9. (OS-15)

24 Cairns W, Malone R (1999) Octreotide as an agent for the relief of malignant ascites in palliative care patients. *Palliative Medicine.* **13**(5): 429–30. (CS-3)

25 Twycross R, Wilcock A (2001) Alimentary symptoms. In: *Symptom Management in Advanced Cancer.* Radcliffe Medical Press, Oxford. (Ch)

26 Pockros PJ, Reynolds TB (1986) Rapid diuresis in patients with ascites from chronic liver disease: the importance of peripheral edema. *Gastroenterology.* **90**: 1827–33. (OS-14)

27 Saravanan R, Cramp ME (2002) Investigation and treatment of ascites. *Clinical Medicine (Journal of the Royal College of Physicians of London).* **2**: 310–13. (R)

28 Sungaila I, Bartle WR, Walker SE *et al.* (1992) Spironolactone pharmacokinetics and pharmaco-dynamics in patients with cirrhotic ascites. *Gastroenterology.* **102**: 1680–5. (OS-9)

29 Regnard C, Mannix K (1995) Management of ascites. In: *Flow Diagrams in Advanced Cancer and Other Diseases.* Edward Arnold, London. pp. 36–8. (Ch)

Bleeding

Clinical decision and action checklist

1 Is there a risk of bleeding?
2 Is the patient hypotensive?
3 Is a coagulation disorder present?
4 Is the bleeding site visible?
5 Is the source of bleeding internal?

Key points

- Catastrophic, external bleeding is rare.[1]
- Control of external bleeding is usually possible.
- Exclude coagulation disorders.

Severe hemorrhage

Since small, repeated bleeds can herald a major bleed, hemorrhage is a common fear, but in reality it is an uncommon problem.[1] Admission may be needed for minor bleeds if the patient and family find these frightening and if they wish treatment. Successful treatment of a major hemorrhage is usually only possible in acute hospital settings in non-malignant conditions.[2]

In any setting, dark green or blue towels soak up the blood loss without appearing red. Perineal pads will help with the management of low gastro-intestinal bleeding. The patient will feel cold because of the hypotension, and will need warm blankets. Such an event is frightening for the patient, who may need rapid sedation intravenously. The touch and closeness of another person is essential. Partner, family and staff will need support after such an experience.

Radiotherapy

This is helpful in many patients with hemoptysis[3] and hematuria.[4] Single treatments are possible in frail patients, and internal radioactive sources (brachytherapy) are being used for esophageal and bronchial bleeding. Intravaginal and intra-uterine sources can also be used to control bleeding from advanced gynecological tumors.[5]

Pharmacological agents

Topical/locally acting drugs

Sucralfate is useful in controlling the bleeding from a gastric carcinoma,[6] or it can be applied topically, directly to the bleeding point if this is visible. A 1% alum solution can reduce bladder hemorrhage (*see* cd-2 in Urinary and sexual problems (p. 153)).[7] Topical tranexamic/aminocaproic acid* reduces bleeding from a rectal carcinoma and other sites.[8] Vasoconstrictors such as adrenaline work for 10–15 minutes but re-bleeding is common as the adrenaline is absorbed.

Systemic drugs

Tranexamic/aminocaproic acid inhibits the breakdown of fibrin clots and is well absorbed orally,[9]

but in hematuria it can produce hard clots that are difficult to remove and can cause obstruction.[10]

Dressings

Some dressings such as calcium alginate are hemostatic. Dressings with very low adherence (e.g. Mepitel) are useful as a base for applying sucralfate. These and moist environment dressings (alginate, hydrogels) can be left in place for up to 7 days, avoiding any disturbance to the fragile bleeding surface.

Heat and cold

Lasers can palliate bleeding from tumors accessible externally or through an endoscope.[11] Diathermy can be helpful, but can make bladder bleeding worse.[7] The effects of cryotherapy are usually brief.

Embolization

This can be useful in controlling bleeding,[12,13] and it has been used in hemoptyses,[13] bleeding from the bladder,[14] prostate,[15] stomach[16] and malignant ulcers.[17] Pain and pyrexia may occur for a few days after embolization. There are risks, especially in the presence of abnormal anatomy,[18] and it needs a radiologist and clinician experienced in the procedure.

Coagulation disorders

These can be caused by platelet deficiency or malfunction, by excessive clotting (e.g. with pancreatic carcinoma), or may be due to widespread microvascular clotting which uses up clotting factors, resulting in a coexistent tendency to bleed (disseminated intravascular coagulation – DIC). If treatment is appropriate, coagulation disorders invariably require admission to hospital under the care of a hematology team. In very advanced disease such treatment is not usually appropriate, but some cases of DIC respond to a simpler regimen of an antifibrinolytic such as tranexamic acid and low dose heparin.[19] The advice of a hematologist remains essential. Fortunately such events are uncommon, and usually occur in the last hours or days of life when distressing bleeding can be managed as described above.

---

* Aminocaproic acid is not available in Canada. In the US topical preparations can be obtained from a compounding pharmacy.

Clinical decision	If YES ⇒ Action
1 Is there a risk of bleeding?	• *If on warfarin:* keep INR to between 1.5 and 3. • *If coagulation disorder (e.g. low platelets):* consider treatment under the advice of a hematologist. • *If rapidly growing and erosive tumor:* keep dark green or blue towel and sedation to hand. Consider referral for radiotherapy or embolization.
2 Is the patient hypotensive?	• *If treatment is appropriate:* see cd-2 in Emergencies: sudden collapse (*see* p. 205). • *If treatment is not appropriate:* If the patient is distressed: give diazepam 5–30 mg titrated IV (if IV access not possible, give midazolam 5–15 mg bucally or into the deltoid muscle). If hemorrhage is visible (ulcer, hemoptysis, hematemesis) – use dark green or blue towels to make the appearance of blood less frightening to patient, partner or family. Place warm blankets over the patient and do not leave him/her unattended.
3 Is a coagulation disorder present?	• Consider: low or abnormal platelets, increased warfarin levels (due to reduced warfarin metabolism or displacement by another drug), disseminated intravascular coagulation, or severe hepatic impairment. • Treatment can be difficult – the advice of a hematologist is essential.
4 Is the bleeding site visible?	• Apply pressure to stop flow. • *Promote clotting:* apply sucralfate suspension or a calcium alginate dressing. • *Prevent rebleeding:* Topical: apply sucralfate under non-adherent dressing (e.g. Mepitel). Dressing can be left in place for several days, although re-bleeding may need a daily application of sucralfate. Systemic: tranexamic acid PO 1 g q8h; aminocaproic acid PO 1 g q6h, max up to PO 30 g/24 h. IV 1 g/h. • Consider: radiotherapy, diathermy or embolization.
5 Is the source of bleeding internal?	• *Hemoptysis:* If minor (streaked sputum) – aminocaproic/tranexamic acid PO 1 g q8h. If troublesome (clots, anemia or frequent bleeds): radiotherapy, laser, or embolization. • *Hematemesis:* Stop gastric irritants, e.g. nonsteroidal anti-inflammatory drugs. If minor (altered blood or positive fecal occult blood): 2 g sucralfate on waking and night. If troublesome (fresh blood, melena or anemia) – 2 g sucralfate q4h + ranitidine 300 mg q12h (or lansoprazole 30 mg PO daily). NB: If source is non-malignant – refer urgently for endoscopy and surgical opinion. • *Mouth or nasopharynx:* If anterior nose: pack with gauze soaked in 1% alum solution or sucralfate suspension. Refer to Ear, Nose and Throat surgeons if re-bleeding occurs. If posterior nose: refer to Ear, Nose and Throat surgeons for packing under observation + diathermy. If oral: use sucralfate suspension (diluted 1:1 with water) as a mouthwash. • *Rectum or vagina:* If minor (streaking only): observe and consider pads. If troublesome (clots, frequent bleeds or anemia) – aminocaproic/tranexamic acid PO 1 g q8h. Consider radiotherapy, topical sucralfate suspension or topical aminocaproic/tranexamic acid. • *Other sources:* Hematuria: *see* cd-2 in *Urinary and sexual problems* (p. 153). Intrapleural or intra-abdominal: exclude coagulation disorder or trauma. Start tranexamic acid PO 1 g q8h.

Adapted from Makin and Regnard[20]
cd = clinical decision

References

B = book; C = comment; Ch = chapter; CS-n = case study-number of cases; CT-n = controlled trial-number of cases; E = editorial; GC = group consensus; I = interviews; Let = letter; LS = laboratory study; MC = multi-center; OS-n = open study-number of cases; R = review; RCT-n = randomized controlled trial-number of cases; RS-n = retrospective survey-number of cases; SA = systematic or meta analysis.

1 Jones DK, Davis RJ (1990) Massive hemoptysis. *BMJ.* **300**: 889–90. (R, 19 refs)

2 Hakanson E, Konstantinov IE, Fransson SG, Svedjeholm R (2002) Management of life-threatening hemoptysis. *BJA: British Journal of Anaesthesia.* **88**(2): 291–5. (CS-2)

3 Bhatt ML, Mohani BK, Kumar L, Chawla S, Sharma DN, Rath GK (2000) Palliative treatment of advanced non small cell lung cancer with weekly fraction radiotherapy. *Indian Journal of Cancer.* **37**(4): 148–52. (OS-47)

4 Onsrud M, Hagen B, Strickert T (2001) 10-Gy single-fraction pelvic irradiation for palliation and life prolongation in patients with cancer of the cervix and corpus uteri. *Gynecologic Oncology.* **82**(1): 167–71. (RS-64)

5 Tan HS (1994) Use of high dose rate gammamed brachytherapy in the palliative treatment of gynaecological cancer. *Annals of the Academy of Medicine, Singapore.* **23**(2): 231–4. (OS-24)

6 Regnard CFB, Mannix K (1990) Palliation of gastric carcinoma hemorrhage with sucralfate. *Palliative Medicine.* **4**: 329–30. (Let, CS-1)

7 Bullock N, Whitaker RH (1985) Massive bladder hemorrhage. *BMJ.* **291**: 1522–3. (E)

8 McElligot E, Quigley C, Hanks GW (1992) Tranexamic acid and rectal bleeding. *Lancet.* **337**: 431. (Let, CS-1)

9 Dean A, Tuffin P (1997) Fibrinolytic inhibitors for cancer-associated bleeding problems. *Journal of Pain and Symptom Management.* **13**(1): 20–4. (CT-16)

10 Schultz M, van der Lelie H (1995) Microscopic hematuria as a relative contraindication for tranexamic acid. *British Journal of Haematology.* **89**(3): 663–4. (CS-3)

11 Ventrucci M, Di Simone MP, Giulietti P, De Luca G (2001) Efficacy and safety of Nd: YAG laser for the treatment of bleeding from radiation proctocolitis. *Digestive & Liver Disease.* **33**(3): 230–3. (OS-9)

12 Broadley KE, Kurowska A, Dick R, Platts A, Tookman A (1995) The role of embolization in palliative care. *Palliative Medicine.* **9**(4): 331–5. (CS-3)

13 Corr P, Blyth D, Sanyika C, Royston D (2001) Efficacy and cost-effectiveness of bronchial arterial embolisation in the treatment of major hemoptysis. *South African Medical Journal.* **91**(10): 861–4. (RS-87)

14 Lang EK, Deutsch JS, Goodman JR *et al.* (1979) Transcatheter embolization of hypogastric branch arteries in the management of intractable bladder hemorrhage. *Journal of Urology.* **121**: 30–6.

15 Appleton DS, Sibley GNA, Doyle PT (1988) Internal iliac artery embolisation of bladder and prostate hemorrhage. *British Journal of Urology.* **61**: 45–7. (OS-8)

16 Blake MA, Owens A, O'Donoghue DP, MacErlean DP (1995) Embolotherapy for massive upper gastrointestinal hemorrhage secondary to metastatic renal cell carcinoma: report of three cases. *Gut.* **37**(6): 835–7. (CS-3)

17 Rankin EM, Rubens RD, Redy JF (1988) Transcatheter embolisation to control severe bleeding in fungating breast cancer. *European Journal of Surgical Oncology.* **14**: 27–32. (OS-9)

18 McQuillan RE, Grzybowska PH, Finlay IG, Hughes J (1996) Use of embolisation in palliative care. *Palliative Medicine.* **10**: 169–72. (Let)

19 Cooper DL, Sandler AB, Wilson LD *et al.* (1992) Disseminated intravascular coagulation and excessive fibrinolysis in a patient with metastatic prostate cancer. *Cancer.* **70**: 656–8. (CS-1)

20 Regnard C, Makin W (1995) Bleeding. In: *Flow Diagrams in Advanced Cancer and Other Diseases.* Edward Arnold, London. pp. 44–7. (Ch)

Bowel obstruction

Clinical decision and action checklist

1 Is there any doubt this is an obstruction?
2 Is constipation the sole cause?
3 Is a physical blockage absent or unlikely?
4 Is thirst present?
5 Is surgery possible?
6 Is nausea and/or vomiting present?
7 Is pain present?
8 Is the obstruction complete and continuous?
9 Is the obstruction partial or intermittent?

Key points

- Inoperable, complete bowel obstruction can be managed at home.
- Nasogastric tubes and IV hydration are not usually needed.

Introduction

Intravenous hydration and nasogastric suction will fail to control the symptoms of inoperable bowel obstruction in approximately 90% of patients.[1,2] Medical management will keep the majority of patients free of nausea and pain,[3] achieving a comfortable phase with the option of doing this at home.[4]

Causes of obstruction

Recurrent abdominal cancer causes multiple blockages,[5] especially with small bowel blockage in ovarian carcinoma.[6–8] *Metastatic obstruction* from outside the abdomen is usually due to spread from primary melanoma, breast or lung.[9] *Constipation* can mimic obstruction and a supine abdominal X-ray will differentiate constipation from other causes of obstruction. *Benign adhesions* may occur in up to 20% of patients with recurrent abdominal cancer,[10,11] and are the commonest cause of small bowel obstruction.[12] *A new primary tumor* can be the cause of obstruction in nearly 10%.[1] *Motility disorders* can cause the same features as a physical blockage.[5]

Management

Surgery: This should always be considered since it may be a simple procedure, but surgery can have a significant mortality and morbidity.[5,13] An understanding surgical opinion is essential.[14]

Stents: These are an option in patients with duodenal or colorectal obstructions who are unfit for surgery.[29]

Dysmotility and ileus: Absent motility (ileus) or abnormal bowel motility (dysmotility) can cause obstructive symptoms. Dysmotility is common in cancer and can be caused by retroperitoneal disease, antimuscarinic drugs or autonomic failure. A trial of a prokinetic is worthwhile, initially given parenterally.

Colic: This can radiate to a variety of sites in the abdomen and elsewhere, but the pain usually has the typical periodic nature of colic, recurring regularly every few minutes (*see* cd-4b in Diagnosing and treating pain (p. 42)). In complete, inoperable obstruction all laxatives should be stopped. The risk of producing an ileus with antispasmodics is not relevant and these can be used to treat the colic. Partial obstruction is different, with a need to preserve bowel motility and yet prevent colic. The use of a laxative with minimal stimulant activity

(docusate), dietary advice (avoiding high fiber foods) and the cautious use of antispasmodics keep symptoms to a minimum.

Proximal obstructions: These are more likely to cause vomiting, but less likely to cause distension. In pancreatic carcinoma most are due to poor motility rather than a physical obstruction,[15] and can be treated as for gastric stasis (*see* Nausea and vomiting (p. 113)). Complete, high obstructions may need gastric aspiration to reduce vomiting and IV hydration to prevent thirst. Gastrostomies have been used to 'vent' gastric contents from high obstructions.[14,16]

Nausea: *See* Nausea and vomiting (p. 113). Nausea (the most distressing symptom) will respond to haloperidol in most patients. A secondary onset of nausea (possibly due to invasion of the small bowel by colonic bacteria) will often respond to methotrimeprazine (not available in the US).

Feeding and hydration: Most patients will absorb sufficient fluid from their upper gut to prevent symptomatic dehydration. Parenteral feeding is often unnecessary, unless it is a preliminary to surgery.[17] Patients with repeated vomiting or high obstructions proximal to the mid-jejunum will need intravenous or subcutaneous hydration to offset the thirst resulting from the rapid dehydration. As patients deteriorate, their fluid intake reduces, and parenteral hydration is not usually needed (*see* Nutrition and hydration problems (p. 119)). A small number with complete obstruction will want to take something orally, and small snacks or drinks are permissible. Most will keep them down, but a few will vomit. This is not an attempt to rehydrate or feed, but attending to the person's comfort.

Nasogastric tubes: These fail to control the symptoms of obstruction in at least 86% of patients,[2] and are ineffective in controlling postoperative vomiting.[18] Antisecretory drugs should be tried first (e.g. hyoscine (hyocyamine in the US), octreotide).[19] Nasogastric suction or drainage has a place in feculant or fecal vomiting. Feculant vomiting is not the vomiting of feces, but of small bowel contents colonized by colonic bacteria in obstructions lasting a week or more. True fecal vomiting (rare) is due to a gastro-colic fistula.

Clinical decision	If YES ⇒ Action
1 Is there any doubt whether this is bowel obstruction?	• Consider other causes of nausea and vomiting (*see* Nausea and vomiting (p. 113)), abdominal distension (e.g. ascites), colic (e.g. contact stimulant laxatives) or altered bowel habit (e.g. constipation).
2 Is constipation the sole cause?	Bowel history, examination and plain abdominal X-ray will help in deciding. • Clear rectum and start laxative (*see* Constipation (p. 75)).
3 Is a physical blockage absent or unlikely?	This may be peristaltic failure (absent or reduced bowel sounds): • Exclude peritonitis, septicemia or recent cord compression. • Stop antiperistaltic drugs (e.g. antimuscarinics) and osmotic laxatives. • Start metoclopramide SC infusion 30–90 mg per 24 hours. In children, domperidone (available from a compounding pharmacy in the US) is safer (*see* Drugs in palliative care for children: starting doses (p. 253)). • Consider adding a stimulant laxative acting on small and large bowel, e.g. bisacodyl. Alternatively try neostigmine SC 1–2.5 mg q6h (but not if the following are present: asthma, cardiac problems, hypotension, peptic ulcer, hypothyroidism, renal problems).
4 Is thirst present?	• Rehydrate orally, SC or IV (*see* Nutrition and hydration problems (p. 119)).
5 Is surgery or stenting possible?	Surgery is possible if the patient agrees and is in good or reasonable nutritional and medical condition. The prognosis is poor if there has been previous abdominal radiotherapy, there are abdominal masses, multiple blockages, rapidly recurring ascites or a small bowel blockage.[7,14,15,20] Referral for stenting is an alternative.[29]
6 Is nausea and/or vomiting present?	• *If poor motility is suspected:* start metoclopramide 10–20 mg SC qid or SC infusion 30–90 mg per 24 hours. In children, domperidone is safer (*see* Drugs in palliative care for children: starting doses (p. 253)). If metoclopramide or domperidone (available from a compounding pharmacy in the US) makes the vomiting worse, reduce the dose. • *If a physical obstruction is likely:* start haloperidol 1–2 mg q8h SC or 5 mg per 24 hours CSCI. Start at half these doses for patients > 70 years of age. For children *see* Drugs in palliative care for children: starting doses (p. 253). • *If nausea and/or vomiting persist:* Replace haloperidol with methotrimeprazine (Canada only) 2.5–5 mg SC once at night. If vomiting persists: **add** octreotide 100–200 microgram SC q8h or SC infusion 100–600 microgram per 24 hours.[21–23] Hyoscine butylbromide (Buscopan) SC infusion 60–120 mg per 24 hours (Canada only; in the US hyoscyamine 0.25–0.5 mg IV/SC q4h PRN) is an alternative but takes up to 3 days to take effect.[24]
7 Is pain present?	• *Colic: see* cd-4b in Diagnosing and treating pain (p. 42). • *Abdominal distension:* acetaminophen 1 g q4h. If this is insufficient, follow the WHO analgesic staircase. • *Celiac plexus pain:* (*see* Pain cd-6, p. 42 and Visceral pain, p. 44) start gabapentin 100 mg q8h (± opioid) and titrate daily until pain controlled.[25] If the pain persists, refer to a pain specialist for a nerve block.
8 Is the obstruction complete and continuous?	• Stop all laxatives. Treat a dry mouth (*see* cd-5 in Oral problems (p. 127)). • If colic is present: start hyoscine butylbromide SC infusion 60–120 mg per 24 hr (Canada only; in the US hyoscyamine 0.25–0.5 mg IV/SC q4h PRN). • Allow oral hydration and feeding, using occasional small snacks, if desired. • Consider high dose dexamethasone (16 mg daily) if short-term relief of obstruction is appropriate.[26,27]
9 Is the obstruction partial or intermittent?	• Stop osmotic and stimulant laxatives. • Start docusate 100 mg PO q8h and titrate to produce a comfortable stool without colic. • Avoid high roughage foods (e.g. peas). Continue oral feeding and hydration in small, frequent snacks. • For intermittent colic use hyoscine (scopolamine) hydrobromide (Canada only) 75–300 microgram sublingually (use injection preparation) or subcutaneously (max 900 micrograms in any 24-hour period). In the US use hyoscyamine (Levsin) 0.125–0.25 mg PO/SL tid-qid PRN.

Adapted from Regnard[28]
cd = clinical decision

References

B = book; C = comment; Ch = chapter; CS-n = case study-number of cases; CT-n = controlled trial-number of cases; E = editorial; GC = group consensus; I = interviews; LS = laboratory study; MC = multi-center; OS-n = open study-number of cases; R = review; RCT-n = randomized controlled trial-number of cases; RS-n = retrospective survey-number of cases; SA = systematic or meta analysis.

1 Glass RL, LeDuc RJ (1973) Small intestinal obstruction from peritoneal carcinomatosis. *American Journal of Surgery.* **125**: 316–17.

2 Bizer LS, Liebling RW, Delany HM, Gliedman ML (1981) Small bowel obstruction: the role of nonoperative treatment in simple intestinal obstruction and predictive criteria for strangulation obstruction. *Surgery.* **89**: 407–13. (RS-405)

3 Frank C (1997) Medical management of intestinal obstruction in terminal care. *Canadian Family Physician.* **43**: 259–65. (R, 29 refs)

4 Platt V (2001) Malignant bowel obstruction: so much more than symptom control. *International Journal of Palliative Nursing.* **7**(11): 547–54. (R, 47 refs)

5 Baines M (1997) The pathophysiology and management of malignant intestinal obstruction. In: D Doyle, GWC Hanks, N MacDonald (eds) *Oxford Textbook of Palliative Medicine* (2e). Oxford University Press, Oxford. pp. 526–34. (Ch)

6 Tunca JC, Buchler DA, Mack EA *et al.* (1981) The management of ovarian-cancer-caused bowel obstruction. *Gynaecological Oncology.* **12**: 186–92.

7 Miller G, Boman J, Shrier I, Gordon PH (2000) Small-bowel obstruction secondary to malignant disease: an 11-year audit. *Canadian Journal of Surgery.* **43**(5): 353–8. (RS-32)

8 Landercasper J, Cogbill TH, Merry WH, Stolee RT, Strutt PJ (1993) Long-term outcome after hospitalization for small-bowel obstruction. *Archives of Surgery.* **128**(7): 765–70. (RS-309)

9 Telerman A, Gerard B, Van den Heule B, Bleiberg H (1985) Gastrointestinal metastases from extra-abdominal tumours. *Endoscopy.* **17**: 99–101. (RS)

10 Ketcham AS, Hoye RC, Pilch YH, Morton DL (1970) Delayed intestinal obstruction following treatment for cancer. *Cancer.* **25**: 406–10.

11 Weiss SM, Skibber JM, Rosato FE (1984) Bowel obstruction in cancer patients: performance status as a predictor of survival. *Journal of Surgical Oncology – Supplement.* **25**(1): 15–17. (RS-95)

12 Miller G, Boman J, Shrier I, Gordon PH (2000) Etiology of small bowel obstruction. *American Journal of Surgery.* **180**(1): 33–6. (RS, 552)

13 Feuer DJ, Broadley KE, Shepherd JH, Barton DPJ (2000) Surgery for the resolution of symptoms in malignant bowel obstruction in advanced gynaecological and gastrointestinal cancer (Cochrane Review). *The Cochrane Library, Issue 2, 2002.* Update Software Ltd, Oxford. www.cochrane.org/cochrane/revabstr/ab002764.htm. (SA)

14 Ripamonti C, Twycross R, Baines M *et al.* (2001) Working Group of the European Association for Palliative Care. Clinical-practice recommendations for the management of bowel obstruction in patients with end-stage cancer. *Supportive Care in Cancer.* **9**(4): 223–33. (GC)

15 Twycross RG, Wilcock A (2001) Alimentary symptoms: obstruction. In: *Symptom Management in Advanced Cancer* (3e). Radcliffe Medical Press, Oxford. pp. 111–15. (Ch)

16 Baines MJ (1994) Management of intestinal obstruction in patients with advanced cancer. *Annals of the Academy of Medicine, Singapore.* **23**(2): 178–82. (R, 30 refs)

17 Mercadante S (1996) Nutrition in cancer patients. *Supportive Care in Cancer.* **4**(1): 10–20. (R)

18 Koukouras D, Mastronikolis NS, Tzoracoleftherakis E, Angelopoulou E, Kalfarentzos F, Androulakis J (2001) The role of nasogastric tube after elective abdominal surgery. *Clinica Terapeutica.* **152**(4): 241–4. (RCT-100)

19 Ripamonti C, Mercadante S, Groff L, Zecca E, De Conno F, Casuccio A (2001) Role of octreotide, scopolamine butylbromide, and hydration in symptom control of patients with inoperable bowel obstruction and nasogastric tubes: a prospective randomized trial. *Journal of Pain and Symptom Management.* **19**(1): 23–34. (RCT)

20 Krebs H, Goplerud D (1987) Mechanical intestinal obstruction in patients with gynecologic disease: a review of 368 patients. *American Journal of Obstetrics and Gynecology.* **157**: 577–83. (RS-368)

21 Khoo D, Hall E, Motson R, Riley J, Denman K, Waxman J (1990) Palliation of malignant intestinal obstruction using octreotide. *European Journal of Cancer.* **30A**: 28–30. (CT-24)

22 Dean A (2001) The palliative effects of octreotide in cancer patients. *Chemotherapy.* **47** Suppl 2: 54–61. (R, 54 refs)

23 Mystakidou K, Tsilika E, Kalaidopoulou O *et al.* (2002) Comparison of octreotide administration vs conservative treatment in the management of inoperable bowel obstruction in patients with far advanced cancer: a randomized, double-blind, controlled clinical trial. *Anticancer Research.* **22**(2B): 1187–92. (RCT-68)

24 Mercadante S, Ripamonti C, Casuccio A, Zecca E, Groff L (2000) Comparison of octreotide and hyoscine butylbromide in controlling gastrointestinal symptoms due to malignant inoperable bowel obstruction. *Supportive Care in Cancer.* **8**(3): 188–91. (RCT-18)

25 Pelham A, Lee MA, Regnard CBF (2002) Gabapentin for coeliac plexus pain. *Palliative Medicine.* **16**: 355–6. (CS-3)

26 Feuer D, Broadley K (1999) Systematic review and meta-analysis of corticosteroids for the resolution of malignant bowel obstruction in advanced gynaecological and gastrointestinal cancers. *Annals of Oncology.* **10**: 1035–41. (SA, 10 refs)

27 Feuer D, Broadley K (2002) Corticosteroids for the resolution of malignant bowel obstruction in advanced gynaecological and gastrointestinal cancers. *The Cochrane Library, Issue 2, 2002.* Update Software Ltd, Oxford. www.cochrane.org/cochrane/revabstr/ab001219.htm. (SA)

28 Regnard C (1995) Bowel obstruction. In: *Flow Diagrams in Advanced Cancer and Other Diseases.* Edward Arnold, London. pp. 29–31. (Ch)

29 Khot P, Lang AW, Murali K, Parker MC (2002) Systematic review of the efficacy and safety of colorectal stents. *British Journal of Surgery.* **89**(9): 1096–102. (R, 48 refs)

Constipation

Advice on children written by Susie Lapwood

Clinical decision and action checklist

1 Is this bowel obstruction?
2 Have feces been easy and comfortable to pass?
3 Ensure privacy.
4 Is there a treatable cause?
5 Is the rectum or stoma full?
6 Is the colon full?
7 Is the constipation persisting?

Key points

- Constipation can mimic some features of advanced disease.
- Give appropriate laxatives regularly and titrate to maintain a comfortable stool. The aim is quality, not quantity!
- Diarrhea can be a symptom of constipation.

Introduction

Constipation is common. It is usually due to analgesics,[1-5] but is also common in many neurological conditions.[1,6-9] Constipation tends to worsen as the illness progresses, but eases in the last days of life.[10,11] It is more common with old age,[12] and is a high risk in those with severe neurological or intellectual disabilities.[13,14]

Symptoms and causes

Symptoms: Feces are usually hard, uncomfortable or difficult to pass, with a sense of incomplete evacuation after defecation. Other symptoms are abdominal pain, flatulence, distension, nausea, vomiting, halitosis, overflow diarrhea, malaise, frequent incontinence and anorexia. It is a cause of distress and may increase agitation in confused patients or precipitate seizures in children with neurological impairment. Assessment may need an abdominal X-ray.[15]

Causes: A dry stool is a hard stool. Factors that reduce water in the stool are dehydration (common in children), reduced bowel transit (drugs, immobility, depression, hypercalcemia, hypothyroidism and neurological gut dysmotility), reduced secretions into the gut (drugs, dehydration) and the inability of the stool to retain water (reduced fiber intake due to anorexia or feeding difficulties). Other causes include painful defecation (local tumor, anal fissure) or a fear of defecation.

Constipating drugs include those that reduce forward peristalsis and increase muscle tone (opioids); those that reduce secretions into the gut (opioids and drugs with antimuscarinic action, including tricyclic antidepressants, hyoscine hydrobromide or butylbromide hyoscyamine, methotrimeprazine) and drugs that reduce all bowel contractions (antimuscarinic drugs).

Treatment

Examination: Rectal examination provides useful information and should always be done gently. However, in children it can be traumatic and should only be done when absolutely necessary, by experienced staff and using the little finger for younger children. Abdominal examination often provides more information in children than in adults.

Opioid-induced constipation does not usually respond to changes in diet; fluids, and laxatives are nearly always needed.[16] Switching to alternative opioids may help and both fentanyl and methadone have been claimed to have a lower incidence of causing constipation.[17-22] Oral naloxone has been used to reverse opioid-induced constipation,[23,24] but the incidence of analgesic reversal is uncertain.[25,26] Naltrexone may be a better alternative as almost none is absorbed from the bowel.[27]

Laxatives: Most common laxatives are well tolerated.[16,28] Apart from the sensation of bloating,[28] lactulose is a safe laxative.[29] In opioid-induced constipation lactulose is as effective as senna,[30] or polyethylene glycol.[31] However, there are problems with using single laxatives: senna causes more adverse effects than lactulose;[32] lactulose can be too sweet for some patients; the evidence of the efficacy of oral docusate alone is lacking;[33] and using polyethylene glycol alone may require large volumes, although it has been tolerated in children[34] and adults.[35] Consequently it is common practice to use a combination of laxatives, usually a contact stimulant (e.g. senna) plus either a softener (e.g. docusate) or an osmotic agent (e.g. lactulose). Commercially available combinations are convenient but much more expensive than two single laxatives given separately. Combinations of senna and lactulose, or senna and docusate are effective.[36]

Laxative dose titration: Proportionately less laxative is required at higher opioid doses.[36,37] Each patient requires individual titration since the dose range is wide.

Patients with colostomies: Gently inserting a gloved finger into the stoma will show if feces are present. If they are present, treat as for feces in rectum (*see* cd-5 opposite). If feces are absent, exclude obstruction and follow the clinical decisions 6 and 7 opposite.

Patients with neurological impairment: There are few adequate trials in patients with paraplegia or cerebral palsy,[7] but rectal stimulation with a bisacodyl suppository will encourage evacuation.[38,39] Evacuation is easier if the feces are made firmer by using a contact laxative alone (e.g. senna). A firmer stool also reduces the risk of accidents due to diarrhea or unexpected defecation.

Clinical decision	If YES ⇒ Action
1 **Is this bowel obstruction?**	• *See* Bowel obstruction (p. 71). Consider abdominal X-ray.
2 **Have feces been easy and comfortable to pass?**	• *If constipation is a risk:* – correct dehydration and ensure good hydration – change to drugs with less constipating action if feasible and possible – encourage mobility and exercise if feasible and possible – review food content and presentation to increase fiber content (*see* cd-7 in Nutrition and hydration problems (p. 121)) – if the risk persists (e.g. starting opioids): start a laxative. • *If the stool frequency is less than usual:* this is common and normal in advanced disease because of reduced fiber intake, but is often misinterpreted as constipation. Reassurance and explanation are needed. • *If this is diarrhea:* exclude overflow diarrhea caused by constipation (an X-ray may be needed). *See* Diarrhea (p. 81).
3 **Ensure privacy:** in a double or four bed room providing help to get to a toilet is preferable to a bedside commode behind curtains transparent to sounds and smells.	
4 **Is there a treatable cause?**	• Examples: constipating drug (change to less constipating drug); hypercalcemia (*see* cd-7b in Emergencies (p. 211)); spinal cord compression (*see* cd-9a in Emergencies (p. 213)); depression (*see* Withdrawal and depression (p. 177)).
5 **Is the rectum or stoma full?**	• *If the feces are hard:* – encourage fluids and start senna plus a softening laxative (docusate or lactulose). – a bisacodyl suppository will increase rectal tone within 45 mins and encourage rectal emptying, but it must be in contact with the rectal wall to be effective.[40,41] A docusate enema (100 mg docusate liquid rectally) may also help in evacuating the rectum and colon.[42] – for colostomies, a suppository is held in place with a gloved finger for 10 min, while an enema is retained using an inflated Foley catheter for 10 min.[38] • *If the feces are soft:* stimulate the colon with senna or bisacodyl PO (10 hour delay). • *If there is no success in emptying the rectum or stoma:* carry out a manual evacuation using topical anesthetic gel and sedative cover (e.g. IV or buccal midazolam).
6 **Is the colon full?**	• *If colic is present:* start docusate 100–300 mg PO q8h. Consider high mineral oil enema. • *If colic is absent:* start regular senna plus docusate or equivalent.
7 **Is the constipation persisting?**	• *If defecation is painful:* exclude or treat anal fissure, painful hemorrhoids or local tumor. • *If opioid-induced:* – consider switching to fentanyl or methadone – consider naloxone at 10% of daily morphine dose, with maximum dose of 5 mg q8h[23,24] • *If neurological gut dysmotility is present* (paraplegia, autonomic insufficiency, children with neurological impairment): consider a weekly dose of bisacodyl. • Consider using polyethylene glycol (Golytely), or a prokinetic agent[43] such as metoclopramide, domperidone (obtained in the US from a Compounding Pharmacy – 10 mg, 20 mg) or erythromycin.[44]

CONTACT LAXATIVES: approximate equivalents (based on contact stimulant content only):
15 ml senna syrup or 3 senna pills plus 300 mg docusate:
approx = 15 ml senna syrup plus 15 ml lactulose syrup.
NB: As the opioid dose is titrated, the laxative dose also needs to increase, but the laxative increases become proportionally smaller until no further increases are required.[36,37]

Adapted from Regnard[45]
cd = **clinical decision**

References

B = book; C = comment; Ch = chapter; CS-n = case study-number of cases; CT-n = controlled trial-number of cases; E = editorial; GC = group consensus; I = interviews; Let = letter; LS = laboratory study; MC = multi-center; OS-n = open study-number of cases; R = review; RCT-n = randomized controlled trial-number of cases; RS-n = retrospective survey-number of cases; SA = systematic or meta analysis.

1 Meuser T, Pietruck C, Radbruch L, Stute P, Lehmann KA, Grond S (2001) Symptoms during cancer pain treatment following WHO-guidelines: a longitudinal follow-up study of symptom prevalence, severity and etiology. *Pain.* **93**(3): 247–57. (OS-593)

2 Edmonds P, Karlsen S, Khan S, Addington-Hall J (2001) A comparison of the palliative care needs of patients dying from chronic respiratory diseases and lung cancer. *Palliative Medicine.* **15**(4): 287–95. (I-636)

3 Walsh D, Donnelly S, Rybicki L (2000) The symptoms of advanced cancer: relationship to age, gender, and performance status in 1000 patients. *Supportive Care in Cancer.* **8**(3): 175–9. (OS-1000)

4 Fallon MT, Hanks GW (1999) Morphine, constipation and performance status in advanced cancer patients. *Palliative Medicine.* **13**(2): 159–60. (OS)

5 Sykes NP (1998) The relationship between opioid use and laxative use in terminally ill cancer patients. *Palliative Medicine.* **12**(5): 375–82. (OS-498)

6 Mitchell SL, Kiely DK, Hamel MB (2004) Dying with advanced dementia in the nursing home. *Archives of Internal Medicine.* **164**(3):321–6. (RS-2492).

7 Wiesel PH, Norton C, Brazzelli M (2003) Management of faecal incontinence and constipation in adults with central neurological diseases. *The Cochrane Library, Issue 3.* Update Software, Oxford (www.cochrane.org). (SA, 53 refs)

8 Krogh K, Christensen P, Laurberg S (2001) Colorectal symptoms in patients with neurological diseases. *Acta Neurologica Scandinavica.* **103**(6): 335–43. (R, 80 refs)

9 Wiesel PH, Norton C, Glickman S, Kamm MA (2001) Pathophysiology and management of bowel dysfunction in multiple sclerosis. *European Journal of Gastroenterology & Hepatology.* **13**(4): 441–8. (R, 86 refs)

10 Mercadante S, Fulfaro F, Casuccio A (2000) The impact of home palliative care on symptoms in advanced cancer patients. *Supportive Care in Cancer.* **8**(4): 307–10. (OS-211)

11 Mercadante S, Casuccio A, Fulfaro F (2000) The course of symptom frequency and intensity in advanced cancer patients followed at home. *Journal of Pain and Symptom Management.* **20**(2): 104–12. (CT-370)

12 Camilleri M, Lee JS, Viramontes B, Bharucha AE, Tangalos EG (2000) Insights into the pathophysiology and mechanisms of constipation, irritable bowel syndrome, and diverticulosis in older people. *Journal of the American Geriatrics Society.* **48**(9): 1142–50. (R, 78 refs)

13 Bohmer CJ, Taminiau JA, Klinkenberg-Knol EC, Meuwissen SG (2001) The prevalence of constipation in institutionalized people with intellectual disability. *Journal of Intellectual Disability Research.* **45**(Pt 3): 212–18. (OS-215)

14 Krogh K, Christensen P, Laurberg S (2001) Colorectal symptoms in patients with neurological diseases. *Acta Neurologica Scandinavica.* **103**(6): 335–43. (R, 80 refs)

15 Bruera E, Suarez-Almanzor M, Velasco A, Bertolino M, MacDonald SM, Hanson J (1994) The assessment of constipation in terminal cancer patients admitted to a palliative care unit: a retrospective review. *Journal of Pain and Symptom Management.* **9**(8): 515–19. (RS-122)

16 Thorpe DM (2001) Management of opioid-induced constipation. *Current Pain & Headache Reports.* **5**(3): 237–40. (R, 7 refs)

17 Mercadante S, Casuccio A, Fulfaro F, Groff L, Boffi R, Villari P, Gebbia V, Ripamonti C (2001) Switching from morphine to methadone to improve analgesia and tolerability in cancer patients: a prospective study. *Journal of Clinical Oncology.* **19**(11): 2898–904. (CT-52)

18 Gourlay GK (2001) Treatment of cancer pain with transdermal fentanyl. *Lancet Oncology.* **2**(3): 165–72. (R, 51 refs)

19 Nugent M, Davis C, Brooks D, Ahmedzai SH (2001) Long-term observations of patients receiving transdermal fentanyl after a randomized trial. *Journal of Pain and Symptom Management.* **21**(5): 385–91. (RCT-73)

20 Radbruch L, Sabatowski R, Loick G, Kulbe C, Kasper M, Grond S, Lehmann KA (2000) Constipation and the use of laxatives: a comparison between transdermal fentanyl and oral morphine. *Palliative Medicine.* **14**(2): 111–19. (MC, CT-46)

21 Ahmedzai S, Brooks D (1997) Transdermal fentanyl versus sustained-release oral morphine

in cancer pain: preference, efficacy, and quality of life. The TTS-Fentanyl Comparative Trial Group. *Journal of Pain and Symptom Management.* **13**(5): 254–61. (MC, RCT)

22 Daeninck PJ, Bruera E (1999) Reduction in constipation and laxative requirements following opioid rotation to methadone: a report of four cases. *Journal of Pain and Symptom Management.* **18**(4): 303–9. (CS-4)

23 Meissner W, Schmidt U, Hartmann M, Kath R, Reinhart K (2000) Oral naloxone reverses opioid-associated constipation. *Pain.* **84**(1): 105–9. (OS-22)

24 Sykes NP (1996) An investigation of the ability of oral naloxone to correct opioid-related constipation in patients with advanced cancer. *Palliative Medicine.* **10**(2): 135–44. (RCT-17)

25 Meissner W, Ullrich K (2002) Naloxone, constipation and analgesia. *Journal of Pain and Symptom Management.* **24**(3): 276–7. (Let)

26 Liu M (2002) Naloxone, constipation and analgesia: author's response. *Journal of Pain and Symptom Management.* **24**(3): 277–9. (Let)

27 Stephenson J (2002) Methylnaltrexone reverses opioid-induced constipation. *Lancet Oncology.* **3**(4): 202. (CT)

28 Xing JH, Soffer EE (2001) Adverse effects of laxatives. *Diseases of the Colon & Rectum.* **44**(8): 1201–9. (R, 107 refs)

29 Hallmann F (2000) Toxicity of commonly used laxatives. *Medical Science Monitor.* **6**(3): 618–28. (R, 110 refs)

30 Agra Y, Sacristan A, Gonzalez M, Ferrari M, Portugues A, Calvo MJ (1998) Efficacy of senna versus lactulose in terminal cancer patients treated with opioids. *Journal of Pain and Symptom Management.* **15**(1): 1–7. (RCT-91)

31 Freedman MD, Schwartz HJ, Roby R, Fleisher S (1997) Tolerance and efficacy of polyethylene glycol 3350/electrolyte solution versus lactulose in relieving opiate induced constipation: a double-blinded placebo-controlled trial. *Journal of Clinical Pharmacology.* **37**(10): 904–7. (RCT-57)

32 Sykes NP (1996) A volunteer model for the comparison of laxatives in opioid-related constipation. *Journal of Pain and Symptom Management.* **11**(6): 363–9. (CT-10)

33 Hurdon V, Viola R, Schroder C (2000) How useful is docusate in patients at risk for constipation? A systematic review of the evidence in the chronically ill. *Journal of Pain and Symptom Management.* **19**(2): 130–6. (SA)

34 Pashankar DS, Bishop WP (2001) Efficacy and optimal dose of daily polyethylene glycol 3350 for treatment of constipation and encopresis in children. *Journal of Pediatrics.* **139**(3): 428–32. (OS-24)

35 Cleveland MV, Flavin DP, Ruben RA, Epstein RM, Clark GE (2001) New polyethylene glycol laxative for treatment of constipation in adults: a randomized, double-blind, placebo-controlled study. *Southern Medical Journal.* **94**(5): 478–81. (RCT-23)

36 Sykes NP (1991) A clinical comparison of laxatives in a hospice. *Palliative Medicine.* **5**: 307–14. (OS)

37 Bennett M, Cresswell H (2003) Factors influencing constipation in advanced cancer patients: a prospective study of opioid dose, dantron dose and physical functioning. *Palliative Medicine.* **17**: 418–22. (OS-20)

38 Fallon M, O'Neill B (1997) ABC of palliative care: constipation and diarrhea. *BMJ.* **315**: 1293–6. (R)

39 Stiens SA, Luttrel W, Binard JE (1998) Polyethylene glycol versus vegetable oil based bisacodyl suppositories to initiate side-lying bowel care: a clinical trial in persons with spinal cord injury. *Spinal Cord.* **36**(11): 777–81. (CT-14)

40 Gosselink MJ, Hop WC, Schouten WR (2000) Rectal tone in response to bisacodyl in women with obstructed defecation. *International Journal of Colorectal Disease.* **15**(5–6): 297–302. (CT-60)

41 Flig E, Hermann TW, Zabel M (2000) Is bisacodyl absorbed at all from suppositories in man? *International Journal of Pharmaceutics.* **196**(1): 11–20. (OS-15)

42 House JG, Stiens SA (1997) Pharmacologically initiated defecation for persons with spinal cord injury: effectiveness of three agents. *Archives of Physical Medicine & Rehabilitation.* **78**(10): 1062–5. (RCT)

43 Halabi IM (1999) Cisapride in management of chronic pediatric constipation. *Journal of Pediatric Gastroenterology & Nutrition.* **28**(2): 199–202. (RCT-73)

44 Sharma SS, Bhargava N, Mathur SC (1995) Effect of oral erythromycin on colonic transit in patients with idiopathic constipation. A pilot study. *Digestive Diseases & Sciences.* **40**(11): 2446–9. (OS-11)

45 Regnard C (1995) Constipation. In: *Flow Diagrams in Advanced Cancer and Other Diseases.* Edward Arnold, London. pp. 11–13. (Ch)

Diarrhea

Clinical decision and action checklist

1 Is the patient dehydrated?
2 Are drugs or diet the cause?
3 Is previous bowel surgery the cause?
4 Is this a secretory diarrhea?
5 Are the stools very dark or very pale?
6 Is the stool mixed with blood or discharge?
7 Is a fistula the cause?
8 Is there clear fluid in the stool?
9 Is the diarrhea persisting?

Key points

- Rehydration is important for comfort.
- Infection should be excluded.
- Constipation with overflow can be a cause.

Introduction

Diarrhea occurs in up to 10% of cancer patients,[1] but up to 38% in AIDS.[2] It is distressing for both patients and carers and causes dehydration, electrolyte disturbances and loss of comfort and dignity.

Treatment

Rehydration: For adults, rehydration powders offer no advantages for those able to maintain oral intake.[3] For children, reduced osmolarity oral solutions are safer and more effective than the traditional WHO formula.[4] Parenteral rehydration is used if the fluid loss is severe and Ringer lactate solution is preferred.[5]

Drugs and diet: A wide range of drugs can cause diarrhea (*see* cd-2 opposite) and the drugs usually need to be stopped. For patients on antibiotics, 5% can develop an infective colitis that will need treatment.[6] Malabsorption and dietary intolerance should be considered since the diet may have to be modified.

Previous surgery can cause diarrhea through a number of mechanisms. Gastrectomy patients can suffer from food being 'dumped' into the bowel, causing nausea, bloating and diarrhea. If the terminal ileum has been resected, bile salts escape into the colon and cause local irritation.

Steatorrhea is due to excessive fat in the stool. Reducing gastric acid with ranitidine or a proton pump inhibitor (PPI) such as lansoprazole or omeprazole improves fat absorption, abolishing steatorrhea in up to 40% of patients with pancreatic insufficiency.[7,8] This is particularly important where alkaline pancreatic secretions are reduced (e.g. pancreatitis, cystic fibrosis) and following small bowel resection (where gastric acid output increases due to raised gastrin). PPIs are more potent gastric acid inhibitors and are often necessary in the Zollinger–Ellison syndrome.

Blood loss into the upper gastrointestinal tract irritates the bowel, producing a loose, dark or black stool (melena stool). Gastric bleeding can be reduced with sucralfate suspension.[9] Blood loss from the small bowel or colon may be reduced with systemic aminocaproic/tranexamic acid. Bleeding from a rectal tumor will lessen with topical sucralfate[10] or topical aminocaproic/tranexamic acid.[11] *See* cd-5 in Bleeding (p. 69).

Loperamide increases water absorption by slowing forward peristalsis. Caution is necessary with infective diarrhea since slowing peristalsis can cause overgrowth of dangerous pathogens and increased absorption of bacterial toxins.

Post-radiotherapy diarrhea can respond to octreotide,[12] acidophilus cultures (active yoghurt) taken orally,[13] or 5HT3 antagonists such as ondansetron.[14] Opioids such as codeine are more effective than bulking agents.[15] If pelvic radiotherapy causes a proctitis, adjust laxatives to keep the stool soft.

Octreotide has been used in AIDS-related diarrhea,[16] cancer,[17] in postgastrectomy dumping,[18] and may also have a role to play in other causes of severe refractory diarrhea,[19,20] although more evidence of efficacy is needed.[21] Side effects of octreotide include steatorrhea.

Helping with the effects of diarrhea

Diarrhea is exhausting and distressing. Any fecal incontinence can create a loss of dignity for the patient and high stress on the carer. At home, washing clothes and sheets becomes a major problem. In any setting odor adds to everyone's distress. It is not surprising, therefore, that persisting diarrhea can have severe effects on image, mood and relationships, which will need support and help.

Clinical decision	If YES ⇒ Action
1 Is the patient dehydrated?	• Oral rehydration formula (e.g. WHO formula) (oral/nasogastric) or Ringer lactate solution (intravenous). Severely dehydrated adults may need as much as 6–8 liters per 24 hours as long as the loss continues.[5]
2 Are drugs or diet the cause?	• *Consider these drugs as a cause:* β-blockers, H_2 blockers (e.g. ranitidine), chemotherapy, diuretics, iron, laxatives, magnesium containing antacids, NSAIDs, octreotide, ondansetron, PPIs (e.g. omeprazole). • *Antibiotic induced colitis:* should be excluded by identifying clostridium toxin in the stool. • *Consider these causes:* malabsorption of carbohydrates, lactose intolerance, disaccharide deficiency, gluten insensitivity. • *Related to nasogastric feeding:* dilute feeds or increase length of feeding time. If the symptoms persist, discuss a change of feed type with the dietician.
3 Is previous bowel surgery the cause?	• *Postgastrectomy* (dumping syndrome): small, frequent snacks. Consider octreotide.[22] • *Intestinal resection* (bile salts irritate colon): cholestyramine 12–16 g daily + ranitidine. • *Blind loop* (causing bacterial overgrowth): tetracycline (or metronidazole) for 2–4 weeks.
4 Is this a secretory diarrhea?	• *Consider infection:* avoid loperamide or atropine. Culture stool if diarrhea persists after 5 days or patient contacts are also affected by diarrhea. • *Diabetic autonomic failure:* clonidine (50–150 microgram/24 hours) may help in diabetes.[19] • *For Zollinger–Ellison syndrome:* high dose ranitidine or omeprazole. • *Tumor secreting vasoactive intestinal peptide* (VIPoma): octreotide (see cd-9 below). • *Carcinoid:* start ranitidine or omeprazole. Consider octreotide SC q8h or CSCI 150–1500 microgram per 24 hours.[23]
5 Are the stools very dark or very pale?	• *If the stools are very pale:* consider whether this is steatorrhea (pale, malodorous stools that are difficult to flush away): start loperamide (2 mg with each loose stool, up to 16 mg daily). For pancreatic insufficiency: enteric coated pancreatin supplement plus lansoprazole. For common bile duct obstruction: ranitidine + enteric coated pancreatin. Consider high dose dexamethasone, bypass surgery or endoscopic stent. • *If the stools are very dark:* If fecal occult blood test negative: consider oral dye (e.g. beetroot) or iron supplements as possible cause. Reassure the patient. If fecal occult test positive: consider upper gastrointestinal blood loss (*see* Bleeding (p. 67)).
6 Is the stool mixed with blood or discharge?	• *Fungating rectal or colonic tumor:* topical corticosteroids (hydrocortisone or betamethasone enema) plus metronidazole 500 mg q12h. Use topical sucralfate or aminocaproic/tranexamic acid to control bleeding close to anal margin. Consider radiotherapy. • *Infection* (e.g. shigella, salmonella, clostridium): identify and treat. • *Inflammation:* assess cause (e.g. Crohn's disease) and treat.
7 Is a fistula the cause?	• *Urine* (vesicocolic or vesicorectal fistula): catheter or desmopressin at night (*See* cd-5 in Urinary and sexual problems (p. 154)). • *Gastrocolic or enterorectal fistula:* consider arranging for a colostomy.
8 Is there clear fluid in the stool?	• *Consider* causes of secretory diarrhea (cd-4 above). • *Mucus* (total bowel obstruction/blind rectum/rectal or colonic tumor secreting mucus): hyoscine butylbromide may help (SC intermittent or infusion 60–300 mg per 24 hours) (in the US hyoscyamine 0.25–0.5 mg IV/SC q4h PRN).
9 Is the diarrhea persisting?	• Exclude: *Constipation* causing spurious diarrhea. *Infection:* send three stool specimens (in AIDS up to six stool specimens may be needed, and for CMV or adenovirus a rectal biopsy or upper GI endoscopy may be required).[24] *Irritable colon:* increase dietary fiber. *Anxiety, fear:* see Anxiety (p. 165). *Fecal incontinence due to neurological or sphincter dysfunction:* consider a colostomy. If time is available, start a bowel management program.[25] *Autonomic failure:* clonidine (50–150 microgram/24 hours) may help in diabetes.[19] • Treat symptomatically: Loperamide 2–4 mg with each loose stool (up to 32 mg daily may be needed in AIDS-related diarrhea). Stop laxatives and magnesium-containing antacids. Consider: hyoscine butylbromide SC infusion 60–300 mg per 24 hours (in the US hyoscyamine 0.25–0.5 mg IV/SC q4h PRN) **or** octreotide SC infusion 150–1500 microgram per 24 hrs. Protective ointment or hydrocolloid dressings to perineum and anal margin. Consider perineal stool-collecting bag if stool volume is large.

Adapted from Regnard and Mannix[26]
cd = clinical decision

References

B = book; C = comment; Ch = chapter; CS-n = case study-number of cases; CT-n = controlled trial-number of cases; E = editorial; GC = group consensus; I = interviews; Let = letter; LS = laboratory study; MC = multi-center; OS-n = open study-number of cases; R = review; RCT-n = randomized controlled trial-number of cases; RS-n = retrospective survey-number of cases; SA = systematic or meta analysis.

1 Walsh TD, O'Shaughnessy C (1989) Diarrhea. In: TD Walsh (ed) *Symptom Control*. Blackwell, Oxford. pp. 99–116. (Ch)

2 Willoughby VR, Sahr F, Russell JB, Gbakima AA (2001) The usefulness of defined clinical features in the diagnosis of HIV/AIDS infection in Sierra Leone. *Cellular & Molecular Biology*. 47(7): 1163–7. (OS-124)

3 Wingate D, Phillips SF, Lewis SJ, Malagelada JR, Speelman P, Steffen R, Tytgat GN (2001) Guidelines for adults on self-medication for the treatment of acute diarrhea. *Alimentary Pharmacology & Therapeutics*. 15(6): 773–82. (R, 79 refs)

4 Hahn S, Kim S, Garner P (2002) Reduced osmolarity oral rehydration solution for treating dehydration caused by acute diarrhea in children. *Cochrane Database of Systematic Reviews*. 1: CD002847. (R, 61 refs)

5 Carpenter CCJ (1996) Cholera. In: DJ Weatherall, JGG Leadingham, DA Warrell (eds) *Oxford Textbook of Medicine on CD-Rom*. Oxford University Press/Publishing BV, Oxford. pp. 576–80. (Ch)

6 Wistrom J, Norrby SR, Myhre EB, Eriksson S, Granstrom G, Lagergren L, Englund G, Nord CE, Svenungsson B (2001) Frequency of antibiotic-associated diarrhea in 2462 antibiotic-treated hospitalized patients: a prospective study. *Journal of Antimicrobial Chemotherapy*. 47(1): 43–50. (OS-2462)

7 DiMagno EP (2001) Gastric acid suppression and treatment of severe exocrine pancreatic insufficiency. *Best Practice & Research in Clinical Gastroenterology*. 15(3): 477–86. (R, 20 refs)

8 Tran TM, Van den Neucker A, Hendriks JJ, Forget P, Forget PP (1998) Effects of a proton-pump inhibitor in cystic fibrosis. *Acta Paediatrica*. 87(5): 553–8. (OS-15)

9 Regnard CFB, Mannix K (1990) Palliation of gastric carcinoma hemorrhage with sucralfate. *Palliative Medicine*. 4: 329–30. (Let, CS-1)

10 Regnard CFB (1991) Control of bleeding in advanced cancer. *Lancet*. 337: 974. (CS-1)

11 McElligot E, Quigley C, Hanks GW (1992) Tranexamic acid and rectal bleeding. *Lancet*. 337: 431. (CS-1)

12 Baillie-Johnson HR (1996) Octreotide in the management of treatment-related diarrhea. *Anti-Cancer Drugs*. 7(Suppl 1): 11–15. (R, 43 refs)

13 Urbancsek H, Kazar T, Mezes I, Neumann K (2001) Results of a double-blind, randomized study to evaluate the efficacy and safety of Antibiophilus in patients with radiation-induced diarrhea. *European Journal of Gastroenterology & Hepatology*. 13(4): 391–6. (RCT-206)

14 Henriksson R, Lomberg H, Israelsson G, Zackrisson B, Franzen L (1992) The effect of ondansetron on radiation-induced emesis and diarrhea. *Acta Oncologica*. 31(7): 767–9. (OS-33)

15 Lodge N, Evans ML, Wilkins M, Blake PR, Fryatt I (1995) A randomized cross-over study of the efficacy of codeine phosphate versus Ispaghula husk in patients with gynaecological cancer experiencing diarrhea during pelvic radiotherapy. *European Journal of Cancer Care*. 4(1): 8–10. (RCT-10)

16 Cello JP, Grendall JH, Basuk P, Simon D, Weiss L, Wittner M, Rood RP, Wilcox CM, Forsmark CE, Read AE (1991) Effect of octreotide on refractory AIDS-associated diarrhea. *Annals of Internal Medicine*. 115: 705–10. (MC, CT-51)

17 Dean A, Bridge D, Lickiss JN (1994) The palliative effects of octreotide in malignant disease. *Annals of the Academy of Medicine, Singapore*. 23(2): 212–15. (R, 38 refs)

18 Mackie CR, Jenkins SA, Hartley MN (1991) Treatment of severe postvagotomy/postgastrectomy symptoms with the somatostatin analogue octreotide. *British Journal of Surgery*. 78: 1338–43. (OS-14)

19 Mercadante S (1995) Diarrhea in terminally ill patients: pathophysiology and treatment. *Journal of Pain and Symptom Management*. 10(4): 298–309. (R, 37 refs)

20 Fried M (1999) Octreotide in the treatment of refractory diarrhea. *Digestion*. 60(Suppl 2): 42–6. (R, 38 refs)

21 Szilagyi A, Shrier I (2001) Systematic review: the use of somatostatin or octreotide in refractory diarrhea. *Alimentary Pharmacology & Therapeutics*. 15(12): 1889–97. (R, 58 refs)

22 Vecht J, Masclee AA, Lamers CB (1997) The dumping syndrome. Current insights into pathophysiology, diagnosis and treatment. *Scandinavian Journal of Gastroenterology: Supplement*. 223: 21–7. (R, 95 refs)

23 Harris AG, Redfern JS (1995) Octreotide treatment of carcinoid syndrome: analysis of published dose-titration data. *Alimentary Pharmacology & Therapeutics*. 9(4): 387–94. (SA, 83 refs)

24 Gane EJ, Thomas MG, Nicholson GI, Lane MR (1992) Upper gastrointestinal endoscopy in patients with human immunodeficiency virus infection: is it worthwhile? *New Zealand Medical Journal*. 105(946): 475–6. (OS-21)

25 Pierce E, Cowan P, Stokes M (2001) Managing faecal retention and incontinence in neurodisability. *British Journal of Nursing*. 10(9): 592–601. (R, 18 refs)

26 Regnard C, Mannix K (1995) The control of diarrhea. In: *Flow Diagrams in Advanced Cancer and Other Diseases*. Edward Arnold, London. pp. 32–5. (Ch)

Dyspepsia

Advice on children written by Susie Lapwood

Clinical decision and action checklist

1 Are any alarm symptoms present?
2 Could this be acid-related dyspepsia?
3 Could this be dysmotility dyspepsia?
4 Could this be gastro-esophageal reflux disease (GERD)?
5 Is the dyspepsia persisting?

Key points

- Dyspepsia can be caused by acid-induced damage, abnormal motility or esophageal reflux.
- Adults and children with severe neurological impairment are particularly prone to dyspepsia.
- 'Alarm' symptoms should usually prompt urgent admission to hospital.
- Prokinetic agents and proton pump inhibitors are important treatments in dyspepsia.

Introduction

Dyspepsia is a common problem that includes a range of upper gastrointestinal symptoms of which upper abdominal pain is the commonest.[1,2] In adults and children with communication difficulties the only symptoms may be food refusal, weight loss or failure to thrive.

Types of dyspepsia

Acid-related (organic) dyspepsia is due to acid-related damage of the stomach or duodenum, e.g. gastric ulcer. NSAIDs and *H. pylori* infection are common causes.[3–5] A common symptom is epigastric pain that is worse at night and relieved by antacids.[2]

Dysmotility (non-ulcer) dyspepsia is due to abnormal motility of the esophagus or of the stomach and duodenum. Gastric stasis and cancer-associated dyspepsia syndrome (CADS) are part of this type of dyspepsia.[6–8] It is more common in neurologically impaired children and often associated with GERD (see next paragraph).[9] In gastro-duodenal dysmotility vomiting relieves pain, but in esophageal dysmotility, pain develops after meals.[2]

Gastro-esophageal reflux disease (GERD) is caused by reflux of gastric contents into the esophagus sufficient to cause local damage and symptoms.[10] It occurs in up to 75% of neurologically impaired children.[9,11] Other causes include hiatus hernia, adoption of a prolonged supine position, and increased intra-abdominal pressure secondary to spasticity, scoliosis or seizures.[12] In adults causes can be due to intrinsic or extrinsic tumor effects, or pressure (e.g. an enlarged liver). Overfeeding, especially through a gastrostomy in neurologically impaired adults and children whose energy needs are less than those of more active patients, can worsen GERD symptoms. Symptoms are intermittent and often non-specific. They may include heartburn (especially on bending and lying flat), dysphagia, epigastric pain, with atypical symptoms of vomiting, dental enamel erosion, respiratory symptoms (e.g. nocturnal and/or post-prandial asthma, aspiration, chest infections), eating-related problems (e.g. irritability, hyperextensive posture, choking, dysphagia) and ear, nose and throat problems (e.g. cough, hoarseness).[12–16] Sandifer's syndrome (neck extension and head rotation during or after meals) can occur in infants or young children and is associated with iron deficiency anemia and severe esophagitis.

Treatment

Alarm symptoms: These symptoms would normally require prompt admission to hospital for investigation and treatment. Some patients will be too ill for transfer or will have made clear their wish to remain at home or hospice. These patients need adequate analgesia, antiemetics, comfort and company for their last days and hours.

Acid-related dyspepsia: First-line treatment is a proton pump inhibitor (PPI).[17] If the patient is vomiting or has swallowing problems, pantoprazole can be given intravenously or through a feeding tube (*see* Drug information (p. 263)). If gastric bleeding is occurring, sucralfate is an effective hemostatic agent.[18–20] Infection with *H. pylori* is common and should be treated if present.[21] NSAIDs are another common cause of mucosal damage and should be stopped or changed to an NSAID less likely to cause damage (*see* Managing the adverse effects of analgesics (p. 53)).

Dysmotility dyspepsia: This often needs a prokinetic agent, which will have to be given by a non-oral route if vomiting is present.[22–24] In standard doses metoclopramide is as effective as domperidone (obtained in the US from a Compounding Pharmacy – 10 mg, 20 mg), but in children domperidone is safer.[25,26] In persistent cases erythromycin can help, but can cause nausea and tolerance may develop.[27–29] Taking meals as frequent snacks rather than large meals may also help. In a patient on tube feeding smaller, more frequent boluses may help. Simethicone (dimethicone) is a defoaming agent that reduces gastric distension.[30,31]

GERD: If dysphagia is a predominant symptom this should be investigated, especially as aspiration occurs silently in up to 40% of patients (*see* Dysphagia (p. 91)). In patients unable to position themselves, repositioning them in a semi-prone position can help. Alginates float on the stomach contents and reduce reflux symptoms.[32] As with dysmotility dyspepsia, prokinetics are an important treatment and altering the size and frequency of meals and feeds can also help.

Persistent dyspepsia

Bile reflux: Substances that bind bile acids can ease this (e.g. cholestyramine).[36]

Infection: In addition to *H. pylori*, infections such as candida, CMV and herpes (zoster or simplex) can cause the same symptoms as dyspepsia. Treatment will resolve the symptoms.

Referral for investigation and treatment: The opinion of a gastroenterologist can be invaluable. In children with persistent GERD, fundoplication +/− pyloroplasty is effective in over 80% but surgery has a high morbidity with 26–59% having post-operative complications, 60–75% getting recurrence of GERD (the higher figure in neurological impairment) and 5–15% needing repeat surgery.[11,33] An effective alternative is to consider a jejunal feeding tube.[34,35]

Clinical decision	If YES ⇒ Action
1 Are any alarm symptoms present?	Any of the following would usually prompt urgent admission to hospital for endoscopy and treatment. Alternative options are: • *Rapid clinical deterioration: see* Emergencies (p. 199). • *Persistent vomiting causing dehydration or electrolyte disturbance: see* Nausea and vomiting (p. 113). • *Hematemesis* (from bleeding ulcer or severe gastritis): *see* cd-5 in Bleeding (p. 69). • *Melena* (upper gastrointestinal hemorrhage): *see* cd-5 in Bleeding (p. 69). • *Persistent and worsening pain* (perforation or other intra-abdominal crisis): *see* cd-5d in Emergencies (p. 207). • *Severe dysphagia* (esophageal obstruction): *see* Dysphagia (p. 91).
2 Could this be acid-related dyspepsia? (e.g. epigastric pain or heartburn worse at night and eased by antacids)	• *If bleeding (hematemesis or melena):* start sucralfate suspension 10 ml q6h. • Start PPI, e.g. omeprazole 20 mg or lansoprazole 30 mg daily. • Stop any drugs causing upper GI mucosal irritation such as iron or an NSAID. • Take blood for serum *H. pylori* immunoassay. If positive, use one week triple therapy of amoxicillin, clarithromycin and a PPI.
3 Could this be a dysmotility dyspepsia? (e.g. pain eased by vomiting or occurring after meals)	• Consider stopping or reducing the dose of antimuscarinic drugs. • Start a prokinetic, e.g. metoclopramide or domperidone (obtained in the US from a Compounding Pharmacy – 10mg, 20 mg) 10 mg q6h. Use domperidone for children (*see* Drugs in palliative care for children: starting doses (p. 253)). If vomiting is present, start metoclopramide 10 mg SC qid, or SC infusion 40 mg/24 hours and change to oral once vomiting is controlled. (If available, a compounding pharmacist can supply suppositories of either metoclopramide or domperidone.) • Consider activated simethicone e.g. Ovol, Phazyme liquid (20–40 mg before meals or feeds) to help trapped gastric air to be brought up. • Reduce the size of meals or feeds and give more frequently.
4 Could this be GERD? (e.g. heartburn or epigastric pain worse on bending or lying flat)	• Start alginate, e.g. Gaviscon 10–20 ml after each meal or feed (*see* Drugs in palliative care for children: starting doses (p. 253)). • Start a prokinetic, e.g. metoclopramide or domperidone (obtained in the US from a Compounding Pharmacy – 10mg, 20 mg) 10 mg q6h. Use domperidone for children (*see* Drugs in palliative care for children: starting doses (p. 253)). • Also consider: If dysphagia and/or aspiration are present: *see* Dysphagia (p. 91). If the patient is unable to move: lie on front or left side, head elevated to 30 degrees. If NG/gastrostomy-fed: alter feeding regime from large bolus to frequent small volume feeds. Continuous feeding can be tried but this sometimes aggravates symptoms.
5 Is the dyspepsia persisting?	• *If infection is present* (*H. pylori*, candida, CMV, herpes): treat the infection. • *If mucosal ulceration is causing pain:* start a mucosal protecting agent (e.g. sucralfate suspension 10 ml q6h–q8h) • *If not on PPI:* start omeprazole 20 mg (PO or through feeding tube) or lansoprazole 30 mg PO daily. Ranitidine is an alternative, but is less effective and can cause problematic rebound nocturnal acid secretion. • *If bile reflux is the problem:* consider cholestyramine 1–2 g after meals. • If dysphagia or NG tube is present: consider gastrostomy. See Dysphagia (p. 91) and Nutrition and hydration problems (p. 119). • *If dysmotility persists:* consider erythromycin 100–250 mg (10 mg/kg in children) q12h. • *If GERD is present:* consider referral for gastroenterological opinion for consideration of a jejunal feeding tube or surgery. • *If symptoms persist:* consider referring for investigation.

cd = clinical decision

References

B = book; C = comment; Ch = chapter; CS-n = case study-number of cases; CT-n = controlled trial-number of cases; E = editorial; GC = group consensus; I = interviews; Let = letter; LS = laboratory study; MC = multicenter; OS-n = open study-number of cases; R = review; RCT-n = randomized controlled trial-number of cases; RS-n = retrospective survey-number of cases; SA = systematic or meta analysis.

1 Meinechie-Schmidt V, Christensen E (1998) Classification of dyspepsia. *Scandinavian Journal of Gastroenterology.* **33**: 1262–72. (CT-7270)

2 Grainger SL, Klass HJ, Rake MO, Williams JG (1994) Prevalence of dyspepsia: the epidemiology of overlapping symptoms. *Postgraduate Medical Journal.* **70**: 154–61. (R, 25 refs)

3 Childs S, Roberts A, Meineche-Scmidt V, de Wit N, Rubin G (2000) The management of *Helicobacter pylori* infection in primary care: a systematic review of the literature. *Family Practice.* **17** (Suppl 2): S6–11. (SA, 59 refs)

4 Hawkey CJ (2000) Non-steroidal anti-inflammatory drug gastropathy. *Gastroenterology.* **119**: 521–35. (R, 143 refs)

5 Weil J, Langamn MJS, Wainwright P, Lawson DH, Rawlins M, Logan RFA, Brown TP, Vessey MP, Murphy M, Colin-Jones DG (2000) Peptic ulcer bleeding: accessory risk factors and interactions with non-steroidal anti-inflammatory drugs. *Gut.* **46**: 27–31. (CT, MC-2000)

6 Nelson K, Walsh T, O'Donovan P, Sheehan F and Falk G (1993) Assessment of upper gastrointestinal motility in the cancer-associated dyspepsia syndrome (CADS). *Journal of Palliative Care.* **9**: 27–31.

7 Armes PJ, Plant HJ, Allbright A, Silverstone T, Slevin ML (1992) A study to investigate the incidence of early satiety in patients with advanced cancer. *British Journal of Cancer.* **65**: 481–4.

8 Bruera E, Catz Z, Hooper R, Lentle B and MacDonald RN (1987) Chronic nausea and anorexia in advanced cancer patients: A possible role for autonomic dysfunction. *Journal of Pain and Symptom Management.* **2**: 19–21.

9 Sullivan PB (1997) Gastro-intestinal problems in the neurologically-impaired child. *Baillière's Clinical Gastroenterology.* **11**(3): 529–46. (R)

10 Vandenplas Y, Ashkenazi A, Belli D, Boige N, Bouquet J, Cadranel S, Cezard JP, Cucchiara S, Dupont C, Geboes K (1993) A proposition for the diagnosis and treatment of gastro-esophageal reflux disease in children: a report from a working group on gastro-esophageal reflux disease. Working Group of the European Society of Paediatric Gastro-enterology and Nutrition (ESPGAN). *European Journal of Pediatrics.* **152**(9): 704–11. (R, 44 refs)

11 Martinez DA, Ginn-Pease ME, Caniano DA (1992) Recognition of recurrent gastroesophageal reflux following antireflux surgery in the neurologically disabled child: high index of suspicion and definitive evaluation. *Journal of Pediatric Surgery.* **27**(8): 983–8. (OS-240)

12 Bagwell CE (1995) Gastro-esophageal reflux in children. *Surgery Annual.* **27**: 133–63. (R)

13 de Caestecker J (2001) ABC of the upper gastrointestinal tract. Oesophagus: heartburn. *BMJ.* **323**: 736–9.

14 Wasowska-Krolikowska K, Toporowska-Kowalska E, Krogulska A (2002) Asthma and gastresophageal reflux in children. *Medical Science Monitor.* **8**(3): RA64–71. (R, 45 refs)

15 Mendell DA, Logemann JA (2002) A retrospective analysis of the pharyngeal swallow in patients with a clinical diagnosis of GERD compared with normal controls: a pilot study. *Dysphagia.* **17**(3): 220–6. (CT-18)

16 Irwin RS, Madison JM (2002) Diagnosis and treatment of chronic cough due to gastroesophageal reflux disease and postnasal drip syndrome. *Pulmonary Pharmacology & Therapeutics.* **15**(3): 261–6. (R, 42 refs)

17 Delaney BC, Innes MA, Deeks J, Wilson S, Oakes R, Moayyedi P, Hobbs FD, Forman D (2000) Initial management strategies for dyspepsia. *Cochrane Database of Systematic Reviews (computer file).* **2**: CD001961.

18 Lam SK (1990) Why do ulcers heal with sucralfate? *Scandinavian Journal of Gastroenterology.* **25** (Suppl 173): 6–16. (R, 106 refs)

19 Caldwell JR, Roth SH, Wu WG, Semble EL, Castell DD, Heller MD, March WH (1987) Sucralfate treatment of nonsteroidal anti-inflammatory drug-induced gastrointestinal symptoms and mucosal damage. *American Journal of Medicine.* **83** (Suppl. 3B): 74–82. (RCT-143)

20 Regnard CFB, Mannix K (1990) Palliation of gastric carcinoma hemorrhage with sucralfate. *Palliative Medicine.* **4**: 329–30. (Let, CS-1)

21 Bazzoli F, Porro G, Bianchi MG, Molteni M, Pazzato P, Zagari RM (2002) Treatment of *Helicobacter pylori* infection. Indications and regimens: an update. *Digestive & Liver Disease.* **34**(1): 70–83. (R, 139 refs)

22 Twycross RG (1995) The use of prokinetic drugs

in palliative care. *European Journal of Palliative Care.* **4**: 141–5. (R)

23 Shivshanker K, Bennett RW, Haynie TP (1983) Tumor-associated gastroparesis: correction with metoclopramide. *American Journal of Surgery.* **145**: 221–5. (OS-10)

24 Kris MG, Yeh SDJ, Gralla RJ, Young CW (1985) Symptomatic gastroparesis in cancer patients. A possible cause of cancer-associated anorexia that can be improved with oral metoclopramide. *Proceedings of the American Society of Clinical Oncology.* **4**: 267.

25 Sanger GJ, King FD (1988) From metoclopramide to selective gut motility stimulants and 5HT3 receptor antagonists. *Drug Design and Delivery.* **3**: 273–95. (R, 143 refs)

26 Loose FD (1979) Domperidone in chronic dyspepsia: a pilot open study and a multicentre general practice crossover comparison with metoclopramide and placebo. *Pharmatherapeutica.* **2**(3): 140–6.

27 Berne JD, Norwood SH, McAuley CE, Vallina VL, Villareal D, Weston J, McClarty J (2002) Erythromycin reduces delayed gastric emptying in critically ill trauma patients: a randomized, controlled trial. *Journal of Trauma-injury Infection & Critical Care.* **53**(3): 422–5. (RCT-68)

28 Booth CM, Heyland DK, Paterson WG (2002) Gastrointestinal promotility drugs in the critical care setting: a systematic review of the evidence. *Critical Care Medicine.* **30**(7): 1429–35. (SA, 70 refs)

29 Costalos C, Gounaris A, Varhalama E, Kokori F, Alexiou N, Kolovou E (2002) Erythromycin as a prokinetic agent in preterm infants. *Journal of Pediatric Gastroenterology & Nutrition.* **34**(1): 23–5. (RCT-20)

30 Bernstein J, Kasich M (1974) A double-blind trial of simethicone in functional disease of the upper gastrointestinal tract. *Journal of Clinical Pharmacology.* **14**: 614–23. (CT)

31 Ogilvie AL, Atkinson M (1986) Does dimethicone increase the efficacy of antacids in the treatment of reflux esophagitis? *Journal of the Royal Society of Medicine.* **79**(10): 584–7. (RCT-45)

32 Mandel KG, Daggy BP, Brodie DA, Jacoby HI (2000) Review article: alginate-raft formulations in the treatment of heartburn and acid reflux. *Alimentary Pharmacology & Therapeutics.* **14**(6): 669–90. (R, 106 refs)

33 Norrashidah AW, Henry RL (2002) Fundoplication in children with gastro-esophageal reflux disease. *Journal of Paediatrics & Child Health.* **38**(2): 156–9. (RS-79)

34 Doede T, Faiss S, Schier F (2002) Jejunal feeding tubes via gastrostomy in children. *Endoscopy.* **34**(7): 539–42. (OS-52)

35 Wales PW, Diamond IR, Dutta S, Muraca S, Chait P, Connolly B, Langer JC (2002) Fundoplication and gastrostomy versus image-guided gastrojejunal tube for enteral feeding in neurologically impaired children with gastro-esophageal reflux. *Journal of Pediatric Surgery.* **37**(3): 407–12. (RS-111)

36 Watters KJ, Murphy GM, Tomkin GH, Ashford JJ (1979) An evaluation of the bile acid binding and antacid properties of hydrotalcite in hiatus hernia and peptic ulceration. *Current Medical Research Opinion.* **6**: 85–7. (OS-25)

Dysphagia

Clinical decision and action checklist

1 Is there doubt about the need for hydration and/or feeding?
2 Is a complete obstruction present?
3 Is aspiration occurring?
4 Is infection the cause?
5 Are drugs the cause?
6 Is pain present?
7 Does the patient feel the problem is at the level of the chest or abdomen?
8 Does the patient feel the problem is at the level of the mouth or throat?
9 Is the problem persisting?

Key points

- Careful assessment may uncover problems with simple solutions.
- The advice of a specialist speech therapist is invaluable.

Introduction

Dysphagia is difficulty in transferring food and drink from the mouth to the stomach. It is seen in 12–23% of cancer patients,[1,2] but is much more common (up to 60%) in patients with neurological disease such as amyotrophic lateral sclerosis, multiple sclerosis, dementia, Parkinson's disease and severe cerebral palsy.[3–7] It is also more common in old age.[8,9] Anything that alters the anatomy or the control of swallowing can affect the oral, pharyngeal and esophageal phases.[10]

History and examination: Localization by the patient is accurate in over 90% of cases.[11] Food consistencies are unreliable indicators,[12] and the gag reflex is of little value.[13,14] Some of the assessment can be done at the bedside.[13,15,16] The oral to pharyngeal transit time (OPT) is important for oropharyngeal causes and is the time from the first movement of the tongue to the last movement of the larynx, measured by placing one finger below the jaw and one over the larynx.[13,16] In the *dry test swallow*, the patient is asked to swallow without fluid, and in the *wet test swallow* the test is repeated with 5 ml water. The OPT is usually less than one second. Speaking immediately after swallowing will uncover laryngeal penetration by the 'gargle' quality to the voice, or by coughing. Some laryngeal penetration by liquids is common,[10] and in 40% aspiration beyond the vocal cords is minor with no symptoms.[11] This challenges the usual view that aspiration is always a serious, life-threatening event. Symptomless aspiration indicates a risk of more serious aspiration and a possible need for non-oral feeding. The advice of a specialist speech and language therapist for oropharyngeal causes is essential.[17]

Investigations: Oropharyngeal dysphagia is best assessed by videofluoroscopy or nasal endoscopy under the advice of a specialist speech and language therapist.[18–21] A barium swallow is of minimal value and may cause barium aspiration. For esophageal causes endoscopy is essential and manometry can diagnose motility problems.[18]

Drug causes: Drugs causing extrapyramidal disorders (antimuscarinic drugs, metoclopramide, haloperidol), increased lower esophageal tone (metoclopramide, domperidone (obtained in the US from a compounding pharmacy – 10 mg, 20 mg)), altered upper esophageal tone (dantrolene), or mucosal damage (cytotoxics, nonsteroidal anti-inflammatory drugs).

Candidosis:[22] This can involve any part of the gastrointestinal tract. Infection below the pharynx may only produce local pain. Vomiting or diarrhea and signs of oral candidosis are present in only 50% of patients with esophageal candidosis.[23] For treatment *see* cd-3 in Oral problems (p. 127).

Treatment

Supportive measures: Small portions of attractive food are essential,[24] while some patients will need the advice of a physiotherapist and/or occupational therapist for posture and physical aids.[25]

Dexamethasone reduces peritumor edema, improves neurological function when perineural tumor invasion has occurred,[26] and may reduce bulbar palsy caused by direct tumor invasion of the skull base.

Radiotherapy can be given as a single intracavity dose. In esophageal carcinoma it can relieve dysphagia in up to 54% of patients for a median of 4 months.[27] External beam treatment over several sessions can also relieve dysphagia.

Dilatation is effective in malignant obstruction but only lasts a few weeks.[28]

Laser can be used as first line and has advantages over intubation.[15,29–31]

Stenting: Small, metal stents are increasingly being used.[32–36] Covered stents are necessary if a fistula is present.[32] Laser and stenting can be combined with good effect.[37]

Non-oral feeding will be necessary in patients with long oropharyngeal transit times (diagnosed clinically), those with more than 10% of swallowed material aspirated (diagnosed radiologically) and those who require more nutrition than they can manage orally. Nasogastric (NG) feeding is poorly tolerated by patients even with fine bore tubes,[38] does not increase survival,[39,40] and may even worsen aspiration.[38] Percutaneous gastrostomy (PEG) has advantages over nasogastric feeding,[10,41] with less aspiration.[42] It can have a lower complication rate in some patients,[43] but not in senile dementia.[44] It can be inserted through an endoscope or under X-ray control if access is not possible with an endoscope.[45–48] Major complications of PEG are infrequent (< 3%) but minor problems (blockage, leakage, local infection) occur in up to one third.[49] Neither NG tube nor PEG feeding greatly reduce the sensation of hunger,[50,51] although hunger is not common in advanced disease.

Persisting dysphagia: Other causes need to be considered such as neurological, dental and environmental problems, dyspepsia due to esophageal dysmotility, dyspepsia caused by gastro-esophageal reflux disease and causes of chronic dysphagia.[18]

Clinical decision	If YES ⇒ Action
1 Is there doubt about the need for hydration and/or feeding?	*See* also Nutrition and hydration problems (p. 119). • *If the prognosis is short (day by day deterioration):* hydrate and feed for comfort or pleasure (moistening the mouth may be all that is needed). • *If dysphagia is due to exhaustion caused by cancer:* only consider non-oral hydration or feeding if active cancer treatment is planned.
2 Is a complete obstruction present?	• *If the prognosis is short (day by day deterioration):* consider high dose dexamethasone 16 mg IV daily (or SC in divided doses) if short-term improvement would be helpful. • *If the prognosis is longer (week by week deterioration or slower):* start IV or SC hydration and refer for urgent endoscopy. If stenting is not possible, consider referral for a feeding gastrostomy.[43]
3 Is aspiration occurring?	NB: 40% of patients with aspiration due to oropharyngeal dysphagia can only be picked up on videofluoroscopy or fiberoptic endoscopy in the presence of a specialist speech therapist. • *If there are no symptoms:* no immediate action is needed, but non-oral feeding may need to be considered. • *If gastro-esophageal reflux is suspected: see* Dyspepsia (p. 85). • *If a tracheo-esophageal fistula is suspected:* refer to the gastroenterologists for a covered wall stent.[32] • *If symptoms are troublesome* (e.g. in 60% the symptoms are choking, coughing, copious secretions, or frequent chest infections): consider stenting for esophageal lesions or a feeding gastrostomy (NB: nasogastric tubes may worsen aspiration).
4 Is infection the cause?	• *Candidiasis: see* cd-3 in Oral problems (p. 127). • *Viral* (e.g. herpes zoster, herpes simplex, CMV): treat according to local antiviral policy.
5 Are drugs the cause?	See the notes opposite for examples of drugs that may cause dysphagia. • Reduce dose, change or stop drug.
6 Is pain present?	• *For oral pain: see* cd-4 in Oral problems (p. 127). • *For head or neck cancer pain with a rapid onset* (i.e. developing over a few hours): consider occult infection and start metronidazole and flucloxacillin. In the US, cephalexin (Keflex) is generally used. • *Soft tissue pain:* use WHO analgesic ladder (*see* Choosing an analgesic (p. 45)). • *Esophageal spasm:* consider nifedipine 5–15 mg q8h PO. • *Esophageal mucosal pain:* – treat any infection present (e.g. candidosis, herpes, CMV) – for protection, try sucralfate suspension 10 ml as required – if still troublesome, use a 'Pink Lady' (Lidocaine Viscous 2% 10 ml with Mylanta 20 ml).
7 Does the patient feel the problem is at the level of the chest or abdomen?	• *In cancer:* consider dexamethasone 6 mg once daily PO or SC to temporarily open the lumen. • Arrange barium swallow (but if aspiration is suspected, ask for a small volume gastrograffin swallow). If an abnormality is found on X-ray, refer to the gastroenterologists for endoscopy and manometry.
8 Does the patient feel the problem is at the level of the mouth or throat?	• Exclude oral problems: *see* Oral problems (p. 125). • Check the oral to pharyngeal transit time (OPT) (= time from the first movement of the tongue to the last movement of the larynx). If the OPT is greater than 1 sec, refer to a specialist speech and language therapist who can carry out a fuller assessment, and advise on management. OPT of > 10 secs means non-oral feeding is needed.
9 Is the problem persisting?	• Consider the following causes: *Dyspepsia:* For esophageal dysmotility with gastric stasis symptoms *see* cd-3 in Dyspepsia (p. 87). *Lambert–Eaton myesthenic syndrome* (LEMS) – seen in 3% of lung cancers:[52] *See* cd-5 in Fatigue, drowsiness, lethargy and weakness (p. 104). *Pseudobulbar palsy* (e.g. motor neurone disease): refer to ENT team for consideration of a cricopharyngeal myotomy.[53] *Stroke:* refer to or consult the stroke team.[54] *Dental problems* (e.g. missing teeth or dentures): refer to dentist.[55–57] *Environmental:* good food presentation, privacy and adequate staffing are necessary if dysphagic patients are to keep up their fluid and nutritional intake.[58]

Adapted from Regnard[59]
cd = clinical decision

References

B = book; C = comment; Ch = chapter; CS-n = case study-number of cases; CT-n = controlled trial-number of cases; E = editorial; GC = group consensus; I = interviews; LS = laboratory study; MC = multi-center; OS-n = open study-number of cases; R, n refs = review, number of references; RCT-n = randomized controlled trial-number of cases; RS-n = retrospective survey-number of cases; SA = systematic or meta analysis.

1 Twycross RG, Lack SA (1986) *Control of Alimentary Symptoms in Far Advanced Cancer.* Churchill Livingstone, Edinburgh. (Ch)

2 Sykes NP, Baines M, Carter RL (1988) Clinical and pathological study of dysphagia conservatively managed in patients with advanced malignant disease. *Lancet.* **2**: 726–8. (OS-33)

3 Saunders C, Walsh TD, Smith M (1981) *A Review of 100 Cases of Motor Neurone Disease in a Hospice.* Edward Arnold, London. (RS)

4 O'Brian T, Kelly M, Saunders C (1992) Motor neurone disease: a hospice perspective. *BMJ.* **304**: 471–3. (R)

5 Fuh JL, Lee RC, Lin CH, Wang SJ, Chiang JH, Liu HC (1997) Swallowing difficulty in Parkinson's disease. *Clinical Neurology and Neurosurgery.* **99**: 106–12. (CT-109)

6 Thomas FJ, Wiles CM (1999) Dysphagia and nutritional status in multiple sclerosis. *Journal of Neurology.* **246**: 677–82. (OS-78)

7 Wasson K, Tate H, Hayes C (2001) Food refusal and dysphagia in older people with dementia: ethical and practical issues. *International Journal of Palliative Nursing.* **7**(10): 465–71. (R)

8 Rademaker AW, Pauloski BR, Colangelo LA, Logemann JA (1998) Age and volume effects on liquid swallowing function in normal women. *Journal of Speech, Language and Hearing Research.* **41**: 275–84. (OS-167)

9 Kayser-Jones J, Pengilly K (1999) Dysphagia among nursing home residents. *Geriatric Nursing.* **20**: 77–82. (OS-82)

10 Regnard CFB (2003) Dysphagia, dyspepsia and hiccups. In: K Calman, D Doyle, GWC Hanks (eds) *Oxford Textbook of Palliative Medicine* (3e). Oxford University Press, Oxford. (Ch)

11 Logemann JA (1983) *Evaluation and Treatment of Swallowing Disorders.* College Hill Press, San Diego. (B)

12 Logemann JA (1985) Aspiration in head and neck surgical patients. *Annals of Otology, Rhinology and Laryngology.* **94**: 373–6.

13 Farell Z, O-Neill D (1999) Towards better screening and assessment of oropharyngeal swallow disorders in the general hospital. *Lancet.* **354**: 355–6.

14 Hughes TA, Wiles CM (1996) Palatal and pharyngeal reflexes in health and in motor neurone disease. *Journal of Neurology, Neurosurgery and Psychiatry.* **61**: 96–8. (CT-214)

15 Murray J (1999) *Manual of dysphagia assessment in adults.* Singular Publishing Group, San Diego.

16 Magnus V (2001) Dysphagia training for nurses in an acute hospital setting – a pragmatic approach. *International Journal of Language and Communication Disorders.* **36**(Suppl): 375–8. (R, 6 refs)

17 Poertner LC, Coleman RF (1998) Swallowing therapy in adults. *Otolaryngologic Clinics of North America.* **31**: 561–79. (R, 31 refs)

18 Leslie P, Carding PN, Wilson JA (2003) Investigation and management of chronic dysphagia. *BMJ.* **326**: 433–6. (R, 40 refs)

19 Langmore SE (2001) *Endoscopic Evaluation and Management of Swallowing Disorders.* Thieme, New York.

20 Bastian RW (1993) The videoendoscopic swallowing study: an alternative and partner to the videofluoroscopic swallowing study. *Dysphagia.* **8**: 359–67. (R)

21 Perie S, Laccourreye L, Flahault A, Hazebroucq V, Chaussade S, St Guily J (1998) Role of videoendoscopy in assessment of pharyngeal function in oropharyngeal dysphagia: comparison with videofluoroscopy and manometry. *Laryngoscope.* **108**: 1712–16. (OS-34)

22 Trier JS, Bjorkman DJ (1984) Esophageal, gastric and intestinal candidiasis. *American Journal of Medicine.* **77**: 39–43. (R)

23 Sheft DJ and Shrago G (1970) Esophageal moniliasis, the spectrum of the disease. *Journal of the American Medical Association.* **213**: 1859–62. (R)

24 Unsworth J (1994) *Coping with the Disability of Established Disease.* Chapman & Hall Medical, London. (B)

25 Hargrove R (1980) Feeding the severely dysphagic patient. *Journal of Neurosurgical Nursing.* **12**: 102–7. (R)

26 Carter RL, Pittam MR, Tanner NSB (1982) Pain and dysphagia in patients with squamous carcinomas of the head and neck: the role of perineural spread. *Journal of the Royal Society of Medicine.* **75**: 598–606. (OS)

27 Brewster AE, Davidson SE, Makin WP, Stout R, Burt PA (1995) Intraluminal brachytherapy using the high dose rate microselectron in the palliation of carcinoma of the oesophagus. *Clinical Oncology.* **7**: 102–5. (OS-197)

28 Aste H, Munizzi F, Martines H, Pugliese V (1985) Esophageal dilation in malignant dysphagia. *Cancer.* **11**: 2713–15. (OS-38)

29 Carter R, Smith JS, Anderson JR (1992) Laser recanalization *versus* endoscopic intubation in the palliation of malignant dysphagia: a randomized

prospective study. *British Journal of Surgery.* **79**: 1167–70. (RCT-40)

30 Lewis-Jones CM, Sturgess R, Ellershaw JE (1995) Laser therapy in the palliation of dysphagia in esophageal malignancy. *Palliative Medicine.* **9**: 327–30. (R, 15 refs)

31 Tietjen TG, Pankaj JP, Kalloo AN (1994) Management of malignant esophageal stricture with esophageal dilatation and esophageal stents. *The Esophagus.* **4**: 851–62. (R, 45 refs)

32 Mason R (1996) Palliation of malignant dysphagia: an alternative to surgery. *Annals of the Royal College of Surgeons of England.* **78**: 457–62. (RCT-474)

33 Sanyka C, Corr P, Haffejee A (1999) Palliative treatment of esophageal carcinoma – efficacy of plastic versus self-expandable stents. *South African Medical Journal.* **89**: 640–3. (RCT-40)

34 Birch JF, White SA, Berry DP, Veitch PS (1998) A cost-benefit comparison of self-expanding metal stents and Atkinson tubes for the palliation of obstructing esophageal tumours. *Diseases of the Esophagus.* **11**: 172–6. (RS-50)

35 Ell C, Hochberger J, May A, Fleig WE, Hahn EGH (1994) Coated and uncoated self-expanding metal stents for malignant stenosis in the upper GI tract: preliminary clinical experiences with wallstents. *American Journal of Gastroenterology.* **89**: 1496–500. (OS-23)

36 Tytgat GNJ, Tytgat S (1994) Esophageal endoprosthesis in malignant stricture. *Journal of Gastroenterology.* **29**: 80–4. (R, 23 refs)

37 Singhvi R, Abbasakoor F, Manson JM (2000) Insertion of self-expanding metal stents for malignant dysphagia: assessment of a simple endoscopic method. *Annals of the Royal College of Surgeons of England.* **82**: 243–8. (OS-50)

38 Scott AG, Austin HE (1994) Nasogastric feeding in the management of severe dysphagia in motor neurone disease. *Palliative Medicine.* **8**: 45–9. (CT-31)

39 Mitchell SL, Kiely DK, Lipsitz LA (1997) The risk factors and impact on survival of feeding tube placement in nursing home residents with severe cognitive impairment. *Archives of Internal Medicine.* **157**: 327–32. (OS-1386)

40 Finucane TE, Bynum JPW (1996) Use of tube feeding to prevent aspiration pneumonia. *The Lancet.* **348**: 1421–4. (R, 28 refs)

41 Park RHR, Allison MC, Lang J *et al.* (1992) Randomised comparison of percutaneous gastrostomy and nasogastric tube feeding in patients with persisting neurological dysphagia. *BMJ.* **304**: 1406–9. (RCT-40)

42 Dwolatzky T, Berezovski S, Friedmann R, Paz J, Clarfield AM, Stessman J, Hamburger R, Jaul E, Friedlander Y, Rosin A, Sonnenblick M (2001) A prospective comparison of the use of nasogastric and percutaneous endoscopic gastrostomy tubes for long-term enteral feeding in older people. *Clinical Nutrition.* **20**(6): 535–40. (CT-122)

43 Hull MA, Rawlings J, Murray J, Murray FE, Field J, McIntyre AS, Mahida YR, Hawkey CJ, Allison SP (1993) Audit of outcome of long-term enteral nutrition by percutaneous endoscopic gastrostomy. *Lancet.* **341**: 869–72. (OS-49)

44 Sanders DS, Carter MJ, D'Silva J, James G, Bolton RP, Bardhan KD (2000) Survival analysis in percutaneous endoscopic gastrostomy feeding: a worse outcome in patients with dementia. *American Journal of Gastroenterology.* **95**(6): 1472–5. (OS-361)

45 Ashby M, Game P, Devitt P, Britten-Jones R, Brooksbank M, Davy M and Keam E (1991) Percutaneous gastrostomy as a venting procedure in palliative care. *Palliative Medicine.* **5**: 147–50.

46 Boyd KJ, Beeken L (1994) Tube feeding in palliative care: benefits and problems. *Palliative Medicine.* **8**: 156–8. (CS-1)

47 Laing B, Smithers M, Harper J (1994) Percutaneous fluoroscopic gastrostomy: a safe option? *Medical Journal of Australia.* **161**: 308–10. (RS-70)

48 Myssiorek D, Siegel D, Vambutas A (1998) Fluoroscopically placed gastrostomies in the head and neck patient. *Laryngoscope.* **108**: 1557–60. (OS-35)

49 Keeley P (2002) Feeding tubes in palliative care. *European Journal of Palliative Care.* **9**(6): 229–31. (R, 19 refs)

50 Stratton RJ, Stubbs RJ, Elia M (1998) Interrelationship between circulating leptin concentrations, hunger, and energy intake in healthy subjects receiving tube feeding. *Jpen: Journal of Parenteral & Enteral Nutrition.* **22**(6): 335–9. (CT-6)

51 Stratton RJ, Elia M (1999) The effects of enteral tube feeding and parenteral nutrition on appetite sensations and food intake in health and disease. *Clinical Nutrition.* **18**(2): 63–70. (R, 79 refs)

52 Elrington G (1992) The Lambert-Eaton myesthenic syndromes. *Palliative Medicine.* **6**: 9–17. (R)

53 Leighton SEJ, Burton MJ, Lund WS, Cochrane GM (1994) Swallowing in motor neurone disease. *Journal of the Royal Society of Medicine.* **87**: 801–5. (OS-92)

54 Daniels SK, Foundas AL (1999) Lesion localization in acute stroke patients with risk of aspiration. *Journal of Neuroimaging.* **9**(2): 91–8. (OS-54)

55 Hildebrandt GH, Dominguez L, Schork MA, Loesche WJ (1997) Functional units, chewing, swallowing and food avoidance among the elderly. *Journal of Prosthetic Dentistry.* **77**: 588–95. (OS-602)

56 Caruso AJ, Max L (1997) Effects of aging on neuromotor processes of swallowing. *Seminars in Speech and Language.* **18**: 181–92. (R, 68 refs)

57 Aviv JE (1997) Effects of aging on sensitivity of the pharyngeal and supraglottic areas. *American Journal of Medicine.* **103**(5A): 74S–76S. (CT-80)

58 Kayser-Jones J, Schell ES, Porter C, Barbaccia JC, Shaw H (1999) Factors contributing to dehydration in nursing homes: inadequate staffing and lack of professional supervision. *Journal of the American Geriatrics Society.* **47**: 1187–94. (OS-40)

59 Regnard C (1995) Dysphagia. In: *Flow Diagrams in Advanced Cancer and Other Diseases.* Edward Arnold, London. pp. 19–21. (Ch)

Edema and lymphedema

Clinical decision and action checklist

1 Is the skin reddened?
2 Is pain present?
3 Is the prognosis short?
4 Is arterial insufficiency present?
5 Is there abnormal venous drainage?
6 Is this leg edema with a negative Stemmer's sign?
7 Is this midline edema?
8 Can hosiery be fitted?
9 Is bandaging indicated?

Key points

- Low compression stockings are often effective for simple edema.
- Lymphedema cannot be squeezed out or treated with diuretics.
- The cornerstones to lymphedema care are CETS (Containment, Exercise, Truncal massage and Skin care).
- Infection requires prompt treatment, usually with penicillin.

Introduction

Tissue swelling can be mild, but for some patients massive swelling of an arm, leg, head or genitalia can cause discomfort, pain, altered function, reduced mobility, altered body image, sexual difficulties, anxiety and depression.[1,2] The advice of a local lymphedema clinic is essential for moderate to severe lymphedema.

Causes and features

Edema is caused by an excess of tissue fluid due to inflammation, raised capillary pressure (e.g. ventricular failure, venous thrombosis, venous insufficiency, vena caval obstruction), fluid overload (heart failure, inappropriate ADH syndrome), reduced venous and lymphatic return (immobility, paralysis), or reduced protein (e.g. poor nutrition).[3,4] This edema pits easily, fluctuates with posture with a pale, cold skin (except in venous obstruction when it is dusky, warm and may ulcerate over time).

Lymphedema: Primary lymphedema is likely to be genetically inherited.[5–7] Secondary lymphedema in the Northern hemisphere is most commonly due to cancer or its treatment.[8] The skin pits with difficulty, has deep skin folds and changes very little with posture. The skin is pale and cool and in time will thicken – in the legs this makes it impossible to pick up a skin fold over the top of the second toe (Stemmer's sign). Eventually warty tags can develop that can leak and become infected. In post breast cancer arm lymphedema the hand may be spared.[9] *Acute inflammatory episodes* are common in lymphedema and cause a diffuse warmth, redness and pain in the affected area. They are usually caused by streptococcal infection and will often respond to amoxicillin.[10] *Classical cellulitis* due to staphylococcal infection is uncommon in lymphedema. *Lymphangiosarcoma* is a rare complication.[11–13]

Alarm signs: these are an indication for further investigation

Sign	Must exclude
Midline edema	Vena caval obstruction
Rapid onset (hours–days)	Venous thrombosis
Dusky or purplish skin colour	Venous thrombosis
Ulceration	Malignancy
Breathlessness	Heart failure
Distended veins	Venous incompetence

Principles of care: CETS

C Containment[14]

Support bandages (usually multilayer) provide a firm layer without compression against which muscle contraction stimulates lymph flow. These are used for treating severe lymphedema or limbs with shapes that could not fit hosiery.[15] Bandages should be applied by those experienced or trained in their use. They are worn continuously, and reapplied once a day – usually this is only necessary for 2 weeks.

Compression hosiery applies elastic pressure to compress the limb and is used in the initial stages of treatment. Support stockings for legs are available over the counter, but higher compression stockings (> 22 mmHg) and armsleeves (> 20 mmHg) require a prescription. Up to around 30 mmHg is suitable for mild edema, and from 30 mmHg up for lymphedema. Simple tubular supports or anti-embolism stockings should not be used since they are too weak and often roll down to produce a tourniquet effect. Made to measure hosiery is not used routinely but has a place in abnormally shaped limbs or for truncal edema. Garments can usually be taken off at night.

E Exercise[16]

Normal use should be encouraged, ideally while wearing containment or compression. Any exercises should be gentle, and are described in a patient information booklet.[17]

T Truncal massage

Massaging has been shown to stimulate lymph drainage.[18] The basic principle is to clear the way ahead, so that the massage always begins in a healthy quadrant of the trunk, before moving gradually to the affected side.[19,20] *Manual lymph drainage* is an intensive massage technique used for rapid reduction or for more severe cases.[21] *Simple lymphatic drainage* is a simplified form of massage that is done by patients.[17,22] Simple massage takes 15 mins twice daily and ends with a breathing exercise.[17]

S Skin care[23]

This is essential to prevent a portal of entry for infection. This includes protection (e.g. gloves while gardening), prompt cleansing of wounds, avoiding venepuncture or constriction on the affected side, and using moisturizers at night.[17,24,25] At the first suspicion of infection antibiotics should be started (*see* clinical decisions opposite).

Other treatments

The place of pneumatic compression is limited to simple edema.[26] Diuretics can help simple edema, but not lymphedema.[27] Corticosteroids have a role in lymphatic obstruction due to tumor, while benzo-pyrones and TENS have been shown to reduce primary lymphedema.[27,28] Surgery has little place in lymphedema management in Canada and the US. For fluid retention due to inappropriate ADH syndrome *see* cd-7e in Emergencies (p. 213).

Clinical decision	If YES ⇒ Action
1 **Is the skin reddened?** (may be a warm, reddened area of skin)	• If infection is suspected (limb temperature normal or raised, occasionally local pain): Start amoxicillin 500 mg q8h **or** erythromycin 500 mg q6h for 2 weeks (if the infection is severe use the IV route and add flucloxacillin (in the US, cephalexin (Keflex) is generally used) 500 mg q6h). Check for infection (e.g. between toes for fungal infection). Treat infection, e.g. antifungal for tinea pedis, potassium permanganate soaks for infected eczematous reactions. If the infection is worsening, add clindamycin 300–600 mg q6h. • If the redness persists: In legs, exclude lipodermatosclerosis (brown colour and wooden feel to lower legs): no antibiotics necessary. If low-grade infection is suspected: continue maintenance of penicillin V or clarithromycin 250 mg once daily for 3 months. Treating the lymphedema will reduce the risk of infection.
2 **Is pain present?**	• Treat infection (*see* cd-1 above). • Exclude myofascial pains (*see* cd-3c in Diagnosing and treating pain (p. 41)).
3 **Is the prognosis short?** (week by week deterioration or faster)	• Use simple lymphatic massage and low compression support hosiery (*see* notes). • Active or passive movement for stiff joints. • If tumor is compressing or blocking lymphatics: try dexamethasone PO 6 mg once daily.
4 **Could arterial insufficiency be present?** (pale or dusky skin, poor capillary filling)	• Measure systolic pressures in posterior tibial and both brachial arteries with Doppler. Calculate the ankle/brachial (AB) ratio (use higher of the two brachial pressures).[29] *If AB ratio > 1 without insufficiency signs or symptoms:* treat as normal. *If AB ratio between 0.8 and 1:* use only low-pressure support (< 30 mmHg). *If AB ratio < 0.8:* avoid all external pressure. Consider referral to the vascular surgeons.
5 **Is there abnormal venous drainage?** (may be a dusky or bluish skin colour)	• *Peripheral thrombosis:* anticoagulate and wait 8 weeks before applying compression. • *Vena caval obstruction: see* cd-9d in Emergencies (p. 214). Support bandaging or hosiery can be used, but avoid compression pumps. • *Venous incompetence* (causes distended veins that collapse on elevation): consider referral to vascular surgeons for investigation and treatment.
6 **Is this leg edema with a negative Stemmer's sign?** (i.e. able to pick up skin fold over second toe)	Consider other causes of edema (*see* notes opposite for examples). • Treat any causes of fluid retention. • *If the skin is in good condition:* use low-pressure support (10–30 mmHg). Consider the use of a pneumatic compression pump but keep pressures below 40 mmHg. • *If skin is in poor condition:* treat with massage and bandaging as in cd-8 and cd-9 below.

7 **Is this midline edema?** (i.e. limited to the trunk, head or genitalia)	• Exclude vena caval obstruction: *see* cd-9d in Emergencies (p. 214).
	• For lymphatic obstruction due to tumor: try dexamethasone PO 6 mg daily.
	• Massage the trunk at least three times daily, plus:
	   – for *head edema:* sleep propped upright with pillows.
	   – for *abdominal edema:* use a support garment if genitals are free of edema.
	   – for *edema of the genitals and perineum:* use made-to-measure compression pants, tights or scrotal support.

8 **Can hosiery be fitted?** (skin intact and limb is a normal shape)	• Fit compression hosiery: *see* notes opposite. • Encourage normal limb movements and advise on skin care. • Review regularly (initially monthly, then yearly). *NB: Do not use hosiery if the following are present:* severe ventricular failure, AB ratio less than 0.8, absent sensation, any microcirculatory problems (vasculitis, diabetes), or within 8 weeks of a venous thrombosis.
9 **Is bandaging indicated?** (damaged skin, hosiery has failed, or hosiery cannot be fitted)	• Refer to a lymphedema clinic that will advise on CETS (Containment, Exercise, Truncal massage, Skin care). *NB: Do not use bandages if the following are present:* severe ventricular failure, AB ratio less than 0.8, absent sensation, or within 8 weeks of a venous thrombosis.

Adapted from Badger and Regnard[24]
cd = clinical decision

References

B = book; C = comment; Ch = chapter; CS-n = case study-number of cases; CT-n = controlled trial-number of cases; E = editorial; GC = group consensus; I = interviews; LS = laboratory study; MC = multi-center; OS-n = open study-number of cases; R = review; RCT-n = randomized controlled trial-number of cases; RS-n = retrospective survey-number of cases; SA = systematic or meta analysis.

1 Twycross R (2000) Pain in lymphoedema. In: R Twycross, K Jenns, J Todd (eds) *Lymphoedema*. Radcliffe Medical Press, Oxford. pp. 69–88. (Ch)

2 Woods M (2000) Psychosocial aspects of lymphoedema. In: R Twycross, K Jenns, J Todd (eds) *Lymphoedema*. Radcliffe Medical Press, Oxford. pp. 89–96. (Ch)

3 Stanton A (2000) How does tissue swelling occur? The physiology and pathophysiology of interstitial fluid formation. In: R Twycross, K Jenns, J Todd (eds) *Lymphoedema*. Radcliffe Medical Press, Oxford. pp. 11–21. (Ch)

4 Topham EJ, Mortimer PS (2002) Chronic lower limb edema. *Clinical Medicine*. 2(1): 28–31. (R, 4 refs)

5 Brice G, Mansour S, Bell R, Collin JR, Child AH, Brady AF, Sarfarazi M, Burnand KG, Jeffery S, Mortimer P, Murday VA (2002) Analysis of the phenotypic abnormalities in lymphedema-distichiasis syndrome in 74 patients with FOXC2 mutations or linkage to 16q24. *Journal of Medical Genetics*. 39(7): 478–83. (OS-74)

6 Usta M, Dilek K, Ersoy A, Alper E, Ozbek S, Ozdemir B, Filiz G, Yavuz M, Gullulu M, Yurtkuran M (2002) A family with IgA nephropathy and hereditary lymphedema praecox. *Journal of Internal Medicine*. 251(5): 447–51. (CS-4)

7 Erickson RP, Dagenais SL, Caulder MS, Downs CA, Herman G, Jones MC, Kerstjens-Frederikse WS, Lidral AC, McDonald M, Nelson CC, Witte M, Glover TW (2001) Clinical heterogeneity in lymphedema-distichiasis with FOXC2 truncating mutations. *Journal of Medical Genetics*. 38(11): 761–6. (OS)

8 Keeley V (2000) Classification of lymphoedema. In: R Twycross, K Jenns, J Todd (eds) *Lymphoedema*. Radcliffe Medical Press, Oxford. pp. 22–43. (Ch)

9 Stanton AW, Svensson WE, Mellor RH, Peters AM, Levick JR, Mortimer PS (2001) Differences in lymph drainage between swollen and non-swollen regions in arms with breast-cancer-related lymphedema. *Clinical Science*. 101(2): 131–40. (OS)

10 Mortimer P (2000) Acute inflammatory episodes. In: R Twycross, K Jenns, J Todd (eds) *Lymphoedema*. Radcliffe Medical Press, Oxford. pp. 130–9. (Ch)

11 Mulvenna P, Gillham L, Regnard CFB (1995) Lymphangiosarcoma – experience in a lymphedema clinic. *Palliative Medicine*. 9: 55–9. (CS-3)

12 Hildebrandt G, Mittag M, Gutz U, Kunze ML, Haustein UF (2001) Cutaneous breast angiosarcoma after conserving treatment of breast cancer. *European Journal of Dermatology*. 11(6): 580–3.

13 Majeski J, Austin RM, Fitzgerald RH (2000) Cutaneous angiosarcoma in an irradiated breast after breast conservation surgery: association with chronic breast lymphedema. *Journal of Surgical Oncology*. 74(3): 208–12.

14 Todd J (2000) Containment in the management of lymphoedema. In: R Twycross, K Jenns, J Todd (eds) *Lymphoedema*. Radcliffe Medical Press, Oxford. pp. 165–202. (Ch)

15 Badger CM, Peacock JL, Mortimer PS (2000) A randomized, controlled, parallel-group clinical trial comparing multilayer bandaging followed by hosiery versus hosiery alone in the treatment of patients with lymphedema of the limb. *Cancer*. 88(12): 2832–7. (RCT-90)

16 Hughes K (2000) Exercise and lymphoedema. In: R Twycross, K Jenns, J Todd (eds) *Lymphoedema*. Radcliffe Medical Press, Oxford. pp. 140–64. (Ch)

17 Regnard C, Badger C, Mortimer P (2002) *Lymphoedema: advice on treatment* (3e). Beaconsfield Publishers, Beaconsfield. (B)

18 Mortimer PS, Simmonds R, Rezvani M, Robbins M, Hopewell JW, Ryan TJ (1990) The measurement of skin lymph flow by isotope clearance. Reliability, reproductibility, injection dynamics and the effect of massage. *Journal of Investigative Dermatology*. 95: 677–82. (OS)

19 Mortimer PS, Badger C, Hall JG (1997) Lymphoedema. In: D Doyle, GWC Hanks, N MacDonald (eds) *Oxford Textbook of Palliative Medicine* (2e). Oxford University Press, Oxford. pp. 657–65. (Ch)

20 Földi E, Földi M, Clodius L (1989) The lymphedema chaos: a lancet. *Annals of Plastic Surgery*. 22: 505–15. (R)

21 Leduc A, Leduc O (2000) Manual lymph drainage. In: R Twycross, K Jenns, J Todd (eds) *Lymphoedema*. Radcliffe Medical Press, Oxford. pp. 203–16. (Ch)

22 Bellhouse S (2000) Simple lymphatic drainage. In: R Twycross, K Jenns, J Todd (eds) *Lymphoedema*. Radcliffe Medical Press, Oxford. pp. 216–35. (Ch)

23 Linnitt N (2000) Skin management in lymphoedema. In: R Twycross, K Jenns, J Todd (eds) *Lymphoedema*. Radcliffe Medical Press, Oxford. pp. 118–29. (Ch)

24 Badger C, Regnard C (1995) Oedema. In: *Flow Diagrams in Advanced Cancer and Other Diseases*. Edward Arnold, London. pp. 60–3. (Ch)

25 Smith J (1998) The practice of venepuncture in lymphoedema. *European Journal of Cancer Care*. 7(2): 97–8. (OS)

26 Bray T, Barrett J (2000) Pneumatic compression therapy. In: R Twycross, K Jenns, J Todd (eds) *Lymphoedema*. Radcliffe Medical Press, Oxford. pp. 236–43. (Ch)

27 Twycross R (2000) Drug treatment for lymphoedema. In: R Twycross, K Jenns, J Todd (eds) *Lymphoedema*. Radcliffe Medical Press, Oxford. pp. 244–70. (Ch)

28 Waller A, Bercovitch M (2000) Novel treatments: transcutaneous electrical nerve stimulation. In: R Twycross, K Jenns, J Todd (eds) *Lymphoedema*. Radcliffe Medical Press, Oxford. pp. 271–84. (Ch)

29 Stubbing NJ, Bailey P, Poole M (1997) Protocol for accurate assessment of ABPI in patients with leg ulcers. *Journal of Wound Care*. 6: 417–18. (OS-250)

Fatigue, drowsiness, lethargy and weakness

Clinical decision and action checklist

1 Is the prognosis very short (day by day deterioration)?
2 Has the patient's alertness reduced?
3 Is the weakness, lethargy or fatigue all over the body?
4 Is postural dizziness present?
5 Is the weakness localized?
6 Is the problem persisting?

Key points

- Fatigue is the commonest symptom in advanced disease.[1,2]
- Drowsiness, tiredness, lethargy, fatigue and weakness have different meanings for different patients.
- Consider reversible causes, but fatigue, drowsiness, lethargy and weakness are also a part of the natural dying process.
- Dexamethasone is not first-line treatment.

Introduction

Fatigue is the commonest symptom in advanced disease and patients view it as more troublesome than pain, nausea or vomiting.[3–5]

The words patients use

Drowsiness, reduced alertness, tiredness, fatigue, lethargy and weakness have different meanings for different patients and their carers.[4] Many people use some of these terms interchangeably.

Drowsiness: Patients usually link this to a sensation of wanting to sleep.

Reduced alertness may be due to drowsiness but can be due to causes that make patients less aware of their surroundings.

Tiredness is often linked to mild energy loss, although some patients use the term to describe drowsiness.

Fatigue is perceived by patients as more severe and persistent than tiredness.[6] It is accompanied by lack of energy, exhaustion, restlessness, boredom, lack of interest in activities, weakness, dyspnea, pain, altered taste and itching.[6,7] It is different to drowsiness as it does not improve with sleep.[8] The concept of fatigue seems to be a combination of physical sensations (e.g. slowing up), affective sensations (e.g. irritability, loss of interest) and cognitive sensations (e.g. loss of concentration).[9]

Lethargy can be used to describe low mood or depression, but may also be used to describe fatigue or weakness.

Weakness is usually used to describe a loss of physical strength, but patients and carers can use the terms fatigue and weakness interchangeably.[10] Weakness can be generalized over the body or localized. When due to fatigue the weakness is usually perceived as generalized, but the profound muscle loss that can occur in cachexia will also cause a generalized muscle weakness. Localized weakness is invariably due to neurological lesions.

Causes

Dying

Patients deteriorating day by day because of their underlying disease often have fatigue, drowsiness, lethargy or weakness. This is a natural part of dying, but can be an important opportunity to open discussions with patient and family about what is happening.

Reduced alertness

Sudden onset: Reduced alertness occurring in minutes, hours or days needs urgent review. Possible causes are drugs (sedation, respiratory depression), severe infection, hypoglycemia, hypercalcemia, hemorrhage, hypoadrenalism (adrenal insufficiency or steroid withdrawal), hypercapnia (due to chronic respiratory failure), and metabolic crises (especially in children with congenital metabolic disease). Confusional states can be associated with reduced alertness.

Slow onset: Reduced alertness occurring over days or weeks may be due to drug accumulation (e.g. diazepam), hyperglycemia (raised glucose), organ failure (liver or kidney), hypercapnia or slow seizure activity.

Indolent: Tumor load may reduce alertness,[11] while some long-term conditions such as hypothyroidism may gradually reduce alertness.

Generalized fatigue and lethargy

The possibilities include infection, anemia, breathlessness, cachexia, depression, drugs, low sodium (IADH syndrome, chest infection, diuretics), hypercapnia, low potassium (diuretics, corticosteroids), high calcium (due to cancer), low magnesium (poor nutrition or chemotherapy), low oxygen levels (chest infection, pleural effusion, lung metastases), nutritional deficiency, psychological causes (severe anxiety, clinical depression) or recent surgery.[52] In advanced cancer fatigue may be linked to low cortisol levels.[53]

Localized weakness

Proximal weakness (weakness of muscles closest to the trunk) can be caused by corticosteroids, low potassium, thyroid abnormalities, motor neurone disease, osteomalacia or the Lambert–Eaton myesthenic syndrome (LEMS).

Localized muscle weakness: Possibilities are intracerebral causes (CVA, brain metastases), localized nerve compression or damage, spinal cord compression, or peripheral neuropathy.

Chemotherapy and radiotherapy

Both cause generalized fatigue. It peaks 1–2 weeks after chemotherapy,[12] and peaks at the end of a course of radiotherapy,[12,13] diminishing after 3 weeks.[14]

Drugs

These are a common cause of drowsiness and can be missed if they accumulate slowly (e.g. diazepam with a half-life of up to 200 hours) or their rate of elimination alters (e.g. the onset of renal failure in a patient on morphine).

Tumor load

Patients with cancer are more cognitively impaired than healthy controls.[11] Chemicals produced by

Clinical decision	If YES ⇒ Action
1 Is the prognosis very short? (e.g. day by day deterioration)	• Any fatigue, drowsiness, lethargy and weakness is likely to be a natural part of the dying process and no action will be needed.
2 Has the patient's alertness reduced? (i.e. a sensation of wanting to sleep or of reduced awareness)	**Sudden onset** (minutes to hours) **or fast onset** (days): • *Bleeding: see* Bleeding (p. 67). • *Drugs:* many drugs may cause this, not just opioids. If the sedation is unwanted by the patient, reduce or change the drug. If the sedation was rapid, consider partial reversal if an antagonist is available, e.g. naloxone for opioids (for correct procedure *see* cd-3b in Emergencies (p. 205)) or flumazanil for benzodiazepines. Antagonists are short-acting and often need repeated doses or infusions. • *Epilepsy:* minor or major seizures. If the cause is known, start sodium valproate 300 mg q12h (for children 20 mg/kg in divided doses) and titrate to control the symptoms. • *Hypercalcemia: see* cd-7b in Emergencies (p. 211). • *Hypercapnia:* if due to inappropriately high inhaled oxygen concentration then reduce oxygen to 24%. • *Hypoadrenalism* (adrenal insufficiency, steroid withdrawal): hydrocortisone 100 mg IV, then continue with hydrocortisone (20 mg on waking, 10 mg at 4 pm) and fludrocortisone (100–200 microgram on waking). • *Hypoglycemia* (e.g. treated diabetic on little or no diet): *see* cd-7d in Emergencies (p. 213). • *Raised intracranial pressure due to tumor:* try high dose dexamethasone (16 mg daily) and refer for cranial irradiation. Consider an MRI scan to exclude hydrocephalus. • *Respiratory depression or sedation: see* cd-2 and cd-3 in Emergencies (pp. 205–7). • *Septicemia:* take blood cultures and start IV antibiotics according to local policies. **Slow onset** (days to weeks): • *Confusional state: see* Confusional states (delirium and dementia) (p. 171). • *Drug accumulation* (e.g. diazepam, amitriptyline): tolerance to the sedative effect may occur, but otherwise reduce the daily dose or change the drug. • *Hyperglycemia* (e.g. corticosteroids): *see* cd-7c in Emergencies (p. 211). • *Organ failure* (renal, hepatic): treat if possible. • *Poor quality sleep:* treat the cause, consider temazepam 10–40 mg or similar at night. • *Tumor load:* (*see* notes opposite): low dose dexamethasone PO (2–4 mg once daily). • *Hypercapnia:* start 24% oxygen and refer to respiratory physician for advice, especially if non-invasive ventilation is an option (*see* Respiratory problems (p. 131)). • *Subclinical seizure activity:* check for exacerbating factors and review anticonvulsants. **Indolent** (months or longer): • *Hypothyroidism/hypoadrenalism:* evaluate and treat as appropriate. • *Loss of sleep:* exclude anxiety or depression (*see* Anxiety (p. 165) and Withdrawal and depression (p. 177)). • *Tumor load:* low dose dexamethasone PO/SC 2–4 mg once daily.
3 Is the weakness, lethargy or fatigue all over the body? (i.e. a sensation of getting persistently tired without an obvious cause and which does not improve after sleep)	*Screening question for fatigue:* 'Do you get tired for no reason for a good part of the time?'[9] • *Anemia:* transfuse if the hemoglobin <10 g/dl (full benefit takes 72 hours). If transfusion is not possible, consider erythropoietin 10 000 IU SC 3 times weekly or 40 000 IU SC weekly.[15] • *Cardiac failure:* ACE inhibitor (consider giving first dose as an inpatient). • *Chronic infection despite antimicrobials* (e.g. persistent mycobacteria in AIDS): consider low dose corticosteroids in addition to antimicrobials. • *Depression or anxiety: see* Anxiety (p. 165) and Withdrawal and depression (p. 177). • *Drugs* (many drugs – check current monograph): reduce the dose or change the drug. • *Electrolyte abnormalities:* low Na^+ (IADH syndrome, hypoadrenalism, chest infection, diuretics), low K^+ (diuretics, corticosteroids, vomiting) (treat as appropriate) or low Mg^{++}.[16] • *Infection* (viral, bacterial): treat with appropriate antimicrobial. • *Nutritional deficiency* (iron, magnesium, vitamin B, D): there is no evidence that one nutritional supplement is better than any other, so consult a dietician.[17] • *Radiotherapy or chemotherapy:* exclude bone marrow suppression. • *Recent surgery:* ensure adequate nutrition. • *Severe dyspnea: see* Respiratory problems (p. 131). • *Tumor load* (*see* notes opposite): dexamethasone PO/SC 2–4 mg once daily.

Table continued overleaf

4	**Is postural dizziness present?** (i.e. feeling faint on standing)	• Consider causes of reduced blood pressure: *Autonomic failure* (*see* opposite for the symptoms): causes include chronic alcohol abuse, diabetes, cancer (paraneoplastic effect), long bed-rest, Lambert–Eaton myesthenic syndrome (*see* cd-5 below), multiple system atrophy, Parkinson's disease and spinal cord compression. *Cardiopulmonary:* arrhythmia, cardiac tamponade, myocardial infarction, pulmonary embolus and transient ischemic attack. *Drugs:* ACE-inhibitors, amitriptyline, beta-blockers, chemotherapy (cisplatinum, vincrisitine), diuretics and methotrimeprazine. *Endocrine:* adrenocortical insufficiency (primary or due to steroid withdrawal). *Intravascular volume loss:* dehydration, blood loss. *Procedures:* intraspinal local anesthetic, rapid paracentesis in cirrhosis. • Treat the primary cause if possible. • Consider symptomatic treatment that may give short-term benefit: mild compression stockings (20–30 mmHg) and fludrocortisone 50–100 microgram q12h. If the problem persists, consider the α_1 adrenergic agonist midodrine (Amatine) 2.5 mg q8h and titrated up to 10 mg q8h.[42–44]
5	**Is the weakness localized?** (i.e. a local loss of strength)	*With any proximal motor weakness* consider the following as possible causes: • *Corticosteroids:* reduce the dose and consider stopping (the weakness may persist despite stopping). • *Hypokalemia:*[45] correct the cause if possible (e.g. loop diuretic and corticosteroid-induced loss). Increase dietary potassium (fruit drinks, bananas). Correct with IV potassium only if the condition is life-threatening. • *Hypothyroidism or hyperthyroidism:* check thyroid function and treat. • *Lambert–Eaton myesthenic syndrome (LEMS):* see notes opposite for symptoms. If LEMS is suspected, refer to a neurologist for diagnosis (voltage gated calcium channel antibodies) and treatment (3,4-Diaminopyridine, intravenous immunoglobulin, plasma exchange or prednisolone 1.5 mg/kg administered on alternate days).[46,47] • *Motor neurone disease:* involve the occupational therapist. • *Osteomalacia:* confirm the diagnosis (X-rays, alkaline phosphatase), find the cause (consider anticonvulsants, malabsorption) and treat. • *Polymyositis:*[48] check creatinine kinase serum levels. Prednisolone may help (or methylprednisolone in children).[49] Muscle strengthening exercises can be helpful.[50] Consider referral to rheumatologists for advice on further treatment. *With any localized motor weakness* consider: • *Cord compression* – *see* cd-9a in Emergencies (p. 213). • *Intracerebral cause* (cerebrovascular accident, metastases) – if metastases are present, consider high dose dexamethasone (16 mg daily) and refer for cranial irradiation. • *Nerve compression:* dexamethasone PO/SC 6 mg daily. • *Neuropathy:* assess the cause and treat if appropriate (e.g. B_{12} deficiency).
6	**Is the problem persisting?**	• *Treat coexisting physical symptoms* (e.g. pain, dyspnea, nausea, vomiting). • *Exclude an anxiety state or depression:* see Anxiety (p. 165) and Withdrawal and depression (p. 177). • Modify activities:[51] – use rest periods between activities – re-time activities to a time of day when energy is highest – plan regular, gentle exercise – arrange help for low-priority activities – review sleep behaviors and sleep environment. • Ensure food presentation encourages sufficient nutritional intake (*see* Nutrition and hydration problems (p. 119)). • *If a rapid response would help* (e.g. for a special event): try methylphenidate 5 mg in the morning, increasing if necessary to 10–15 mg. A second dose can be given, but no later than lunchtime to avoid insomnia. Higher doses of methylphenidate are sometimes used in the US, often up to 30 mg PO bid.[54] A recent review of the palliative use of methylphenidate in cancer patients recommended doses of up to 1 mg/kg/day.[55] • Modafinil (Provigil) is a stimulant approved in the US for narcolepsy, obstructive sleep apnea and shift work sleep disorder. It can help diminish fatigue, lethargy, sedation in palliative patients. It does not cause tachycardia. Starting doses are usually 100 mg PO qid; may increase up to 200 mg PO qid.[56]

Adapted from Regnard and Mannix[18]
cd = clinical decision

tumors (e.g. tumor necrosis factor) may partly mediate fatigue.[19] Corticosteroids can suppress their production[20] and produce a temporary but worthwhile increase in well-being.[21]

Chronic infection

End-stage AIDS patients may have several organisms or foci of persistent infection (e.g. candida, mycobacteria). Corticosteroids are sometimes used with long-term antimicrobials to suppress the symptoms of infection.[22,23]

Lambert–Eaton myesthenic syndrome (LEMS)

This is an autoimmune disease that causes a proximal weakness (legs worse than arms) that improves after sustained contraction or with cold.[24,25] Patients can have a waddling type of gait when walking. Other symptoms are dysphagia and features of autonomic failure (see below).

Autonomic failure

This has several different causes and is common in advanced disease.[26–28] Symptoms include hypotension (with dizziness on standing or associated with eating), fatigue, syncope, inability to sweat, impotence, bladder symptoms (including incontinence) and gastric stasis.

Disturbed sleep

Sleep may be disturbed by symptoms, anxiety or depression. Disturbed sleep is associated with fatigue.[8]

Treatment

Finding the cause

A sensible initial screen is as follows:

1 If the reduced alertness is sudden, check for hypoxia, hypercapnia, bleeding, cardiac arrhythmia and respiratory depression.
2 Enquire about:
   • sleep patterns and mood
   • recent treatment (radiotherapy, chemotherapy, surgery, drugs started or withdrawn).
3 Examine for:
   • chest or urinary infection
   • local weakness
   • postural hypotension.
4 Take blood for hemoglobin, calcium, liver function, renal function and electrolytes.

Treating the cause

This is possible in a wide range of conditions. In a patient with advanced disease such as cancer or AIDS, it is important not to assume that the fatigue is due to the primary condition. Such patients can develop unrelated treatable conditions, or a treatable condition indirectly caused by the primary condition (e.g. recurrent infection), or an adverse effect of treatment (e.g. corticosteroid-induced diabetes).

Depression and anxiety states

Depression is strongly associated with lethargy and fatigue, while an anxiety state can cause fatigue through constant physical arousal.[29] Both will cause sleep disturbances.

Nutrition

This is important in the earlier stages of any disease, and it is important to ensure that good food presentation encourages sufficient nutritional intake. In the late stages of disease, nutrition becomes more important for pleasure and comfort. See Nutrition and hydration problems (p. 119).

Drugs

In fatigue related to advanced disease without a clear cause, there is little evidence that drugs have any long-term benefit.[30] Dexamethasone 2–4 mg daily can give a short-term improvement for up to 4 weeks.

Persisting problems

It is common for fatigue, drowsiness, lethargy or weakness to persist as part of the underlying condition.

Modifying activities that cause fatigue: Although counter-intuitive, graded and planned aerobic exercise can help patients cope more effectively with fatigue.[31–35] Activities are changed by using rest periods between activities, re-timing activities to a time of day when energy is highest, planning regular gentle exercise, arranging help for low-priority activities, and reviewing sleep behaviours and sleep environment.[36]

Psychostimulants such as methylphenidate are occasionally used to achieve a rapid effect when this is needed for a special event, but anxiety, anorexia and insomnia can occur.[37–41]

Helping the patient and family adjust: If the problems cannot be changed by treatment or altered activities, then much can be done to enable the patient, partner and family to re-adjust to the change through support, altering the environment and therapy such as cognitive behavioural therapy.

References

B = book; C = comment; Ch = chapter; CS-n = case study-number of cases; CT-n = controlled trial-number of cases; E = editorial; GC = group consensus; I = interviews; LS = laboratory study; MC = multi-center; OS-n = open study-number of cases; Q = questionnaire; R = review; RCT-n = randomized controlled trial-number of cases; RS-n = retrospective survey-number of cases; SA = systematic or meta analysis.

1 Donnelly S, Walsh D (1995) The symptoms of advanced cancer. *Seminars in Oncology.* **22**: 67–72. (OS-1000)

2 Winningham ML, Nail LM, Burke MB, Brophy L, Cimprich B, Jones LS, Pickard-Holley S, Rhodes V, St Pierre B, Beck S (1994) Fatigue and the cancer experience: the state of the knowledge. *Oncology Nursing Forum.* **21**(1): 23–36. (R, 45 refs)

3 Stone P, Richardson A, Ream E, Smith AG, Kerr DJ, Kearney N (2000) Cancer-related fatigue: inevitable, unimportant and untreatable? Results of a multi-centre patient survey. Cancer Fatigue Forum. *Annals of Oncology.* **11**(8): 971–5. (MC, Q-576)

4 Håvard Loge J (2003) Unpacking fatigue. *European Journal of Palliative Care.* **10**(2)Suppl: 14–20. (R, 88 refs)

5 Curt GA (2001) Fatigue in cancer. *BMJ.* **322**: 1560. (E, 8 refs)

6 Richardson A, Ream E (1996) The experience of fatigue and other symptoms in patients receiving chemotherapy. *European Journal of Cancer Care.* **5**: 24–30. (OS-100)

7 Gall H (1996) The basis of fatigue: where does it come from? *European Journal of Cancer Care.* **5**: 31–4. (R, 24 refs)

8 Ancoli-Israel S, Moore PJ, Jones V (2001) The relationship between fatigue and sleep in cancer patients: a review. *European Journal of Cancer Care.* **10**(4): 245–55. (R, 66 refs)

9 Kirsh KL, Passik S, Holtsclaw E, Donaghy K, Theobald D (2001) I get tired for no reason: a single item screening for cancer-related fatigue. *Journal of Pain and Symptom Management.* **22**(5): 931–7. (OS-52)

10 Richardson A (1995) Fatigue in cancer patients: a review of the literature. *European Journal of Cancer Care.* **4**: 20–32. (R, 93 refs)

11 Clemons M, Regnard C, Appleton T (1996) Alertness, cognition and morphine in patients with advanced cancer. *Cancer Treatment Reviews.* **22**: 451–68. (OS)

12 Irvine D, Vincent L, Graydon JE, Bubela N, Thompson L (1994) The prevalence and correlates of fatigue in patients receiving treatment with chemotherapy and radiotherapy: a comparison with the fatigue experienced by healthy individuals. *Cancer Nursing.* **17**: 367–78. (CT-101)

13 Hickok JT, Morrow GR, McDonald S, Bellg AJ (1996) Frequency and correlates of fatigue in lung cancer patients receiving radiation therapy: implications for management. *Journal of Pain and Symptom Management.* **11**: 370–7. (RS-50)

14 Greenberg DB, Sawicka J, Eisenthal S *et al.* (1992) Fatigue syndromes due to localised radiation. *Journal of Pain and Symptom Management.* **7**: 38–45.

15 Yount S, Lai JS, Cella D (2002) Methods and progress in assessing the quality of life effects of supportive care with erythropoietin therapy. *Current Opinion in Hematology.* **9**(3): 234–40. (R, 51 refs)

16 Brogan G, Exton L, Kurowska A, Tookman A (2000) The importance of low magnesium levels in palliative care: two case reports. *Palliative Medicine.* **14**: 59–61. (CS-2)

17 Stratton RJ, Elia M (2000) Are oral nutritional supplements of benefit to patients in the community? Findings from a systematic review. *Current Opinion in Clinical Nutrition & Metabolic Care.* **3**(4): 311–15. (SA)

18 Regnard C, Mannix K (1995) Weakness and fatigue. In: *Flow Diagrams in Advanced Cancer and Other Diseases.* Edward Arnold, London. pp. 64–7. (Ch)

19 Cicoira M, Bolger AP, Doehner W, Rauchhaus M, Davos C, Sharma R, Al-Nasser FO, Coats AJ, Anker SD (2001) High tumour necrosis factor-alpha levels are associated with exercise intolerance and neurohormonal activation in chronic heart failure patients. *Cytokine.* **5**(2): 80–6. (OS)

20 Chikanza IC (2002) Mechanisms of corticosteroid resistance in rheumatoid arthritis: a putative role for the corticosteroid receptor beta isoform. *Annals of the New York Academy of Sciences.* **966**: 39–48. (R, 60 refs)

21 Mercadante S, Fulfaro F, Casuccio A (2001) The use of corticosteroids in home palliative care. *Supportive Care in Cancer.* **9**(5): 386–9. (OS-376)

22 Castro M (1998) Treatment and prophylaxis of *Pneumocystis carinii* pneumonia. *Seminars in Respiratory Infections.* **13**(4): 296–303. (R, 65 refs)

23 Dorman SE, Heller HM, Basgoz NO, Sax PE (1998) Adjunctive corticosteroid therapy for patients whose treatment for disseminated Mycobacterium avium complex infection has failed. *Clinical Infectious Diseases.* **26**(3): 682–6. (OS-12)

24 Maddison P, Lang B, Mills K, Newsom-Davis J

(2001) Long term outcome in Lambert-Eaton myaesthenic syndrome without lung cancer. *Journal of Neurology, Neurosurgery & Psychiatry.* **70**(2): 212–17. (RS-47)

25 Elrington G (1992) The Lambert-Eaton myaesthenic syndromes. *Palliative Medicine.* **6**: 9–17. (R)

26 Goldstein DS, Holmes CS, Dendi R, Bruce SR, Li ST (2002) Orthostatic hypotension from sympathetic denervation in Parkinson's disease. *Neurology.* **58**(8): 1247–55. (CT-57)

27 Bruera E (1989) Autonomic failure in patients with advanced cancer. *Journal of Pain and Symptom Management.* **4**(3): 163–6. (CS)

28 Bruera E, Chadwick S, Fox R, Hanson J, MacDonald N (1986) Study of cardiovascular autonomic insufficiency in advanced cancer patients. *Cancer Treatment Reports.* **70**(12): 1383–7. (CT-63)

29 Ko DT, Hebert PR, Coffey CS, Sedrakyan A, Curtis JP, Krumholz HM (2002) Beta-blocker therapy and symptoms of depression, fatigue, and sexual dysfunction. *JAMA.* **288**(3): 351–7. (R, 46 refs)

30 Stone P (2002) The measurement, causes and effective management of cancer-related fatigue. *International Journal of Palliative Nursing.* **8**(3): 120–8. (R, 77 refs)

31 Nail LM (2002) Fatigue in patients with cancer. *Oncology Nursing Forum.* **29**(3): 537–46. (R, 92 refs)

32 Mock V, Dow KH, Meares CJ, Grimm PM, Dienemann JA, Haisfield-Wolfe ME, Quitasol W, Mitchell S, Chakravarthy A, Gage I (1997) Effects of exercise on fatigue, physical functioning, and emotional distress during radiation therapy for breast cancer. *Oncology Nursing Forum.* **24** (6): 991–1000. (CT-46)

33 MacVicar MG, Winningham ML, Nickel JL (1989) Effects of aerobic interval training on cancer patients' functional capacity. *Nursing Research.* **38**(6): 348–51. (RCT-50)

34 Schwartz AL, Mori M, Gao R, Nail LM, King ME (2001) Exercise reduces daily fatigue in women with breast cancer receiving chemotherapy. *Medicine & Science in Sports & Exercise.* **33**(5): 718–23. (OS-61)

35 Porock D, Kristjanson LJ, Tinelly K, Duke T, Blight J (2000) An exercise intervention for advanced cancer patients experiencing fatigue: a pilot study. *Journal of Palliative Care.* **16**(3): 30–6. (OS-11)

36 Johnston MP, Coward DD (2001) Cancer-related fatigue: nursing assessment and management: increasing awareness of the effect of cancer-related fatigue. *AJN, American Journal of Nursing.* **Suppl**: 19–22. (R, 24 refs)

37 Homsi J, Walsh D, Nelson K (2000) Psychostimulants in supportive care. *Supportive Care in Cancer.* **8**: 385–97.

38 Sugawara Y, Akechi T, Shima Y, Okuyama T,

Akizuki N, Nakano T, Uchitomi Y (2002) Efficacy of methylphenidate for fatigue in advanced cancer patients: a preliminary study. *Palliative Medicine.* **16**: 261–3. (OS-14)

39 Breitbart W, Rosenfeld B, Kaim M, Funesti-Esch J (2001) A randomized, double-blind, placebo-controlled trial of psychostimulants for the treatment of fatigue in ambulatory patients with human immunodeficiency virus disease. *Archives of Internal Medicine.* **161**(3): 411–20. (RCT-144)

40 Dein S, George R (2002) A place for psychostimulants in palliative care? *Journal of Palliative Care.* **18**(3): 196–9. (R, 27 refs).

41 Wilwerding MB, Loprinzi CL, Mailliard JA, O'Fallon JR, Miser AW, van Haelst C, Barton DL, Foley JF, Athmann LM (1995) A randomized, crossover evaluation of methylphenidate in cancer patients receiving strong narcotics. *Supportive Care in Cancer.* **3**(2): 135–8. (RCT)

42 Perez-Lugones A, Schweikert R, Pavia S, Sra J, Akhtar M, Jaeger F, Tomassoni GF, Saliba W, Leonelli FM, Bash D, Beheiry S, Shewchik J, Tchou PJ, Natale A (2001) Usefulness of midodrine in patients with severely symptomatic neurocardiogenic syncope: a randomized control study. *Journal of Cardiovascular Electrophysiology.* **12**(8): 935–8. (RCT-61)

43 Wright RA, Kaufmann HC, Perera R, Opfer-Gehrking TL, McElligott MA, Sheng KN, Low PA (1998) A double-blind, dose-response study of midodrine in neurogenic orthostatic hypotension. *Neurology.* **51**(1): 120–4. (CT-25)

44 Kaufmann H, Saadia D, Voustianiouk A (2002) Midodrine in neurally mediated syncope: a double-blind, randomized, crossover study. *Annals of Neurology.* **52**(3): 342–5. (RCT-12)

45 Rastergar A, Soleimani M (2001) Hypokalemia and hyperkalemia. *Postgraduate Medical Journal.* **77**(914): 759–64. (R, 21 refs)

46 Bain PG, Britton TC, Jenkins JH, Thompson PD, Rothwell JC, Thomas PK, Brooks DJ, Marsden CD (1996) Effects of intravenous immunoglobulin on muscle weakness and calcium channel auto-antibodies in the Lambert-Eaton myesthenic syndrome. *Neurology.* **47**: 678–83. (RCT-9)

47 Newsom-Davis J (2001) Lambert-Eaton Myasthenic Syndrome. *Current Treatment Options in Neurology.* **3**(2): 127–31. (R)

48 Hilton-Jones D (2001) Inflammatory muscle diseases. *Current Opinion in Neurology.* **14**(5): 591–6. (R, 36 refs)

49 Reed AM (2001) Myositis in children. *Current Opinion in Rheumatology.* **13**(5): 428–33. (R, 60 refs)

50 Lawson Mahowald M (2001) The benefits and limitations of a physical training program in patients with inflammatory myositis. *Current Rheumatology Reports.* **3**(4): 317–24. (R, 50 refs)

51 Yarbro CH (1996) Interventions for fatigue. *European Journal of Cancer Care.* **5**: 35–8. (R, 15 refs)

52 Hwang SS, Chang VT, Rue M, Kasimis B (2003) Multidimensional independent predictors of cancer-related fatigue. *Journal of Pain and Symptom Management.* **26**: 604–14.

53 Lundström S, Fürst CJ (2003) Symptoms in advanced cancer: relationship to endogenous cortisol levels. *Palliative Medicine.* **17**: 503–8. (OS-23)

54 Breitbart W, Rosenfeld B, Kaim M, Funesti-Esch J (2001) A randomized, double blind, placebo controlled trial of psychostimulants for the treatment of fatigue in ambulatory patients with human immunodeficiency virus disease. *Archives of Internal Medicine.* **12**: 411–20.

55 Rozans M, Dreischbach A, Lertora JJ, Kahn MJ (2002) Palliative use of methylphenidate in patients with cancer: a review. *Journal of Clinical Oncology.* **1**: 335–9.

56 Miller MM, Harsh J, Hirshkowitz M *et al.* (2000) Long-term efficacy and safety of modafinil for the treatment of daytime sleepiness associated with narcolepsy. *Sleep Medicine.* **1**: 231–43.

Malignant ulcers and fistulae

Clinical decision and action checklist

1 Can the local malignancy be treated?
2 Is the wound bleeding?
3 Is the wound causing psychosocial effects?
4 Is the odor troublesome?
5 Is the exudate or discharge troublesome?
6 Is the wound painful?
7 Is the wound itchy?

Key points

- Each malignant ulcer requires individual assessment.
- Healing may be possible, but comfort is the primary aim.
- Malignant ulcers can have a major impact on body image and the ability to cope.

Introduction

A malignant ulcer can cause disfigurement, altered function, discharge and odor. Its effects may be very visible, as in a head and neck cancer, obvious when it causes odor or discharge, or hidden with psychological symptoms. The psychosocial effects of such wounds are at least as great as their physical effects.[1–3] They can have a profound effect on how patients perceive themselves, causing anxiety, depression and social isolation. Sexuality can be seriously affected, but professionals do not often elicit this.[4] Social relationships can suffer so that reduced contact worsens the low self-esteem. The fact that many malignant ulcers cannot be removed or healed adds to the despair.

Managing the effects of an ulcer

Treating a malignancy

If the area has not previously received a maximum radiation dose then more radiotherapy may be possible. Chemotherapy or hormone therapy can be useful in sensitive tumors.[5,6] Surgery has a limited role for localized lesions.[7]

Odor

Treating the odor: Malignant ulcers are colonized by anaerobic bacteria.[8] Systemic metronidazole can be effective and reactions with alcohol are rare.[9] Topical 0.8% metronidazole gel can help,[10,11] but is expensive, may make a wound too wet, and can be ineffective on large wounds.[12] It is useful when systemic metronidazole is not tolerated or is ineffective. Attempts to mask a smell with perfumes soon fail as the patient associates the new odor with the unpleasant one.

Isolating the odor may be possible with specific dressings.[12,13] Charcoal dressings are only effective for a few hours. Colostomy bags can be used for fistulae. Dressings that absorb exudate can help, such as hydrogels and polyurethane foam dressings.[14] Food wrap can be placed over dressings to provide an additional barrier to odor.

Managing exudate and discharge

This may be exudate from a wound, discharge caused by infection, or leakage from a fistula.

Wound exudate: Unlike acute wounds that need to be kept moist, exudate from chronic wounds needs to be removed.[15] The key is well-fitting dressings that can absorb fluid and allow its evaporation.[16] The ability of alginates to absorb fluid is limited, but polyurethane foam dressings (e.g. Lyofoam Extra, Allevyn) allow evaporation and the removal of more fluid.[17] If an exudate is severe, plastic food wrap can be used over

dressings to protect clothes. Use barrier preparations to protect the surrounding skin (*see* table).

Vaginal and rectal discharges: These can be due to local ulcerating carcinomas. They may become less offensive with antiseptic douches/lavage, e.g. povidone-iodine. Corticosteroids (rectally or vaginally) will reduce local inflammation and pain. Regularly changed tampons can control vaginal discharges if there is no discomfort on insertion. Perineal and perianal skin often needs protection from the continual moisture with barrier preparations (*see* table).

Fistulae: Some malignant ulcers are associated with an enterocutaneous fistula (an abnormal link between a hollow organ and the skin). They occur most commonly with Crohn's disease, but also occur with abdominal cancers.[18] Colostomy bags can be fitted over the fistula if the surrounding area is flat – the pediatric types are easier to fit because of a softer flange. If the area around the wound is uneven, the irregularities can be made smooth with fillers such as Stomahesive or Adapt paste, allowed to dry and covered with a hydrocolloid dressing (e.g. Comfeel, Duoderm, Signal).[19]

Fistulae with the oral cavity: It may be worthwhile considering a latex mould,[20] or self-polymerizing silicone materials such as those used in dentistry. Silicone materials are more versatile and longer lasting and a local dentist or dental school would advise.[21]

Rectovaginal fistulae may cause stool to pass vaginally. A firmer stool is less likely to enter the fistula, and reducing the laxative or giving a low dose of loperamide will produce a firmer stool.

Octreotide is helpful in patients with postoperative small bowel fistulae,[22–25] and may be useful in other fistulae. There may be a delay of 2–3 days before the output reduces.

Clinical decision	If YES ⇒ Action
1 Can the local malignancy be treated?	• Refer to an oncologist for advice. *If the tumor is radiosensitive and further local radiation is possible:* discuss the option of radiotherapy with the patient. Do not use metal-containing topical agents (e.g. silver sulfadiazine (Flamazine, Silvadene, Dermazin)) during treatment. *If the tumor is chemosensitive:* discuss the option of chemotherapy with the patient. • Consider surgery if the tumor is localized, the patient agrees, and the patient is fit for surgery.
2 Is the wound bleeding?	• *see* cd-4 in Bleeding (p. 69).
3 Is the wound causing psychosocial effects?	• Improve the cosmetic appearance if possible: treat any odor (*see* cd-4 below), fill the defect with dressings. Consider using self-polymerizing silicone materials (the nearest dental school can advise). • Elicit problems: e.g. adjustment issues, social isolation, relationships, sexual issues. • Enable the patient to cope with altered image through active listening. Consider referral for cognitive behavioural therapy. • *See* also Anger (p. 161), Anxiety (p. 165) and Withdrawal and depression (p. 177).
4 Is the odor troublesome?	• Start metronidazole 250 mg PO tid for 5–7 days, then continue with 500 mg PO qd. If adverse effects are a problem, use topical metronidazole gel. • Use hydrogels (e.g. Intrasite, Duoderm Gel) or polyurethane foam dressings (e.g. Allevyn, Lyofoam Extra) to help clear debris. • Charcoal dressings may help for a few hours. Avoid perfumes. • If the odor persists, cover the dressings with a layer of food wrap to trap odor.
5 Is the exudate or discharge troublesome?	• *If the exudate or discharge is from the wound:* Absorb the discharge: use conformable polyurethane foam dressing (e.g. Lyofoam Extra, Allevyn). If exudate soaks through, cover dressing with food wrap to protect the patient's clothes. Protect the surrounding skin: use a barrier preparation (e.g. zinc ointments or simethicone cream) or a barrier application[12] (e.g. Critic aid). Reduce any inflammation: potent topical corticosteroid (e.g. Dermovate, Temovate (clobetasol), Cutivate (fluticasone)) once daily for one week. Rectal or vaginal discharge: if infection is present, treat with topical antimicrobials (systemic if necessary) and antiseptic douches or lavage (e.g. povidone-iodine). Inflammation can be reduced with a potent topical corticosteroid (e.g. betamethasone 0.1%). If the area is too sensitive to apply cream, reduce the local pain by applying for a few days beclomethasone inhaler used as a spray. • *If a fistula is present:* Reduce the volume of the discharge: – for a distal small bowel fistula try loperamide 8–24 mg/24 hours in divided doses.[26] – for a higher upper gastrointestinal fistula try hyoscine butylbromide (in the US use hyoscyamine (Levsin) 0.25–0.5 mg IV/SC q4h PRN, 0.125–0.25 mg SL q4h PRN) 60–120 mg/24 hours by intermittent SC or SC infusion. – if the discharge persists, try octreotide 100–200 microgram q8h or 300–600 microgram/24 hours by SC infusion. Alternatively, and if the prognosis is 2 weeks or more, try lanreotide 30 mg IM once every 14 days. In the US use Sandostatin LAR Depot, long-acting octreotide given as 20 mg IM q4 weeks. Divert the discharge: use a stoma bag if adhesion on a flat surface is possible. Consider surgical diversion, e.g. colostomy, urostomy.
6 Is the wound painful?	• Only at dressing changes: Change the dressing: stop using hydrocolloid dressings[27] or dressings with adhesive.[28] Consider using non-adherent, soft silicone net dressings next to the ulcer (e.g. Mepitel).[29,30] Protect the surrounding skin with a barrier cream (e.g. simethicone-containing cream) or a barrier application[12] (e.g. Cavilon 'No Sting Barrier Film'). • Predose with SL fentanyl or sufentanil (*see* cd-5 in Diagnosing and treating pain (p. 42)). • *At any time:* consider topical morphine[31–34] (*see* cd-9 in Diagnosing and treating pain (p. 43)). Review the systemic analgesia and consider ketamine or spinal analgesia.
7 Is the wound itchy?	• Remove allergen: exclude allergy to dressing or topical agent. • Reduce inflammation: NSAID or use topical steroid (e.g. Dermovate, Temovate (clobetasol), Cutivate (fluticasone)) daily for 1 week. • Consider using TENS on intact skin between wound and spine.[12]

Adapted from Saunders and Regnard[35]
cd = clinical decision

References

B = book; C = comment; Ch = chapter; CS-n = case study-number of cases; CT-n = controlled trial-number of cases; E = editorial; GC = group consensus; I = interviews; LS = laboratory study; MC = multi-center; OS-n = open study-number of cases; Q-n = questionnaire-number of respondents; R = review; RCT-n = randomized controlled trial-number of cases; RS-n = retrospective survey-number of cases; SA = systematic or meta analysis.

1 Ivetic O, Lyne PA (1990) Fungating and ulcerating malignant lesions: a review of the literature. *Journal of Advanced Nursing.* **15**(1): 83–8. (R, 42 refs)

2 Bird C (2000) Managing malignant fungating wounds. *Professional Nurse.* **15**(4): 253–6. (R, 28 refs)

3 Schulz V, Triska OH, Tonkin K (2002) Malignant wounds: caregiver-determined clinical problems. *Journal of Pain and Symptom Management.* **24**(6): 572–7. (Q-136)

4 Rice AM (2000) Clinical review. Sexuality in cancer and palliative care 1: effects of disease and treatment. *International Journal of Palliative Nursing.* **6**(8): 392–7. (R, 49 refs)

5 Dauphin S, Katz S, el Tamer M, Wait R, Sohn C, Braverman AS (1997) Chemotherapy is a safe and effective initial therapy for infected malignant breast and chest wall ulcers. *Journal of Surgical Oncology – Supplement.* **66**(3): 186–8. (OS-33)

6 Heirler F, de la Motte S, Popp W (1995) Influence of metronidazole and tamoxifen in a case of otherwise untreated ulcerous breast carcinoma. *European Journal of Gynaecological Oncology.* **16**(6): 448–52. (CS-1)

7 Sanders R, Goodacre TE (1989) When radiotherapy offers no more: the surgical management of advanced breast malignancy. *Annals of the Royal College of Surgeons of England.* **71**(6): 349–53. (RS-47)

8 Rotimi VO, Durosinmi-Etti FA (1984) The bacteriology of infected malignant ulcers. *Journal of Clinical Pathology.* **37**(5): 592–5. (OS-70)

9 Visapaa JP, Tillonen JS, Kaihovaara PS, Salaspuro MP (2002) Lack of disulfram-like reaction with metronidazole and ethanol. *Annals of Pharmacotherapy.* **36**(6): 971–4.

10 Newman V, Allwood M, Oakes RA (1989) The use of metronidazole gel to control the smell of malodorous lesions. *Palliative Medicine.* **3**: 303–5.

11 Finlay IG, Bowszyc J, Ramlau C, Gwiezdzinski Z (1996) The effect of topical 0.75% metronidazole gel on malodorous cutaneous ulcers. *Journal of Pain and Symptom Management.* **11**(3): 158–62. (OS-47)

12 Grocott P (1999) The management of fungating wounds. *Journal of Wound Care.* **8**(5): 232–4. (R, 24 refs)

13 Grocott P (1995) The palliative management of fungating malignant wounds. *Journal of Wound Care.* **4**(5): 240–2. (R, 36 refs)

14 Kelly N (2002) Malodorous fungating wounds: a review of current literature. *Professional Nurse.* **17**(5): 323–6. (R, 40 refs)

15 Parnham A (2002) Moist wound healing: does the same theory apply to chronic wounds? *Journal of Wound Care.* **11**(4): 143–6. (R, 36 refs)

16 Grocott P (1998) Exudative management in fungating wounds. *Journal of Wound Care.* **7**(9): 445–8. (CS-3)

17 Grocott P (2000) The palliative management of fungating malignant wounds. *Journal of Wound Care.* **9**(1): 4–9. (OS-45)

18 Metcalf C (1999) Enterocutaneous fistulae. *Journal of Wound Care.* **8**: 141–2. (R, 10 refs)

19 Pringle WK (1995) The management of patients with enterocutaneous fistulae. *Journal of Wound Care.* **4**: 211–13. (R, 6 refs)

20 Grocott P (1992) The latest on latex. *Nursing Times.* **88**: 61–2. (R, 6 refs)

21 Walls AWG, Regnard CFB, Mannix KA (1994) The closure of an abdominal fistula using self-polymerising silicone rubbers – a case study. *Palliative Medicine.* **8**: 59–62. (CS-1)

22 Alivizatos V, Felekis D, Zorbalas A (2002) Evaluation of the effectiveness of octreotide in the conservative treatment of postoperative enterocutaneous fistulas. *Hepato-Gastroenterology.* **49**(46): 1010–12. (RS-39)

23 Gonzalez-Pinto I, Gonzalez EM (2001) Optimising the treatment of upper gastrointestinal fistulae. *Gut.* **49** (Suppl. 4): 22–31. (R, 81 refs)

24 Yeo CJ, Cameron JL, Lillemoe KD, Sauter PK, Coleman J, Sohn TA, Campbell KA, Choti MA (2000) Does prophylactic octreotide decrease the rates of pancreatic fistula and other complications after pancreaticoduodenectomy? Results of a prospective randomized placebo-controlled trial. *Annals of Surgery.* **232**(3): 419–29. (RCT, 211)

25 Mercadante S (1994) The role of octreotide in palliative care. *Journal of Pain and Symptom Management.* **9**(6): 406–11. (R, 37 refs)

26 Twycross R, Wilcock A (2001) Skin care. In: *Symptom Management in Advanced Cancer* (3e). Radcliffe Medical Press, Oxford.

27 Jones V, Milton T (2000) When and how to use hydrocolloid dressings. *Nursing Times Plus.* **96**: 5–7. (R)

28 Collier M (2000) Tissue viability. Management of patients with fungating wounds. *Nursing Standard.* **15**(11): 46, 48–50, 52. (R, 17 refs)

29 Gotschall CS, Morrison MI, Eichelberger MR (1998) Prospective randomized study of the efficacy of Mepitel on partial thickness scalds in children. *Journal of Burn Care Rehabilitation.* **19**: 279–83. (RCT)

30 Taylor R (1999) Use of a silicone net dressing in severe mycosis fungoides. *Journal of Wound Care.* **8**(9): 429–30. (CS-1)

31 Back IN, Finlay I (1995) Analgesic effect of topical opioids on painful skin ulcers. *Journal of Pain and Symptom Management.* **10**: 493.

32 Krajnik M, Zylicz Z (1997) Topical morphine for cutaneous cancer pain. *Palliative Medicine.* **11**: 325–6. (CS-6)

33 Twillman RK, Long TD, Cathers TA, Mueller DW (1999) Treatment of painful skin ulcers with topical opioids. *Journal of Pain and Symptom Management.* **17**(4): 288–92. (CS-9)

34 Briggs M, Nelson EA (2003) Topical agents or dressings for pain in venous leg ulcers (Cochrane review). In: *The Cochrane Library, Issue 3.* Oxford: Update software. (Also on www.update-software.com/abstracts/ab001177.htm)

35 Saunders J, Regnard C (1995) Malignant ulcers. In: *Flow Diagrams in Advanced Cancer and Other Diseases.* Edward Arnold, London. pp. 57–9. (Ch)

Nausea and vomiting

Clinical decision and action checklist

1 If vomiting, make available a large bowl, tissues and water.
2 Is the patient troubled mainly by vomiting?
3 Could the cause be drugs, toxins or biochemical?
4 Is the nausea or vomiting worse on movement?
5 Is gastritis present?
6 Could fear or anxiety be contributing?
7 Is the nausea or vomiting persisting?

Key points

- Antiemetic choice depends on the cause.
- A single antiemetic is sufficient in two-thirds of patients.[1]
- Any added antiemetics should have a different action.[2]
- Gastric motility disorders have specific signs and symptoms.

Introduction

Nausea and vomiting occur in up to 50% of patients with cancer,[3,4] and both are common in AIDS,[5] and end-stage heart failure.[6,7] Most patients find it very distressing.[8] Assessment of the cause will depend on knowledge of the underlying disease, history and examination. Commonly overlooked causes are hypercalcemia,[9] pharyngeal stimulation by copious sputum, gastric stasis and drugs other than opioids. In one third of patients there is more than one cause of emesis.[2]

Features and causes

Gastric stasis is common.[10] It is suggested by large volume vomiting with esophageal reflux, epigastric fullness, early satiation or hiccups.

Total outflow obstruction produces a similar picture but with rapid dehydration.

'Squashed stomach syndrome': This occurs when the gastric cavity is reduced by gastric tumour or by external compression. Symptoms are similar to gastric stasis but with low volume vomiting.

'Floppy stomach syndrome': Here gastric tone is absent, resulting in a very distended stomach, discomfort and very small volume vomits.

Regurgitation produces vomits of undigested material that test negative to acid.

Other causes of nausea and vomiting have non-specific patterns.

Treatment

Receptor basis for treating nausea and vomiting[11–14]

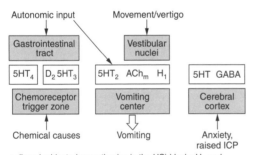

- dimenhydrinate (promethazine in the US) blocks H₁ and ACh_m receptors
- haloperidol blocks D₂ receptors
- methotrimeprazine blocks D₂, H₁, 5HT₂ and ACh_m receptors
- metoclopramide blocks D₂ and stimulates 5HT₄ receptors
- domperidone blocks D₂ receptors
- ondansetron blocks 5HT₃ receptors

H_1 = histamine 1; D_2 = dopamine 2; $5HT_3$ = serotonin receptors; ACh_m = muscarinic cholinergic.

Choosing an antiemetic

Key antiemetics: These are dimenhydrinate (promethazine in the US)*,[13] haloperidol,[15,54] metoclopramide (or domperidone in children (obtained in the US from a compounding pharmacy))[16,17] and methotrimeprazine (Canada only) or prochlorperazine (US).[18,19] The receptors likely to be involved dictate the choice of antiemetic[11]

(see figure on this page and clinical decisions opposite).

Other antiemetics: 5HT₃ antagonists are helpful in radiotherapy and chemotherapy.[20] Cannabinoids have been used, such as dronabinol for GI metastases[21] and nabilone for chemotherapy.[22] Ondansetron has sometimes been helpful in emesis due to AIDS and cancer,[23] and in multiple sclerosis.[24]

Associated management

Bucket, tissues and water: A decent-sized bowl is essential to avoid the distress to patients of soiling their clothes and bedsheets. Also available should be tissues to wipe the mouth and water or juice to rinse the mouth.

Parenteral hydration: 500–1000 ml/24 hours may help to reduce persistent nausea.[25,26]

Nasogastric suction has no role to play in most causes of nausea and vomiting.[27–31] There are three exceptions where it may help: (1) gastric outflow or duodenal obstruction to reduce high volume vomiting,[32] (2) gastric atony ('floppy stomach'), where a nasogastric tube can be passed easily (even in semi-conscious or unconscious patients) and removed once all the fluid and air have been aspirated and (3) feculant vomiting, to reduce odour.

Acupuncture has good evidence for efficacy in nausea and vomiting,[33–36] but acupuncture-like TENS has not been shown to help.[37] *Acupressure* at the P6 acupuncture point on the wrist may have a role in some patients.[38,39]

Chemotherapy is only helpful in treating nausea and vomiting if there is a good tumor response.[40]

Anxiety and fear can cause nausea and vomiting,[41] especially prior to chemotherapy, for which hypnosis has been used to good effect.[42–44]

Persistent nausea and vomiting

Chemotherapy: A 5HT₃ antagonist is more effective when combined with dexamethasone[45] or haloperidol.

Dexamethasone also can help in persistent nausea due to other causes.[46,47]

Percutaneous gastrostomy is a means of giving enteral nutrition and hydration when oral feeding is not possible, but can have complications.[28,49] It may help in emptying the stomach in persistent vomiting due to gastric outlet obstruction or severe gastric stasis.[48]

Thalidomide may have a role in persistent emesis.[50] (Special access category in North America.)

---

* Dimenhydrinate is available in some formulations in the US.

Clinical decision	If YES ⇒ Action
1 If vomiting, make available a large bowl, tissues and water.	
2 Is the patient troubled mainly by vomiting? (i.e. no nausea or brief nausea relieved by vomiting)	**(a) Large volume vomiting** (with heartburn, hiccups, fullness or early satiation): • *If dehydrating rapidly* consider *total gastric outflow obstruction* – will need NG tube and IV hydration for comfort. If tumor is the cause, high dose dexamethasone (16 mg SC daily) may help clear the obstruction, but if persisting refer for stenting.[51,52] • *If not dehydrating rapidly:* This is probably *gastric stasis* due to drugs (*see* notes), partial outflow obstruction (local tumor, hepatomegaly, ascites, disordered motility of duodenum) or autonomic failure: start metoclopramide 10 mg SC q6h or 40–100 mg SC infusion per 24 hours. For children use domperidone (*see* Drugs in palliative care for children: starting doses (p. 253)). Maintain on oral route 10–20 mg q6h. In the US, a medication commonly used in children for nausea and vomiting is dimenhydramine (Benadryl) 5 mg/kg/day divided q4–6h IV/PO. It is commonly used in hospitals and for outpatients. • *If gastric stasis is still a problem:* consider erythromycin 100–250 mg q12h, but this can itself cause troublesome nausea.[53] • *If there is still no improvement*, consider a percutaneous gastrostomy. **(b) Regurgitation** (unaltered food or drink vomited within minutes of ingestion, litmus test is negative to acid): *see* Dysphagia (p. 91). **(c) Distended stomach** ('Floppy stomach syndrome'). May contain fluid, air or both. Using brief nasogastric suction will bring rapid relief, even in unconscious patients. **(d) Compressed stomach** ('Squashed stomach syndrome'): The features are the same as gastric stasis but vomits are small. Treat as for gastric stasis in cd-2a above. **(e) Raised intracranial pressure**: dimenhydrinate 25–50 mg PO or 50–100 mg PR q8h, or 25 mg SC q6–8h. *If due to intracranial tumor:* start high dose dexamethasone (16 mg/day) and refer to clinical oncologist for cranial irradiation.
3 Could the cause be drugs, toxins or biochemical?	• *Area postrema stimulation* (bacterial toxins, most drugs, hypercalcemia, uremia): low dose haloperidol 1.5–3 mg PO or SC once at night. • *5HT₃ receptor stimulation* (e.g. antibiotics, cytotoxic drugs, SSRI antidepressants): ondansetron 4–8 mg q8h SC or PO. With cytotoxic drugs add haloperidol.[54] • *Gastrointestinal mucosal irritation* (antibiotics, cytotoxic drugs, iron supplements, NSAIDs, tranexamic acid): change drug if possible. For gastritis use sucralfate 2 g q12h or lansoprazole 30 mg in the morning (omeprazole in children). • *Gastric stasis* (antimuscarinic drugs including amitriptyline, hyoscine, and opioids): treat as in cd-2a above.
4 Is the nausea or vomiting worse on movement?	• *Mechanical distortion of a distended stomach or bowel:* for gastric stasis treat as in cd-2a above. For bowel or liver distension use dimenhydrinate 25–50 mg PO or 50–100 mg PR q8h, or 25 mg SC q6–8h. • *Motion sickness:* hyoscine hydrobromide (scopolamine) transdermally (more than one patch may be needed). • *Other causes* (e.g. middle ear infection, vestibular viral neuronitis (e.g. zoster), ototoxic drugs, tumor at cerebello-pontine angle, Ménière's disease): dimenhydrinate (or promethazine in the US) 25–50 mg PO or 50–100 mg PR q8h, or 25 mg SC q6–8h.

Table continued overleaf

5 Is gastritis present?	• *If on NSAID:* start PPI cover (e.g. lansoprazole or omeprazole). Do not use ranitidine or cimetidine since these are less effective at protecting against gastric NSAID damage.[55,56] If there is no response, stop the NSAID.
	• *If not on ulcer healing drug:* start ranitidine 300 mg q12h or lansoprazole 30 mg in the morning (omeprazole in children).
	• *If nausea or vomiting persists*: start metoclopramide 10 mg SC q6h or 40–100 mg SC infusion per 24 hours. For children use domperidone (Canada) or diphenhydramine (US, available from a compounding pharmacy) (*see* Drugs in palliative care for children: starting doses (p. 253)). Maintain on oral route 10–20 mg q6h.
	• *If anxiety is contributing*: see cd-6 below.
6 Could fear or anxiety be contributing?	• *See* Anxiety (p. 165).
	• Explanation and effective antiemetic therapy may help.
	• Consider lorazepam 0.5 mg SL 2–4 hours prior to chemotherapy.
	• Persistent emesis may respond to hypnosis,[57] or behavioral therapy.[58]
7 Is the nausea or vomiting persisting?	• Start methotrimeprazine (Canada only) 3–6 mg PO or 6.25 mg SC at bedtime, on its own or in addition to other antiemetics. In US use prochlorperazine (Compazine) 10 mg PO IV q6h or 25 mg PR q6h.
	• If dehydrated, moderate rehydration of 500–1000 ml/24 hours may help.[25]
	• Other antiemetics: consider adding ondansetron 4 mg q8h,[23,24] dexamethasone PO/SC 4 mg once daily,[46,47]or olanzepine 2.5 mg q12h.[59]

Adapted from Regnard and Comiskey[60]
cd = clinical decision

References

B = book; C = comment; Ch = chapter; CS-n = case study-number of cases; CT-n = controlled trial-number of cases; E = editorial; GC = group consensus; I-n = interviews-number of cases; LS = laboratory study; MC = multi-center; OS-n = open study-number of cases; R = review; RCT-n = randomized controlled trial-number of cases; RS-n = retrospective survey-number of cases; SA = systematic or meta analysis.

1 Hanks GW (1982) Antiemetics for terminal cancer patients. *Lancet.* **i**: 1410.
2 Lichter I (1993) Which antiemetic? *Journal of Palliative Care.* **9**: 42–50.
3 Morita T, Tsunoda J, Inoue S, Chihara S (1999) Contributing factors to physical symptoms in terminally-ill cancer patients. *Journal of Pain and Symptom Management.* **18**(5): 338–46. (OS-350)
4 Vainio A, Auvinen A (1996) Prevalence of symptoms among patients with advanced cancer: an international collaborative study. *Journal of Pain and Symptom Management.* **12**(1): 3–10. (OS-1840)
5 Newshan G, Sherman DW (1999) Palliative care: pain and symptom management in persons with HIV/AIDS. *Nursing Clinics of North America.* **34**(1): 131–45.

6 Davies N, Curtis M (2000) Providing palliative care in end-stage heart failure. *Professional Nurse.* **15**(6): 389–92. (R, 31 refs)
7 McCarthy M, Lay M, Addington-Hall J (1996) Dying from heart disease. *Journal of the Royal College of Physicians of London.* **30**(4): 325–8. (I-600)
8 Addington-Hall J, Altmann D (2000) Which terminally ill cancer patients in the United Kingdom receive care from community specialist palliative care nurses? *Journal of Advanced Nursing.* **32**(4): 799–806. (I-2074)
9 Lamy O, Jenzer-Closuit A, Burckhardt P (2001) Hypercalcemia of malignancy: an undiagnosed and undertreated disease. *Journal of Internal Medicine.* **250**(1): 73–9. (OS-71)
10 Bentley A, Boyd K (2001) Use of clinical pictures in the management of nausea and vomiting, a

prospective audit. *Palliative Medicine.* **15**(3): 247–53. (OS-40)

11 Peroutka SJ, Snyder SH (1982) Antiemetics: Neurotransmitter receptor binding predicts therapeutic actions. *Lancet.* **i**: 658–9. (R)

12 Sanger GJ (1993) The pharmacology of anti-emetic agents. In: *Emesis in Anti-cancer Therapy: Mechanisms and Treatment.* Chapman and Hall, London. pp. 179–210. (Ch)

13 Twycross RG, Wilcock A, Charlesworth S (2002) *PCF2: Palliative Care Formulary.* Radcliffe Medical Press, Oxford. (B)

14 Mannix KA (2002) Palliation of nausea and vomiting. In: K Calman, D Doyle, GWC Hanks (eds) *Oxford Textbook of Palliative Medicine* (3e). Oxford University Press, Oxford. (Ch)

15 Mickle J (1998) The use of haloperidol to treat nausea. *Oncology Nursing Forum.* **25**(8): 1309.

16 Wilson J, Plourde JY, Marshall D, Yoshida S, Chow W, Harsanyi Z, Pearen S, Darke A (2002) Long-term safety and clinical effectiveness of controlled-release metoclopramide in cancer-associated dyspepsia syndrome: a multicentre evaluation. *Journal of Palliative Care.* **18**(2): 84–91. (OS-48)

17 Bruera E, Belzile M, Neumann C, Harsanyi Z, Babul N, Darke A (2000) A double-blind, cross-over study of controlled-release metoclopramide and placebo for the chronic nausea and dyspepsia of advanced cancer. *Journal of Pain and Symptom Management.* **19**(6): 427–35. (RCT-26)

18 Twycross RG *et al.* (1997) The use of low dose levomepromazine (methotrimeprazine) in the management of nausea and vomiting. *Progress in Palliative Care.* **5**(2): 49–53.

19 Skinner J, Skinner A (1999) Levomepromazine for nausea and vomiting in advanced cancer. *Hospital Medicine (London).* **60**(8): 568–70. (R, 10 refs)

20 Priestman TJ (1996) Controlling the toxicity of palliative radiotherapy: the role of 5-HT3 antagonists. *Canadian Journal of Oncology.* **Suppl 1**: 17–22. (R)

21 Gonzales-Rosales F, Walsh D (1997) Palliative care rounds. Intractable nausea and vomiting due to gastrointestinal mucosal metastases relieved by tetrahydrocannabinol (dronabinol). *Journal of Pain and Symptom Management.* **14**(5): 311–14. (CS-1)

22 Tramer MR, Carroll D, Campbell FA, Reynolds DJ, Moore RA, McQuay HJ (2001) Cannabinoids for control of chemotherapy induced nausea and vomiting: quantitative systematic review. *BMJ.* **323**(7303): 16–21. (R, 38 refs)

23 Currow DC, Coughlan M, Fardell B, Cooney NJ (1997) Clinical note. Use of ondansetron in palliative medicine. *Journal of Pain and Symptom Management.* **13**(5): 302–7. (RS-16)

24 Macleod AD (2000) Ondansetron in multiple sclerosis. *Journal of Pain and Symptom Management.* **20**(5): 388–91. (CS-2)

25 Ripamonti C, Mercadante S, Groff L, Zecca E, De Conno F, Casuccio A (2000) Role of octreotide, scopolamine butylbromide, and hydration in symptom control of patients with inoperable bowel obstruction and nasogastric tubes: a prospective randomized trial. *Journal of Pain and Symptom Management.* **19**(1): 23–34. (CT-17)

26 Cerchietti L, Navigante A, Sauri A, Palazzo F (2000) Clinical trial. Hypodermoclysis for control of dehydration in terminal-stage cancer. *International Journal of Palliative Nursing.* **6**(8): 370–4. (CT-42)

27 Ripamonti C, Panzeri C, Groff L, Galeazzi G, Boffi R (2001) The role of somatostatin and octreotide in bowel obstruction: pre-clinical and clinical results. *Tumori.* **87**(1): 1–9. (R, 82 refs)

28 Ripamonti C, Twycross R, Baines M, Bozzetti F, Capri S, De Conno F, Gemlo B, Hunt TM, Krebs HB, Mercadante S, Schaerer R, Wilkinson P (2001) Working Group of the European Association for Palliative Care. Clinical-practice recommendations for the management of bowel obstruction in patients with end-stage cancer. *Supportive Care in Cancer.* **9**(4): 223–33. (R)

29 Frank C (1997) Medical management of intestinal obstruction in terminal care. *Canadian Family Physician.* **43**: 259–65. (SA, 29 refs)

30 Cheatham ML, Chapman WC, Key SP, Sawyers JL (1995) A meta-analysis of selective versus routine nasogastric decompression after elective laparotomy. *Annals of Surgery.* **221**(5): 469–76; discussion 476–8. (SA)

31 Koukouras D, Mastronikolis NS, Tzoraceleftherakis E, Angelopoulou E, Kalfarentzos F, Androulakis J (2001) The role of nasogastric tube after elective abdominal surgery. *Clinica Terapeutica.* **152**(4): 241–4. (RCT-100)

32 Upadhyay V, Sakalkale R, Parashar K, Mitra SK, Buick RG, Gornall P, Corkery JJ (1996) Duodenal atresia: a comparison of three modes of treatment. *European Journal of Pediatric Surgery.* **6**(2): 75–7. (RS-33)

33 Wang SM, Kain ZN (2002) P6 acupoint injections are as effective as droperidol in controlling early postoperative nausea and vomiting in children. *Anesthesiology.* **97**(2): 359–66. (CT-186)

34 Kaptchuk TJ (2002) Acupuncture: theory, efficacy, and practice. *Annals of Internal Medicine.* **136**(5): 374–83. (R, 113 refs)

35 Carlsson CP, Axemo P, Bodin A, Carstensen H, Ehrenroth B, Madegard-Lind I, Navander C (2000) Manual acupuncture reduces hyperemesis gravidarum: a placebo-controlled, randomized, single-blind, crossover study. *Journal of Pain and Symptom Management.* **20**(4): 273–9. (RCT-33)

36 Johnstone PA, Polston GR, Niemtzow RC, Martin PJ (2002) Integration of acupuncture into the oncology clinic. *Palliative Medicine.* **16**(3): 235–9. (OS-123)

37 Gadsby JG, Franks A, Jarvis P, Dewhurst F (1997) Acupuncture-like transcutaneous electrical nerve stimulation within palliative care: a pilot study. *Complementary Therapies in Medicine.* **5**(1): 13–18. (RCT-15)

38 Dundee JW, McMillan C (1991) Positive evidence for P6 acupuncture antiemesis. *Postgraduate Medical Journal.* **67**: 417–22. (R, 53 refs)

39 Stern RM, Jokerst MD, Muth ER, Hollis C (2001) Acupressure relieves the symptoms of motion sickness and reduces abnormal gastric activity. *Alternative Therapies in Health & Medicine.* **7**(4): 91–4. (RCT-25)

40 Geels P, Eisenhauer E, Bezjak A, Zee B, Day A (2000) Palliative effect of chemotherapy: objective tumor response is associated with symptom improvement in patients with metastatic breast cancer. *Journal of Clinical Oncology.* **18**(12): 2395–405. (RCT-300)

41 Watson M, Meyer L, Thomson A, Osofsky S (1998) Psychological factors predicting nausea and vomiting in breast cancer patients on chemotherapy. *European Journal of Cancer.* **34**(6): 831–7. (OS-100)

42 Morrow GR, Roscoe JA, Kirshner JJ, Hynes HE, Rosenbluth RJ (1998) Anticipatory nausea and vomiting in the era of 5-HT3 antiemetics. *Supportive Care in Cancer.* **6**(3): 244–7. (R, 43 refs)

43 Eckert RM (2001) Understanding anticipatory nausea. *Oncology Nursing Forum.* **28**(10): 1553–8; quiz 1559–60. (R, 44 refs)

44 Marchioro G, Azzarello G, Viviani F, Barbato F, Pavanetto M, Rosetti F, Pappagallo GL, Vinante O (2000) Hypnosis in the treatment of anticipatory nausea and vomiting in patients receiving cancer chemotherapy. *Oncology.* **59**(2): 100–4. (OS-16)

45 Roila F, Aapro M, Stewart A (1998) Optimal selection of antiemetics in children receiving cancer chemotherapy. *Supportive Care in Cancer.* **6**(3): 215–20. (R, 39 refs)

46 Bruera E, Seifert L, Watanabe S, Babul N, Darke A, Harsanyi Z, Suarez-Almazor M (1996) Chronic nausea in advanced cancer patients: a retrospective assessment of a metoclopramide-based antiemetic regimen. *Journal of Pain and Symptom Management.* **11**(3): 147–53. (RS-100)

47 Hardy JR, Rees E, Ling J, Burman R, Feuer D, Broadley K, Stone P (2001) A prospective survey of the use of dexamethasone on a palliative care unit. *Palliative Medicine.* **15**(1): 3–8. (OS-106)

48 Watson JP, Mannix KA, Matthewson K (1997) Percutaneous endoscopic gastroenterostomy and jejunal extension for gastric stasis in pancreatic carcinoma. *Palliative Medicine.* **11**: 407–10.

49 Mathus-Vliegen LM, Koning H (1999) Percutaneous endoscopic gastrostomy and gastrojejunostomy: a critical reappraisal of patient selection, tube function and the feasibility of nutritional support during extended follow-up. *Gastrointestinal Endoscopy.* **50**(6): 746–54. (OS-286)

50 Peuckmann V, Fisch M, Bruera E (2000) Potential novel uses of thalidomide: focus on palliative care. *Drugs.* **60**(2): 273–92. (R, 120 refs)

51 Johnston SD, McKelvey ST, Moorehead RJ, Spence RA, Tham TC (2002) Duodenal stents for malignant duodenal strictures. *Ulster Medical Journal.* **71**(1): 30–3. (CS-4)

52 Uthappa MC, Ho SM, Boardman P (2003) Role of metallic stents in palliative care. *Progress in Palliative Care.* **11**(1): 3–9. (R, 29 refs)

53 Zatman TF, Hall JE, Harmer M (2001) Gastric residual volume in children: a study comparing efficiency of erythromycin and metoclopramide as prokinetic agents. *BJA: British Journal of Anaesthesia.* **86**(6): 869–71. (RCT-80)

54 Bregni M, Siena S, Di Nicola M, Bonadonna G, Gianni AM (1991) Tropisetron plus haloperidol to ameliorate nausea and vomiting associated with high-dose alkylating agent cancer chemotherapy. *European Journal of Cancer.* **27**(5): 561–5. (RCT-32)

55 Graham DY, Agrawal NM, Campbell DR, Haber MM, Collis C, Lukasik NL, Huang B (2002) NSAID-Associated Gastric Ulcer Prevention Study Group. Ulcer prevention in long-term users of nonsteroidal anti-inflammatory drugs: results of a double-blind, randomized, multi-center, active- and placebo-controlled study of misoprostol vs lansoprazole. *Archives of Internal Medicine.* **162**(2): 169–75. (MC, RCT-537)

56 Twycross R (1994) The risks and benefits of corticosteroids in advanced cancer. *Drug Safety.* **11**(3): 163–78. (R)

57 Marchioro G, Azzarello G, Viviani F, Barbato F, Pavanetto M, Rosetti F, Pappagallo GL, Vinante O (2000) Hypnosis in the treatment of anticipatory nausea and vomiting in patients receiving cancer chemotherapy. *Oncology.* **59**(2): 100–4. (OS-16)

58 Redd WH, Montgomery GH, DuHamel KN (2001) Behavioral intervention for cancer treatment side effects. *Journal of the National Cancer Institute.* **93**(11): 810–23. (R, 106 refs)

59 Passik SD, Lundberg J, Kirsh KL, Theobald D, Donaghy K, Holtsclaw E, Cooper M, Dugan W (2002) A pilot exploration of the antiemetic activity of olanzapine for the relief of nausea in patients with advanced cancer and pain. *Journal of Pain and Symptom Management.* **23**(6): 526–32. (OS-15)

60 Regnard C, Comiskey M (1995) Nausea and vomiting. In: *Flow Diagrams in Advanced Cancer and Other Diseases.* Edward Arnold, London. pp. 14–18. (Ch)

Nutrition and hydration problems

Advice on children written by Justin Amery

Clinical decision and action checklist

1 Is the prognosis short (day by day deterioration)?
2 Is the patient anxious or withdrawn?
3 Is there a request to withdraw hydration and/or feeding?
4 Are physical symptoms present?
5 Is the feeding tube blocked?
6 Could drugs be the cause?
7 Is the food presentation or environment a problem?
8 Is anorexia persisting?
9 Is thirst still present?

Key points

- Consider reversible causes before starting an appetite stimulant.
- Reduced intake is normal at the end of life.

Introduction

Hunger and thirst make us eat and drink for survival. But we also eat out of habit, boredom, pleasure, satisfaction or comfort, and because we choose to make it a social activity. Advanced disease can severely reduce our ability, need or desire to eat and drink.

Decisions

The decision lies with the patient, and sometimes with the carers. Every situation is different and fixed policies are indefensible,[1] especially as data on the advantages or disadvantages of hydration are lacking.[2,3] In Canada and the US, non-oral feeding would fall into the category of medical treatment and, depending on clinical condition, prognosis and other factors, would not always be legally obligatory to provide. As with any treatment decisions, consent of the patient (or of the legally authorized substitute decision-maker/healthcare proxy, as the case may be) must be considered and, in cases of patients lacking capacity and where no prior wishes have been expressed or are known, the best interests of the patient (including a weighing of the benefits and burdens to the patient) must be taken into account (see Making ethical choices (p. 185), and Decisions around competency (p. 189)).

In patients who are comatose and comfortable, dehydration causes few symptoms,[2] but dehydration can cause or contribute to an agitated confusional state in some patients.[4,5] Thirst may only need sips of water or may need parenteral rehydration.[6,7] Hunger is not usually a problem in the terminal stages,[7] and unwanted feeding by any route may increase distress.[8] Family, friends or staff may feel a need to continue hydration or feeding and they will need explanation and support.[9] Occasionally, the relatives or parents persist with the request for hydration or feeding in a dying adult or child, even though the patient is comfortable. In such circumstances it is reasonable to hydrate since hydration subcutaneously or feeding through an existing PEG tube is unlikely to cause discomfort whilst refusing their request may complicate their bereavement.

Managing reduced hydration and feeding

Oral hydration and feeding

Environment: In health we have the choice of eating when, what, where and with whom we choose. Illness greatly reduces that choice.[10] Problems will result from inflexible mealtimes or crowded eating areas.

Food presentation: The key is food presentation,[11] with a pleasant atmosphere, variety, and food that is attractive, the correct temperature and an appropriate portion size for the patient. An alcoholic drink before meals is more effective poured from bottle to glass rather than dispensed in calibrated plastic pots.

Patients may develop taste abnormalities and may prefer sweeter, colder and spicier foods, while others cannot tolerate the bitterness of urea in red meats.[12,13] The skills of an enthusiastic chef and the advice of a dietician can be invaluable.

Equipment: If necessary the patient should be assessed by a physiotherapist and occupational therapist for seating and advice on utensils.

Communication: Mealtimes are a time for communication, especially if the carer pays attention, is responsive, is at face-to-face level, gives eye contact, asks simple questions, creates choices, uses simple language about the meal, and allows the patient to use all sensory information such as looking, smelling and touching.

Enriching the diet: This can be done in many ways,[14] but there is no evidence that one type of supplement is better than any other.[15] Neutral flavour types are most versatile since they can be added to many different foods.

Non-oral hydration and feeding

Non-oral hydration is most conveniently given subcutaneously (hypodermoclysis).[16] The suprascapular area is safe and convenient, and up to 100 ml/hour can be infused without hyaluronidase.[17–19] Unlike the intravenous route, subcutaneous cannulae can be left in place for 7–10 days without problems. Other non-oral routes are discussed in Dysphagia (p. 91). In the last days of life, non-oral feeding offers no advantages.

Persistent anorexia

Cachexia: This is a syndrome of weight loss (fat and skeletal muscle), anorexia, anemia, fatigue and edema. It is seen in cancer, AIDS, heart failure, rheumatoid arthritis, chronic respiratory disease and liver cirrhosis.[20–24] It is very different to starvation and is due to a cytokine-mediated inflammatory response to the underlying illness.[25]

Drug treatments: Anorexia may be linked to low cortisol levels[26] and dexamethasone or prednisolone can improve anorexia.[27–29] Progestins are effective,[30] and megestrol acetate 800 mg daily has the same effect on anorexia as 3 mg dexamethasone daily,[31] but is much more expensive.[32] Cachexia in cancer can be modified by 1–3 g daily of the fatty acid eicosapentaenoic acid (EPA).[33] Concentrated omega-3 fish oils are widely available and contain 15–20% EPA. Thalidomide may also have a role.[34,35] (Special access category in North America.)

Support and reassurance: In many patients, the anorexia is part of the advanced illness and is more of a concern to carers.[36] It is helpful to support the patient to adapt to the reduced intake to reduce their fear, and reassure the partner and family it is not their failure to care.

Clinical decision	If YES ⇒ Action
1 Is the prognosis short? (i.e. day by day deterioration)	• *If hydration or feeding would help* (e.g. thirst, hunger or confusion due to dehydration): hydrate and feed for comfort or pleasure (may include IV or SC hydration). • *If hydration or feeding is unnecessary* (e.g. comatose and comfortable): ensure the partner, family and staff understand the situation. If the family or partner feel a need to continue hydration and/or feeding, the family will need help to understand the situation. If they remain firm in their belief, try to negotiate maintenance hydration IV or SC (*see* notes).
2 Is the patient anxious or withdrawn?	• Help the patient manage anxiety or low mood: *see* Anxiety (p. 165) and Withdrawal and depression (p. 177).

3   Is there a request to
withdraw hydration and/
or feeding?
	• If this is from a person competent for this decision:
	  – ensure good oral hygiene (*see* Oral problems (p. 125))
	  – prevent skin pressure damage (*see* Skin problems (p. 139)).
	• If this is about an adult or child who is not competent for this decision: *see* Decisions around competency (p. 189).

4 Are physical symptoms present?	• *Swallowing problems*: *see* Dysphagia (p. 91). • *Constipation*: *see* Constipation (p. 75). • *Nausea and vomiting*: *see* Nausea and vomiting (p. 113). • *Infection*: treat infection with appropriate antibiotics. • *Odor*: *see* cd-4 in Malignant ulcers and fistulae (p. 111). • *Breathlessness*: *see* Respiratory problems (p. 131). • *Weakness*: exclude reversible causes of weakness (*see* Fatigue, drowsiness, lethargy and weakness (p. 101)). • *Disabled*: regular help with feeding and drinking (ask occupational therapist for advice).
5 Is the feeding tube blocked?	• Check the tube is in the correct position. • Try flushing the tube with 30 ml of warm water, followed if necessary by 30 ml of carbonated water. If still blocked put in 30 ml of pineapple juice and leave for 1 hour before flushing again (annanase will dissolve any protein material). • Avoid drugs that interact with feeds (*see* Drug interactions (pp. 249–50)).
6 Could drugs be the cause?	Consider drugs that cause nausea (e.g. opioids, metronidazole, trimethoprim), mucosal irritation (e.g. NSAIDs, chemotherapy, antibiotics), delayed gastric emptying (e.g. opioids, amitriptyline) or drugs with a central appetite suppressant effect (e.g. opioids, amphetamines): • Reduce the dose, change drug, or stop.
7 Is the food presentation or environment a problem?	**Food:** • Ensure the food is presented attractively on small plates. • Keep portions small, have snacks available, use calorie and protein additives that add little bulk (e.g. Ensure). Vary food consistency, temperature, and taste. • Add 'neutral flavour' supplements to soups, potatoes or desserts. • Ask advice from a dietician and from catering staff. **Environment:** • Ensure a pleasant atmosphere (coffee or baking smells, company without crowding, attractive table cover, possibly alcohol before meals, avoid frying smells). • *If the patient is embarrassed* (e.g. unavoidable dribbling): ensure privacy. • *If cultural food is required* (e.g. Kosher food): ensure this is available.
8 Is anorexia persisting?	• Consider central depression of appetite due to pain (*see* Diagnosing and treating pain (p. 39)). • Consider altered taste due to: *Nutritional deficiency* (zinc, vitamin B complex): supplement might help.[13] *Drugs* (phenytoin, flurazepam). *Dry mouth* (dyspnea, drugs, radiotherapy, chemotherapy): *see* cd-5 in Oral problems (p. 127). *Related conditions* (diabetes, chronic infection, renal failure). • *If all else is inappropriate or fails to improve appetite:* treat empirically with an appetite stimulant, e.g. dexamethasone PO 4 mg once daily,[29] medroxyprogesterone 400 mg daily[37] or megestrol acetate (Megace) 160 mg PO bid to 800 mg PO od (once daily dosing most commonly used in the US). • *If cachexia is present:* consider adding EPA 0.5–1 g/day (found in omega-3 concentrated fish oil).
9 Is thirst still present?	• Moisten mouth frequently. • Consider non-oral hydration: if needed for 3 weeks or less: use IV route or subcutaneous infusion into the suprascapular area (*see* notes). The nasogastric route is a less well tolerated alternative. If needed for 1 month or more: consider percutaneous gastrostomy.[38] *See* also Dysphagia (p. 91).

Adapted from Regnard and Mannix[39]
cd = clinical decision

References

C = comment; Ch = chapter; CS-n = case study-number of cases; CT-n = controlled trial-number of cases; E = editorial; GC = group consensus; I = interviews; Let = letter; LS = laboratory study; MC = multi-center; OS-n = open study-number of cases; R = review; Rep = report; RCT-n = randomized controlled trial-number of cases; RS-n = retrospective survey-number of cases; SA = systematic or meta analysis; Th = thesis.

1 Joint working party of the National Council for Hospice and Palliative Care Services and the ethics committee of the Association for Palliative Medicine of Great Britain and Ireland (1997) Artificial hydration (AH) for people who are terminally ill. *European Journal of Palliative Care.* **4**: 124. (Rep)

2 Dunphy K, Finlay I, Rathbone G, Gilbert J, Hicks F (1995) Rehydration in palliative and terminal care: if not – why not? *Palliative Medicine.* **9**(3): 221–8. (R, 32 refs)

3 Burge FI (1996) Dehydration and provision of fluids in palliative care. What is the evidence? *Canadian Family Physician.* **42**: 2383–8. (SA, 14 refs)

4 Fainsinger RL, Bruera E (1997) When to treat dehydration in a terminally ill patient? *Supportive Care in Cancer.* **5**: 205–11. (R, 54 refs)

5 Lawlor PG, Gagnon B, Mancini IL, Pereira JL, Hanson J, Suarez-Almazor ME, Bruera ED (2000) Occurrence, causes, and outcome of delirium in patients with advanced cancer: a prospective study. *Archives of Internal Medicine.* **160**(6): 786–94. (OS-104)

6 Morita T, Tei Y, Tsunoda J, Inoue S, Chihara S (2001) Determinants of the sensation of thirst in terminally ill cancer patients. *Supportive Care in Cancer.* **9**(3): 177–86. (OS-88)

7 McCann RM, Hall WJ, Groth-Juncker A (1994) Comfort care for terminally ill patients. The appropriate use of nutrition and hydration. *JAMA.* **272**(16): 1263–6. (OS-32)

8 Winter SM (2000) Terminal nutrition: framing the debate for the withdrawal of nutritional support in terminally ill patients. *American Journal of Medicine.* **109**(9): 723–6. (R, 30 refs)

9 Parkash R, Burge F (1997) The family's perspective on issues of hydration in terminal care. *Journal of Palliative Care.* **13**(4): 23–7. (I)

10 Matthews D, Gibson L, Regnard C, Kindlen M (2004) Maintaining the environment for eating and drinking. In: C Regnard (ed) *CLiP (Current Learning in Palliative Care). Helping the Patient with Advanced Disease: a workbook.* Radcliffe Medical Press, Oxford. (Ch)

11 Williams J, Copp G (1990) Food presentation and the terminally ill. *Nursing Standard.* **4**: 29–32.

12 DeWys D (1978) Changes in taste sensation and feeding behaviour in cancer patients: a review.

Journal of Human Nutrition. **32**: 447–53. (R, 16 refs)

13 Moody C (1997) Taste acuity, appetite and zinc status in patients with terminal cancer: BSc thesis in Food and Human Nutrition. University of Newcastle upon Tyne (Department of Biological and Nutritional Sciences). (Th)

14 Matthews D, Gibson L, Regnard C, Kindlen M (2004) Enriching the diet. In: C Regnard (ed) *CLiP (Current Learning in Palliative Care). Helping the Patient with Advanced Disease: a workbook.* Radcliffe Medical Press, Oxford. (Ch)

15 Stratton RJ, Elia M (2000) Are oral nutritional supplements of benefit to patients in the community? Findings from a systematic review. *Current Opinion in Clinical Nutrition & Metabolic Care.* **3**(4): 311–15. (R, 37 refs)

16 Fainsinger RL, MacEachern T, Miller MJ, Bruera E, Spachynski K, Kuehn N, Hanson J (1994) The use of hypodermoclysis for rehydration in terminally ill cancer patients. *Journal of Pain and Symptom Management.* **9**: 298–302. (CT-100)

17 Bruera E, Neumann CM, Pituskin E, Calder K, Hanson J (1999) A randomized controlled trial of local injections of hyaluronidase versus placebo in cancer patients receiving subcutaneous hydration. *Annals of Oncology.* **10**(10): 1255–8. (RCT-21)

18 Regnard CFB (1996) Comparison of concentrations of hyaluronidase. *Journal of Pain and Symptom Management.* **12**: 147. (Let)

19 Bruera E (1996) Comparison of concentrations of hyaluronidase: author's response. *Journal of Pain and Symptom Management.* **12**: 148. (Let)

20 Anker S, Sharma R (2002) The syndrome of cardiac cachexia. *International Journal of Cardiology.* **85**(1): 51. (R)

21 Berry C, Clark AL (2000) Catabolism in chronic heart failure. *European Heart Journal.* **21**(7): 521–32. (R, 187 refs)

22 Walsmith J, Roubenoff R (2002) Cachexia in rheumatoid arthritis. *International Journal of Cardiology.* **85**(1): 89. (R)

23 Plauth M, Schütz E (2002) Cachexia in liver cirrhosis. *International Journal of Cardiology.* **85**(1): 83. (R)

24 Schols A (2002) Pulmonary cachexia. *International Journal of Cardiology.* **85**(1): 101. (R)

25 Strasser F, Bruera E (2002) Mechanism of cancer

cachexia: progress on disentangling a complex problem. *Progress in Palliative Care.* **10**(4): 161–7. (R, 55 refs)

26 Lündstrom S, Fürst CJ (2003) Symptoms in advanced cancer: relationship to endogenous cortisol levels. *Palliative Medicine.* **17**: 503–8. (OS-23)

27 Mercadante S, Fulfaro F, Casuccio A (2001) The use of corticosteroids in home palliative care. *Supportive Care in Cancer.* **9**(5): 386–9. (OS-376)

28 Hardy JR, Rees E, Ling J, Burman R, Feuer D, Broadley K, Stone P (2001) A prospective survey of the use of dexamethasone on a palliative care unit. *Palliative Medicine.* **15**(1): 3–8. (OS-106)

29 Willox JC, Corr J, Shaw J, Richardson M, Calman KC, Drennan M (1984) Prednisolone as an appetite stimulant in patients with cancer. *BMJ.* **288**: 27. (RCT)

30 Maltoni M, Nanni O, Scarpi E, Rossi D, Serra P, Amadori D (2001) High-dose progestins for the treatment of cancer anorexia-cachexia syndrome: a systematic review of randomised clinical trials. *Annals of Oncology.* **12**(3): 289–300. (SA, 50 refs)

31 Loprinzi CL, Kugler JW, Sloan JA, Mailliard JA, Krook JE, Wilwerding MB, Rowland KM Jr, Camoriano JK, Novotny PJ, Christensen BJ (1999) Randomized comparison of megestrol acetate versus dexamethasone versus fluoxymesterone for the treatment of cancer anorexia/cachexia. *Journal of Clinical Oncology.* **17**(10): 3299–306. (RCT)

32 Twycross R, Wilcock A (2001) Alimentary symptoms. In: *Symptom Management in Advanced Cancer* (3e). Radcliffe Medical Press, Oxford. (Ch)

33 Barber MD, Fearon KC, Tisdale MJ, McMillan DC, Ross JA (2001) Effect of a fish oil-enriched nutritional supplement on metabolic mediators in patients with pancreatic cancer cachexia. *Nutrition & Cancer.* **40**(2): 118–24. (OS-20)

34 Davis MP, Dickerson ED (2001) Thalidomide: dual benefits in palliative medicine and oncology. *American Journal of Hospice & Palliative Care.* **18**(5): 347–51. (R, 56 refs)

35 Jatoi A, Loprinzi CL (2001) An update: cancer-associated anorexia as a treatment target. *Current Opinion in Clinical Nutrition & Metabolic Care.* **4**(3): 179–82. (R, 17 refs)

36 Poole K, Froggatt K (2002) Loss of weight and loss of appetite in advanced cancer: a problem for the patient, the carer or the health professional? *Palliative Medicine.* **16**(6): 499–506. (SA, 53 refs)

37 Downer S, Joel S, Allbright A, Plant H, Stubbs L, Talbot D, Slevin M (1993) A double blind placebo controlled trial of medroxyprogesterone acetate (MPA) in cancer cachexia. *British Journal of Cancer.* **67**: 1102–5. (RCT-60)

38 Hull MA, Rawlings J, Murray FE, Field J, McIntyre AS, Mahida YR, Hawkey CJ, Allison SP (1993) Audit of outcome of long-term enteral nutrition by percutaneous endoscopic gastrostomy. *Lancet.* **341**: 869–72. (OS-49)

39 Regnard C, Mannix K (1995) Reduced hydration and feeding. In: *Flow Diagrams in Advanced Cancer and Other Diseases.* Edward Arnold, London. pp. 25–8. (Ch)

Oral problems

Clinical decision and action checklist

1 Is oral health at risk?
2 Is an ulcer present?
3 Is the mouth dirty?
4 Is the mouth painful?
5 Is the mouth dry?
6 Is there too much saliva?

Key points

- A healthy mouth has an intact mucosa and is clean, moist and pain-free.
- Regular mouth care will prevent many oral problems.
- Candidosis and dry mouth are the two commonest problems.

Introduction

Poor oral hygiene may be due to a reduced fluid intake, mouth breathing when asleep and reduced host immunity. Maintaining oral hygiene is very important to reduce infections and treatment-induced mucositis.[1-3] A soft toothbrush will gently clean coated tongues and teeth, but foam sticks or gauze are less effective.[4-6] Irrigation with warm water or 0.9% saline will help removal of oral debris, and is soothing and non-traumatic.[7] Some other solutions have problems such as an unpleasant taste, exhausting the salivary glands, or causing damage to the teeth or the mucosa.[6-9] The frequency of oral care depends on the circumstances (*see* cd-1 in the table on p. 127).

Managing oral problems

Apthous ulcers

These painful, shallow ulcers are common and can be associated with autoimmune diseases, immunodeficiency and deficiency of iron, folate or vitamin B$_{12}$.[10] Topical corticosteroids or tetracycline can help. Thalidomide (special access category in North America) has a role in treating persistent ulceration in adults and children and has been shown to be well tolerated, although its potential for causing birth defects remains.[11–15]

Candidosis

This may present as white semi-adherent plaques, a red tongue or angular chelitis. It may be present in stomatitis secondary to radiation or chemotherapy, or related to the use of dentures.[16–18] The type of candidosis depends on the candida species and local immunity.[19] Candida is in the mouths of up to two-thirds of cancer and AIDS patients, especially those with a dry mouth and dentures,[20–22] but there is no association with using systemic steroids or antibiotics.[20,23] Cross-infection does not easily occur by way of cups and cutlery but may occur by way of carers' hands.[24] Prophylactic nystatin does not reduce the incidence of positive mouth swabs,[24] but in AIDS patients long-term therapy with systemic antifungals may be necessary.

Antifungals: All candida species are sensitive to nystatin or amphotericin, but to be effective patients must take them q6h for up to 10 days and avoid eating or drinking for 30 minutes.[25] Ketoconazole 200 mg once daily rapidly clears candidal plaques,[26] is more convenient to the patient and cheaper than one week with nystatin. Serious adverse effects with ketoconazole are rare,[27] and low-dose ketoconazole long-term is well tolerated.[28] (In the US, though, ketoconazole PO/IV is not commonly used in the palliative care setting due to its potential for hepatotoxicity (Black Box warning) and interactions with H$_2$ blockers, proton pump inhibitors, and other medications often used in palliative patients.)[63] Fluconazole is effective in a single dose,[26] making it useful in patients with a short prognosis, but is more expensive than other antifungals. Fluconazole is used for longer-term prophylaxis in AIDS patients, with itraconazole as second line.[29] Systemic antifungals interact with several drugs used in palliative care (*see* Drug interactions (pp. 241–242)). Topical ketoconazole is a more effective alternative than nystatin.[30]

Chlorhexidine also has antifungal activity[31] but it inactivates nystatin if used together.[32] Up to 24% of strains are resistant to some systemic antifungals, but the risk of resistance developing may be reduced if short courses are used.[33,34]

Children: With topical antifungals in babies it is usual to treat both the mouth and perineum at the same time. In older children, single dose fluconazole is often used.

Dry mouth

This is very common in advanced cancer and drugs are a common cause.[35–38]

Artificial salivas: Glycerin dehydrates the mucosa[39] and should be avoided. All acidic salivas should be avoided. Moi-Stir (Canada only), Saliva Substitute (US) and Salivart have a pH between 6.5 and 7.5 and are acceptable. But these salivas only last 10–15 minutes and may be little better than placebo,[40] and frequent sprays with water may be just as effective.

Chewing gum is as effective as artificial salivas.[41]

Pilocarpine in low doses is as effective as artificial saliva in low doses in cancer patients, but it can cause sweating, dizziness and rhinorrhoea.[42] The evidence for improvement with pilocarpine after radiotherapy is conflicting.[43,44] Pilocarpine 4% eye drops taken orally are one-tenth the cost of pilocarpine tablets,[45] and lower doses can be used. Bethanocol may be a better alternative.[46]

Acupuncture may help in resistant cases.[47]

Oral pain relief

Some topical agents can offer mucosal protection. Carmellose (Orabase) paste is an effective protective for local lesions. There is no evidence that benzydamine, sucralfate or chlorhexidine ease oral pain.[48–50] Choline salicylate gel can help but can cause pain on application. In the US, gel preparation can be obtained via a Compounding Pharmacy. Lidocaine (cream, gel or spray) can help acutely painful lesions at the expense of numbness, but toxicity has been reported with frequent use.[51] In very severe pain, systemic analgesia is required. Topical opioids may help, but in very severe pain systemic opioids are required. Ketamine may have a role in extensive mucositis.[64]

Neurologically impaired children

Teething can present in unusual ways in these children, such as an increase in seizures. Dental caries is also common in this population and regular oral hygiene and checks are important.

Clinical decision	If YES ⇒ Action

1 **Is oral health at risk?** (any patient with advanced disease, neurological impairment and/or undergoing anticancer treatment)	• Twice daily: brush the teeth with fluoride-containing toothpaste and rinse with a fluoride mouthwash.
	• Throughout the day: rinse the mouth regularly with water or 0.9% saline, and provide adequate hydration. Clear debris from teeth and tongue with a soft toothbrush. Frequency of oral care:[52]
	  (a) general care: 4–6-hourly (after meals)
	  (b) prevention of oral problems: 2-hourly
	  (c) patients at high risk or with severe problems (e.g. oxygen therapy, oral infections, coma, severe mucositis, dehydration, immunosuppression, diabetes): hourly.

2 **Is an ulcer present?**	• *Viral* (zoster or herpes simplex): oral acyclovir 200 mg q4h for 1 week (400 mg if immunosuppressed). • *Apthous ulcers:* exclude deficiencies of iron, folate and B$_{12}$. Try topical corticosteroid (triamcinolone in Orabase[53,54]) or tetracycline mouthwash[55] (disperse the contents of a 250 mg capsule in water, rinse for 2 mins then swallow q6h). Persistent and severe ulcers may respond to thalidomide 50–300 mg/day (in children 1 mg/kg/week to 1 mg/kg/day). Check precautions for prescribing thalidomide.[56] (Special access category in North America.) • *Malignant ulcers:* Anaerobic infection causing halitosis – *see* cd-3 below. For bleeding use sucralfate suspension 1 g (5 ml) diluted with 5 ml water as a mouthwash (also *see* Bleeding (p. 67)).

3 **Is the mouth dirty?**	• Clean the tongue: gently brush with a soft toothbrush. Chewing pineapple (fresh or tinned, unsweetened) may help remove debris.
	Clean the mucosa: helped by rinsing frequently with water or 0.9% saline.
	• *If candidosis is the cause* (white patches, thick debris):
	  1 Try nystatin or amphotericin suspension. Treat any dryness (*see* cd-5 below). In babies treat the mouth and perineum simultaneously.
	  2 If topical antifungals are not tolerated or there is no response, start ketoconazole (not commonly used in the US) 200 mg once daily for 5 days. For a longer course or in children use fluconazole 50 mg daily.[57,58] If systemic antifungals are not tolerated, consider ketoconazole 40 mg q12h as a mouthwash. If compliance is difficult, give fluconazole 150 mg as a single dose.
	• *If halitosis is due to local tumor:* start metronidazole 250 mg PO tid for 5–7 days, then continue with 500 mg PO qd. If adverse effects are a problem, rinse the mouth with metronidazole suspension 400 mg (10 ml) and spit out.

4 **Is the mouth painful?**	• *If the pain is localized:* Topical analgesia: choline salicylate gel (0.5 ml or less topically). Available as Teejel in Canada. In the US, gel preparation can be obtained via a compounding pharmacy. Protection: carmellose paste (Orabase). Exclude candida: a red, painful mouth may be caused by acute or chronic erythematous candidosis in the absence of white patches. • *If the pain is extensive:* Topical analgesia: benzocaine lozenges (Bionet), lidocaine spray, gel or cream, or acetaminophen suspension as a mouthwash. Consider: topical morphine (5 mg morphine in hydrogel).[59–61] Alternatively, start or increase systemic oral morphine.

5 **Is the mouth dry?** (dry mucosa, difficulty swallowing and talking)	• Treat the cause if possible (e.g. drugs, dehydration, oral infection, anxiety).
	• Use local measures such as frequent sprays or sips of cold water, sucking ice-cubes or applying petroleum jelly to lips. Avoid acidic solutions (e.g. fruit juices, 'Oral Balance'). Chewing gum may help.
	• Consider:
	  1 Artificial salivas, e.g. Moi-Stir, Moisturel, Salivart.
	  2 Pilocarpine 4% eye drop solution; 2–3 drops or 5 mg tablets PO q8h. Bethanecol 10–25 mg PO q8h if side-effects are a problem. Do not use pilocarpine or bethanecol in patients with bowel obstruction, asthma, glaucoma, cardiovascular disease or COPD.

6 **Is there too much saliva?** (leakage from the mouth)	• *If there is difficulty clearing saliva: see* Dysphagia (p. 91).
	• Try hyoscine hydrobromide/scopolamine sublingually (Canada only) (75–150 mcg q8–12h) or transdermally (scopolamine patch, US and Canada (1.5 mg/72 hrs)). For doses in children *see* Drugs in palliative care for children: starting doses (p. 253). For thick secretions, *see* cd-4 in Respiratory problems (p. 133).
	• Radiotherapy to salivary glands – 1 Gy followed if needed 4 weeks later by a further 1 Gy.

Adapted from Regnard and Fitton[62]
cd = clinical decision

References

B = book; C = comment; Ch = chapter; CS-n = case study-number of cases; CT-n = controlled trial-number of cases; E = editorial; GC = group consensus; I = interviews; Let = letter; LS = laboratory study; MC = multi-center; OS-n = open study-number of cases; R = review; RCT-n = randomized controlled trial-number of cases; RS-n = retrospective survey-number of cases; SA = systematic or meta analysis.

1 Cheng KK, Molassiotis A, Chang AM, Wai WC, Cheung SS (2001) Evaluation of an oral care protocol intervention in the prevention of chemotherapy-induced oral mucositis in paediatric cancer patients. *European Journal of Cancer.* **37**(16): 2056–63. (CT-42)

2 Larson PJ, Miaskowski C, MacPhail L, Dodd MJ, Greenspan D, Dibble SL, Paul SM, Ignoffo R (1998) The PRO-SELF Mouth Aware program: an effective approach for reducing chemotherapy-induced mucositis. *Cancer Nursing.* **21**(4): 263–8. (R, 44 refs)

3 Xavier G (2000) The importance of mouth care in preventing infection. *Nursing Standard.* **14**(18): 47–51. (R, 16 refs)

4 Sammon P, Page C, Shepherd G (1987) Oral hygiene. *Nursing Times.* **83**: 25–7.

5 Howarth H (1977) Mouth care procedures for the very ill. *Nursing Times.* **73**(10): 354–5.

6 Evans G (2001) A rationale for oral care. *Nursing Standard.* **15**(43): 33–6. (R, 43 refs)

7 Miller M, Kearney N (2001) Oral care for patients with cancer: a review of the literature. *Cancer Nursing.* **24**(4): 241–54. (R, 100 refs)

8 Pritchard P, Walker VA (1984) Mouth care. In: P Pritchard, VA Walker (eds) *Manual of Clinical Nursing Policies and Procedures: the Royal Marsden Hospital.* Harper and Row, London. pp. 273–84. (Ch)

9 Davis W, Winter P (1980) The effect of abrasion on enamel and dentine after exposure to dietary acid. *British Dental Journal.* **148**: 11–12, 253–6. (OS)

10 Scully C, Shotts R (2000) ABC of oral health: mouth ulcers and other causes of orofacial soreness and pain. *BMJ.* **321**: 162–5. (R)

11 Grover JK, Vats V, Gopalakrishna R, Ramam M (2000) Thalidomide: a re-look. *National Medical Journal of India.* **13**(3): 132–41. (R, 150 refs)

12 Jacobson JM, Greenspan JS, Spritzler J, Ketter N, Fahey JL, Jackson JB, Fox L, Chernoff M, Wu AW, MacPhail LA, Vasquez GJ, Wohl DA (1997) Thalidomide for the treatment of oral aphthous ulcers in patients with human immunodeficiency virus infection. National Institute of Allergy and Infectious Diseases AIDS Clinical Trials Group. *New England Journal of Medicine.* **336**(21): 1487–93. (RCT-20)

13 Kari JA, Shah V, Dillon MJ (2001) Behçet's disease in UK children: clinical features and treatment including thalidomide. *Rheumatology.* **40**(8): 933–8. (RS-10)

14 Wohl DA, Aweeka FT, Pomerantz R, Cherng DW *et al.* (2002) Safety, tolerability, and pharmacokinetic effects of thalidomide in patients infected with human immunodeficiency virus: AIDS Clinical Trials Group 267. *Journal of Infectious Diseases.* **185**(9): 1359–63. (CT-36)

15 Peuckmann V, Fisch M, Bruera E (2000) Potential novel uses on the use on thalidomide: focus on palliative care. *Drugs.* **60**: 273–93. (R)

16 Sammon P, Page C, Shepherd G (1987) Oral hygiene. *Nursing Times.* **83**: 25–7. (Ch)

17 Dorko E, Jenca A, Pilipcinec E, Danko J, Svicky E, Tkacikova L (2001) Candida-associated denture stomatitis. *Folia Microbiologica.* **46**(5): 443–6. (OS-240)

18 Bagg J (2003) Oral candidosis: how to treat a common problem. *European Journal of Palliative Care.* **10**(2): 54–6. (R, 23 refs)

19 Reichart PA, Samaranayake LP, Philipsen HP (2000) Pathology and clinical correlates in oral candidiasis and its variants: a review. *Oral Diseases.* **6**(2): 85–91. (R, 51 refs)

20 Davies AN, Brailsford S, Broadley K, Beighton D (2002) Oral yeast carriage in patients with advanced cancer. *Oral Microbiology & Immunology.* **17**(2): 79–84. (OS-120)

21 Campisi G, Pizzo G, Milici ME, Mancuso S, Margiotta V (2002) Candidal carriage in the oral cavity of human immunodeficiency virus-infected subjects. *Oral Surgery, Oral Medicine, Oral Pathology, Oral Radiology & Endodontics.* **93**(3): 281–6. (OS-83)

22 Finlay IG (1986) Oral symptoms and candida in the terminally ill. *BMJ.* **292**: 592–3. (OS)

23 Torres SR, Peixoto CB, Caldas DM, Silva EB, Akiti T, Nucci M, de Vzeda M (2002) Relationship between salivary flow rates and candida counts in subjects with xerostomia. *Oral Surgery, Oral Medicine, Oral Pathology, Oral Radiology & Endodontics.* **93**(2): 149–54.

24 Burnie JP, Odds FC, Lee W, Webster C, Williams JD (1985) Outbreak of systemic *Candida albicans* in intensive care unit caused by cross-infection. *BMJ.* **290**: 746–8. (OS-55)

25 Boon JM, Lafeber HN, Mannetje AH, van Olphen AH, Smeets HL, Toorman J, van der Vlist GJ (1989) Comparison of ketoconazole with nystatin in the treatment of newborns and infants with oral candidosis. *Mycosis.* **32**: 312–15. (OS-35)

26 Regnard CFB (1994) Single dose fluconazole versus five day ketoconazole in oral candidiasies. *Palliative Medicine.* **8**: 72–3. (OS-100)

27 Hay RJ (1985) Ketoconazole: a reappraisal. *BMJ.* **290**: 260–1. (E)

28 Harris KA, Weinberg V, Bok RA, Kakefuda M, Small EJ (2002) Low dose ketoconazole with replacement doses of hydrocortisone in patients with progressive androgen independent prostate cancer. *Journal of Urology.* **168**(2): 542–5. (OS-28)

29 Ball K, Sweeney MP, Baxter WP, Bagg J (1998) Fluconazole sensitivities of *Candida* species isolated from the mouths of terminally ill cancer patients. *American Journal of Hospice & Palliative Care.* **15**(6): 315–19. (OS-30)

30 Cornejo LS, Lopez de Blanc S, Femopase F, Azcurra A, Calamari S, Battellino LJ, Dorronsoro de Cattoni ST (1998) Evolution of saliva and serum components in

patients with oral candidosis topically treated with Ketoconazole and Nystatin. *Acta Odontologica Latinoamericana.* **11**(1): 15–25. (RCT-20)

31 Ellepola AN, Samaranayake LP (2001) Adjunctive use of chlorhexidine in oral candidoses: a review. *Oral Diseases.* **7**(1): 11–17. (R, 74 refs)

32 Barkvoll P, Attramadal A (1989) Effect of nystatin and chlorhexidine digluconate on *Candida albicans. Oral Surgery, Oral Medicine and Oral Pathology.* **67**(3): 279–81. (OS)

33 Davies A, Brailsford S, Broadley K, Beighton D (2002) Resistence amongst yeasts isolated from the oral cavities of patients with advanced cancer. *Palliative Medicine.* **16**(3): 527–31. (OS-70)

34 Bagg J, Sweeney MP, Lewis MAD, Jackson MS, Coleman D, Al Mosaid A, Baxter W *et al.* (2003) High prevalence of non-albicans yeasts and detection of anti-fungal resistence in the flora of patients with advanced cancer. *Palliative Medicine.* **17**: 477–81. (OS-207)

35 Sweeney MP, Bagg J, Baxter WP, Aitchison TC (1998) Oral disease in terminally ill cancer patients with xerostomia. *Oral Oncology.* **34**(2): 123–6. (OS-70)

36 Mercadante S (2002) Dry mouth and palliative care. *European Journal of Palliative Care.* **9**(5): 182–5. (R, 10 refs)

37 Davies AN, Broadley K, Beighton D (2002) Salivary gland hypofunction in patients with advanced cancer. *Oral Oncology.* **38**(7): 680–5. (OS-120)

38 Davies AN, Broadley K, Beighton D (2001) Xerostomia in patients with advanced cancer. *Journal of Pain and Symptom Management.* **22**(4): 820–5. (OS-120)

39 Van Drimmelen J, Rollins HF (1969) Evaluation of a commonly used oral hygiene agent. *Nursing Research.* **18**: 327–32.

40 Sweeney MP, Bagg J, Baxter WP, Aitchison TC (1997) Clinical trial of a mucin-containing oral spray for treatment of xerostomia in hospice patients. *Palliative Medicine.* **11**: 225–32. (RCT-31)

41 Oneschuk D, Hanson J, Bruera E (2000) A survey of mouth pain and dryness in patients with advanced cancer. *Supportive Care in Cancer.* **8**(5): 372–6. (RCT)

42 Davies AN, Daniels C, Pugh R, Sharma K (1998) A comparison of artificial saliva and pilocarpine in the management of xerostomia in patients with advanced cancer. *Palliative Medicine.* **12**(2): 105–11. (MC, RCT)

43 Haddad P, Karimi M (2002) A randomized, double-blind, placebo-controlled trial of concomitant pilocarpine with head and neck irradiation for prevention of radiation-induced xerostomia. *Radiotherapy & Oncology.* **64**(1): 29. (RCT-60)

44 Warde P, O'Sullivan B, Aslanidis J, Kroll B, Lockwood G, Waldron J, Payne D, Bayley A, Ringash J, Kim J, Liu FF, Maxymiw W, Sprague S, Cummings BJ (2002) A Phase III placebo-controlled trial of oral pilocarpine in patients undergoing radiotherapy for head-and-neck cancer. *International Journal of Radiation Oncology, Biology, Physics.* **54**(1): 9–13. (RCT-130)

45 Twycross RG, Wilcock A, Charlesworth S (2002) *PCF2: Palliative Care Formulary* (2e). Radcliffe Medical Press, Oxford. (B)

46 Davies AN (June 2003) *Oral Medicine.* Lecture given at Advanced Course in Pain and Symptom Management. Newcastle upon Tyne. Organized by Oxford International Centre for Palliative Care.

47 Johnstone PA, Peng YP, May BC, Inouye WS, Niemtzow RC (2001) Acupuncture for pilocarpine-resistant xerostomia following radiotherapy for head and neck

malignancies. *International Journal of Radiation Oncology, Biology, Physics.* **50**(2): 353–7. (OS-18)

48 Chiara S, Nobile MT, Vincenti M, Gozza A, Pastrone I, Rosso M, Rosso R (2001) Sucralfate in the treatment of chemotherapy-induced stomatitis: a double-blind, placebo-controlled pilot study. *Anticancer Research.* **21**(5): 3707–10. (RCT-40)

49 Loprinzi CL, Ghosh C, Camoriano J, Sloan J, Steen PD, Michalak JC, Schaefer PL, Novotny PJ, Gerstner JB, White DF, Hatfield AK, Quella SK (1997) Phase III controlled evaluation of sucralfate to alleviate stomatitis in patients receiving fluorouracil-based chemotherapy. *Journal of Clinical Oncology.* **15**(3): 1235–8. (RCT-131)

50 Worthington HV, Clarkson JE, Eden OB (2002) Interventions for treating oral mucositis for patients with cancer receiving treatment. *Cochrane Database of Systematic Reviews.* **1**: CD001973. (SA, 30 refs)

51 Yamashita S, Sat S, Kakiuchi Y, Miyabe M, Yamaguchi H (2002) Lidocaine toxicity during frequent viscous lidocaine use for painful tongue ulcer. *Journal of Pain and Symptom Management.* **24**(6): 543–5. (CS-1)

52 Krishnasamy M (1995) Oral problems in advanced cancer. *European Journal of Cancer Care.* **4**: 173–7. (R, 100 refs)

53 Zegarelli EV, Kutschner AH, Silvers HF *et al.* (1960) Triamcinalone acetonide in the treatment of acute and chronic lesions of the oral mucous membranes. *Oral Surgery.* **13**: 170–5.

54 Miles DA, Bricker SL, Razmus TF, Potter RH (1993) Triamcinolone acetonide versus chlorhexidine for treatment of recurrent stomatitis. *Oral Surgery, Oral Medicine, Oral Pathology.* **75**(3): 397–402. (RCT-20)

55 Graykowski EA, Kingman A (1978) Double blind trial of tetracycline in recurrent aphthous ulceration. *Journal of Oral Pathology.* **7**: 376–82. (CT-25)

56 Twycross R, Wilcock A, Charlesworth S, Dickman A (2003) Thalidomide. In: *PCF2: Palliative Care Formulary.* Radcliffe Medical Press, Oxford. pp. 237–9 (also on www.palliativedrugs.com).

57 Patton LL, Bonito AJ, Shugars DA (2001) A systematic review of the effectiveness of antifungal drugs for the prevention and treatment of oropharyngeal candidiasis in HIV-positive patients. *Oral Surgery, Oral Medicine, Oral Pathology, Oral Radiology & Endodontics.* **92**(2): 170–9. (SA, 33 refs)

58 Samonis G, Rolston K, Karl C, Miller P, Bodey GP (1990) Prophylaxis of oropharyngeal candidiasis with fluconazole. *Reviews of Infectious Diseases.* **12**(Suppl3): S369–73. (RCT-112)

59 Back IN, Finlay I (1995) Analgesic effect of topical opioids on painful skin ulcers. *Journal of Pain and Symptom Management.* **10**: 493. (Let)

60 Krajnik M, Zylicz Z (1997) Topical morphine for cutaneous cancer pain. *Palliative Medicine.* **11**: 325–6. (CS-6)

61 Twillman RK, Long TD, Cathers TA, Mueller DW (1999) Treatment of painful skin ulcers with topical opioids. *Journal of Pain and Symptom Management.* **17**(4): 288–92. (CS-9)

62 Regnard C, Fitton S (1995) Mouth care. In: *Flow Diagrams in Advanced Cancer and Other Diseases.* Edward Arnold, London. pp. 22–4. (Ch)

63 *Physicians' Desk Reference* (2004) 58th Edition, pp. 1757–9.

64 Slatkin NE, Rhiner M (2003) Topical ketamine in the treatment of mucositis pain. *Pain Med.* **4**: 298–303.

Respiratory problems

Clinical decision and action checklist

1 If the patient is breathless, call for help and start simple measures.
2 Is the patient hypoxic or hypercapnic?
3 Has the problem developed rapidly?
4 Are airway secretions causing distress?
5 Is infection present?
6 Are hiccups present?
7 Has the breathlessness developed slowly?
8 Is a dry cough present?
9 Is the breathlessness persisting?

Key points

- Breathlessness is what the patient says it is.
- Breathlessness can be frightening, and managing the fear is essential.
- Simple measures are often helpful for breathlessness.
- Much treatment is conventional and logical.
- Other symptoms such as cough, secretions and hiccups can be eased.

Introduction

Breathlessness is the commonest respiratory problem. It is common in advanced disease, being present in 94% of chronic lung disease, 83% of heart failure patients and up to 70% of cancer patients, but it is also common in dementia, multiple sclerosis and AIDS.[1-8] Other respiratory problems include airway secretions, cough and hiccups.

Assessment

For many respiratory problems a clear history and bedside examination provide most of the information. Standard dyspnea assessments and tests like spirometry do not reflect the effect of breathlessness on the patient.[9-13] Patients describe breathlessness in their own way.[14] Like pain, breathlessness is what the patient says it is. Apart from emergencies, much of the evaluation is about eliciting the patient's concerns, since fear, anxiety and low mood are common companions to breathlessness (*see* Helping the person to share their problems (p. 17)).

Urgent management

Breathlessness is the commonest respiratory problem requiring urgent help. For details of causes and treatments *see* cd-6 in Emergencies (pp. 209 and 211). Simple measures can be offered by any carer (*see* cd-1 opposite).[15-18] It needs a minimum of two carers, one to ensure that the assessment of the cause begins, and the other to start the simple measures to help the patient. Mild facial cooling reduces breathlessness and discomfort.[19,20] Sitting upright increases peak ventilation and reduces airway obstruction.[21-23] Relaxing and dropping the shoulders improves ventilation by reducing the 'hunching' that occurs with anxiety. This can be helped by a carer gently massaging the shoulders whilst standing behind or to one side. This gives the carer a helpful role, is comforting to the patient and avoids the increase in anxiety caused by eye-to-eye contact. Being with a patient is essential during the fear of breathlessness.

Hypoxia is not always accompanied by cyanosis and a pulse oximeter is invaluable to confirm hypoxia in the absence of cyanosis.[24] If the oxygen saturation (S_aO_2) is 90% or less, a trial of oxygen is indicated. The highest concentration available should be used, unless chronic hypercapnia is present (*see* hypercapnia below).

Airway obstruction needs urgent treatment. Stridor due to local tumor blocking the trachea is uncommon but is an emergency (*see* cd-6g in Emergencies (p. 211)). Generalized bronchoconstriction will respond to inhaled bronchodilators using a spacer device. Nebulizers deliver much larger doses that may cause adverse effects, but a nebulizer may be needed in weak patients or for severe bronchospasm. The use of mouthpieces with nebulizers is better tolerated and more effective than face masks.[25] Bronchodilators will have little effect on breathlessness caused by widespread intrapulmonary cancer.

Hypercapnia: This is most commonly seen in chronic respiratory failure due to conditions such as neuromuscular disease (e.g. motor neurone disease, muscular dystrophy) or primary respiratory disease (e.g. COPD – chronic obstructive pulmonary disease). Some of these patients are dependent on some hypoxia to stimulate respiration. If they are given oxygen above 24% their hypercapnia will worsen and they will go into rapid respiratory failure. If in doubt, it is best to restrict oxygen in these patients to 24%.

Heart failure needs urgent treatment even when the prognosis is very limited (hours or days), since the consequent agitation and bronchial secretions will be distressing to patient, family and staff. A common cause is a terminally ill patient being nursed flat, and such patients will be less breathless sitting upright or lying at a 45° angle.

Pulmonary emboli can cause distressing pain and breathlessness. The standard practice is to anticoagulate,[26] but in patients with advanced malignancy full anticoagulation causes new problems with bleeding or unstable anticoagulation control.[27] A compromise is to use low molecular weight heparin that, in low doses, needs no monitoring and can be given once daily.[28] Preventing recurrent emboli with an inferior vena caval filter can help a few patients, although much of the evidence for this is based on small numbers.[29]

Thick airway secretions need to be loosened. If nebulized saline is insufficient, alternatives are oral (if aged >14 years) or nebulized N-acetylcysteine[30] or nebulized Dornase alfa.[31]

Loose airway secretions at the end of life can be a problem in 23% of patients in the last hours, or occasionally days, of their life.[32] Most comatose patients seem unaware of its presence, but it is distressing for relatives and staff[33] and the family will need reassurance. Antimuscarinic drugs will help secretions due to accumulation of saliva, but are probably less helpful for secretions due to lung pathology.[34] Hyoscine butylbromide (Canada) (hyoscyamine in US) is cheap, widely available, but short-acting. Hyoscine hydrobromide is more sedating and longer lasting.[35] In the US it is available as scopolamine transdermal patch. An injection preparation, i.e. scopolamine SC, can be obtained but it is not readily available and not widely used. Glycopyrrolate may not act as quickly as hyoscine hydrobromide, but is cheaper and less sedating.[36,37] Antimuscarinic drugs only reduce 50% of secretions and gentle suction may be needed. Parenteral antibiotics can ease distressing sputum due to a chest infection at the end of life,[38] and infected secretions will respond to a single injection of a long-acting, broad-spectrum cephalosporin.[39-41]

Clinical decision	If YES ⇒ Action
1	**If the patient is breathless, call for help and start simple measures:** • sit the patient upright and increase air movement over the patient's face (fan, open window) • encourage the patient to relax and lower the shoulders since this reduces the 'hunching' caused by anxiety • explain what is happening and stay with the patient.
2 Is the patient hypoxic or hypercapnic?	• Confirm hypoxia with a pulse oximeter if available (the absence of cyanosis does not exclude hypoxia). If S_aO_2 is < 90% start oxygen (100% via face mask, 24% if previous pulmonary disease with CO_2 retention) for 30 mins. Continue working through the clinical decisions. • *If hypercapnia is present:* exclude drug-induced ventilatory failure (*see* cd-3 in Emergencies (p. 205)). If symptoms are distressing consider referral for investigation and possibility of non-invasive ventilation (*see* notes (p. 135)).
3 Has the problem developed rapidly? (minutes to hours)	**Treatments for most of these causes are in cd-6 in Emergencies (pp. 209 and 211).** • *Airway obstruction:* Rasping or wheeze from the upper airway suggests stridor due to an inhaled object or upper airway compression: *see* cd-6g in Emergencies (p. 211). Edema of the face with distended neck and arm veins suggests SVC obstruction: *see* cd-9d in Emergencies (p. 214). Generalized wheeze on auscultation suggests bronchospasm (e.g. asthma) but in severe cases, wheeze will be absent: *see* cd-6e in Emergencies (pp. 209 and 211). • *Heart failure:* history of breathlessness on lying flat (orthopnea). Crepitations in both lung bases, peripheral edema or both: *see* cd-6d in Emergencies (p. 209). • *Poor ventilation due to pain* (e.g. pleurisy, rib fracture or spinal metastases) causes patients to 'catch' their breath to prevent the pain: *see* cd-3d in Diagnosing and treating pain (p. 41). • *'Air hunger'* causes a gasping type of respiration: Hyperventilation due to diabetic ketoacidosis: *see* cd-7c in Emergencies (p. 211). Terminal gasping in the last stages of life: *see* cd-6b in Emergencies (p. 209). • *Breathlessness due to reduced lung capacity:* Pleural effusion causes increasing breathlessness, trachea sometimes deviated away from the effusion, dullness and reduced air entry on the same side. *See* cd-6f in Emergencies (p. 211). Pneumothorax causes acute breathlessness, trachea deviated towards same side as the collapsed lung, hollow chest on percussion but reduced or absent breath sounds: *see* cd-6c in Emergencies (p. 209). Pericardial effusion causes raised PR, BP is maintained initially, poor pulse volume that reduces on inspiration (an exaggeration of normal), cold skin, pallor: refer urgently for drainage. • *Pulmonary embolism* (breathlessness not relieved by sitting up, increased respiratory rate, chest sounds are normal, there may be chest pain and signs of a peripheral thrombosis): Sudden collapse suggests a massive embolism from which recovery is unlikely. Otherwise: treat symptomatically with oxygen and analgesia (opioids, intercostal block) and check D-dimers to confirm the diagnosis. Start low molecular weight heparin 2000–3000 units SC once daily. If recurrent emboli are suspected, arrange a perfusion scan and consider referral for a vena caval filter. • If the patient is panicking: *see* cd-4 in Emergencies (p. 207). • If anxiety is present: *see* Anxiety (p. 165).
4 Are airway secretions causing distress?	• Start respiratory exercises with a physiotherapist if the patient is well enough. • *If the sputum is thick and difficult to cough up:* use hypertonic saline 6% 4 ml nebulized q12h. Consider propranolol 40 mg q12h.[92,93] Alternatively, try acetylcysteine 200 mg PO q8h (if over 14 years) or nebulized 10% solution or Dornase alfa 2500 U by jet nebulizer once daily. • *If the sputum is thin and loose* (e.g. bronchorrhea due to alveolar cell carcinoma): try hyoscine hydrobromide transdermal patch (Canada) or scopolamine patch (US). If the problem persists, try nebulized terbutaline,[42] or nebulized indomethacin 25 mg in 2 ml 0.9% saline (pH adjusted with sodium bicarbonate) q6h.[43] Octreotide SC may be an alternative systemic treatment. • *If secretions continue to be a problem* consider these causes: aspiration (*see* Dysphagia (p. 91)), chest infection, tracheo-esophageal fistula. • *If there are retained secretions at the end of life:* give glycopyrrolate 0.4 mg SC (or hyoscine hydrobromide/scopolamine 400 microgram SC if sedation needed) q2h PRN, or scopolamine patch in the US. If no improvement, reposition the patient on one side and with upper body elevated. Consider suction with a soft catheter. If the secretions are infected, consider a single dose of 500 mg ceftriaxone SC (mix with 1 ml lidocaine to reduce local pain).[39,41] Repeat only if symptoms recur.

Table continued overleaf

5	**Is infection present?**	• *If the patient is deteriorating day by day due to underlying disease:* No symptoms due to the infection: no action is required. Symptoms due to the infection: treat fever with cooling and acetaminophen 1 g PO or PR, reduce secretions with hyoscine, hyoscyamine, scopolamine or glycopyrrolate, ease pain with analgesics. Persistent symptoms of infection (e.g. profuse sputum): give single dose of 500 mg ceftriaxone SC (mix with 0.5 ml lidocaine to reduce local pain).[39,41] Repeat only if symptoms recur. • *For all other patients:* start amoxicillin or erythromycin PO (if immunocompromised or this is a persistent infection, send sputum for microbiology). If the infection responds poorly or briefly to repeated courses, try colistin (Canada only) 0.5–1 million units nebulized q12h, or gentamicin 80–120 mg nebulized q12h. • *For Pneumocystis carinii* (PCP) in AIDS start high dose co-trimoxazole (20/100 mg/kg q6–8h) for 2 weeks (will cause rash, gastritis and neutropenia), or nebulized pentamidine (600 mg daily) for 3 weeks. If hypoxia is present, add prednisolone 40 mg q12h for 5 days on a reducing dosage. For maintenance use co-trimoxazole 160/800 mg daily.
6	**Are hiccups present?**	• *If gastric stasis or a 'squashed stomach syndrome' is present:* start metoclopramide or domperidone (in US only available from Compound Pharmacies) (*see* cd-2 in Nausea and vomiting (p. 115)). • Treat ascites if present: *see* Ascites (p. 63). • Try simple measures, e.g. rebreathing from paper bag. • *If hiccups are persisting:* start baclofen 5 mg q8h, and titrate if necessary.[83,84] • *If hiccups are severe:* try midazolam 2–10 mg titrated IV.[85] If persistent, alternatives are nifedipine 10 mg q12h, or sodium valproate 200–400 mg q12h.[59]
7	**Has the breathlessness developed slowly?** (days to weeks)	• Exclude ventricular failure, pleural effusion or diaphragmatic splinting (tumor, ascites). • *If anemic:* transfuse if the Hb < 10 g/dl.[86–88] Full benefit takes 72 hours. • *If pulmonary tumor is present:* try dexamethasone 6 mg daily, readjusting to lowest dose that will control symptoms. Consider: chemotherapy or hormone therapy if the tumor is likely to respond. • *If respiratory muscle weakness is present* (e.g. motor neuron disease, muscular dystrophy): refer to respiratory physician for consideration of non-invasive ventilation (NIV). (*See* notes opposite.)
8	**Is a dry cough present?**	• Consider the following as causes of dry cough: aspiration, asthma, drugs (e.g. ACE inhibitors), heart failure, esophageal reflux, persistent infection (e.g. TB). • Treat any chest infection present. • Humidify the room air. Start simple linctus as required. Alternatively, try dextromethorphan (DM) 10 mg (10 ml) q8h or codeine 30–60 mg q6h. • If the cough is persistent and troublesome, one of the following may help: – nifedipine 5–10 mg q8h – lidocaine as a 10% spray in single spray to back of throat (a single spray is unlikely to compromise swallowing) – nebulized lidocaine 5 ml 2% solution over 20 mins (this may compromise swallowing and patients need to fast for one hour after use) – nebulized ipratropium – baclofen 10–20 mg q8h.[89,90] • *If bronchial tumor is present:* try beclomethasone 500 microgram inhaled q6h.
9	**Is the breathlessness persisting?**	• If the agitation or distress are severe: *see* cd-4 in Emergencies (p. 207). • *If the patient is anxious or frightened:* when relaxation is needed give lorazepam 0.5 mg sublingually or 2.5 mg midazolam SC. Sedation is not the aim. • Start oral morphine, or equivalent opioids, titrated as for analgesia. Consider the following: – consider nabilone (Canada only) (if there is no cardiac impairment): 100–500 microgram PO q8h[91] – acupuncture (upper sternum and L14 points in hands)[50,51] – nebulized furosemide 2 mg q6h.[71,72] • Plan future support: – refer to dyspnea clinic if this is available, and promote 'breathing retraining'[75,95] – help the patient to re-adapt to new respiratory capacity, e.g. review demands on mobility. • Manage the consequences of dyspnea: *see* Oral problems (p. 125), Skin problems (p. 139), Anxiety (p. 165) and Constipation (p. 75).

Adapted from Ahmedzai and Regnard[44]
cd = clinical decision

Other treatments and decisions

Pleural effusions: Drainage should be considered if the patient is distressed and the patient agrees. Ideally, the first time an effusion is drained should be in preparation for pleurodesis. Pleurodesis is done with talc, tetracycline or bleomycin and may be performed medically or surgically.[45] A pleuroperitoneal shunt is an alternative in a patient who is deteriorating slowly (month by month).[46,47]

Radiotherapy and chemotherapy: These can help in sensitive tumors but are less successful at treating breathlessness in other tumors.[48,49]

Acupuncture: This may have a role in persistent breathlessness.[50,51]

Respiratory infections: Whether to treat a chest infection in very advanced disease often causes concern. In most cases the disease will progress regardless of antibiotics.[52] If symptoms such as fever, purulent sputum or pleuritic chest pain are present, and the patient is willing and able to take oral medication, oral antibiotics should be used.[53–56] Some patients respond poorly or briefly to repeated antibiotic courses, but further control is possible for some weeks or months with nebulized antibiotics such as colistin (Canada only) or gentamicin.[57,58] In very ill patients, symptoms can be palliated in other ways (*see* clinical decision table).

Hiccups: Gastric stasis can cause hiccups and should be treated. For persistent hiccups most treatments are based on case studies, hence the wide range of drugs reported.[59,60] The current favourite is baclofen, backed by parenteral midazolam if the hiccups persist.[61]

Cough: Simple linctus or humidified air are soothing preparations that can be repeated as often as required. Lidocaine given by way of a jet nebulizer through a mouthpiece is helpful to suppress cough arising anywhere down to the larger bronchi.[25,62,63] It is not always tolerated and may cause numbness of the mouth and throat, temporarily preventing safe eating or drinking. High dose dexamethasone may reduce pleural, pericardial or diaphragmatic irritation by tumor.

Drugs used to treat breathlessness: Apart from bronchodilators and antibiotics, other drugs have a limited role in breathlessness.[64] Opioids can reduce the demand for ventilation without significant respiratory depression in both cancer and end-stage heart failure.[65–68] There is no evidence that high dose opioids decrease survival,[69] but there is evidence for their role in easing breathlessness.[70,94] Opioids can be prescribed in the same way as for pain control (*see* Using opioids (p. 49)). Nebulized opioids have been used in the past but evidence does not support their use.[70,94] Nebulized furosemide may help, even in the absence of heart failure,[71,72] but more evidence is awaited.[73,74]

Breathing retraining involves helping the patient to readapt to their new respiratory capacity through relaxation, positioning, establishing a sense of control, and improving respiratory muscle strength.[75,76,95] It has an important role in dyspnea that persists for several months or more. This is facilitated by specialist physiotherapists and clinical nurse specialists.

Non-invasive ventilation (NIV): At first this seems inappropriate in the context of very advanced disease. But ventilation can significantly improve the quality of life for patients with chronic hypercapnic respiratory failure due to progressive neuromuscular disease (e.g. motor neuron disease, Duchenne's muscular dystrophy) or chronic obstructive pulmonary disease. Symptoms of hypercapnia include morning headaches, daytime lethargy and poor sleep patterns. The technique is now well established and can improve sleep and daytime symptoms.[77–80] Since NIV relies on some of the patient's respiratory function, there will still be a gradual deterioration into respiratory failure, but this is often gentle and peaceful. Indeed, the role of NIV in terminal breathlessness is not clear[80] and it has no role in any respiratory failure accompanying the natural process of dying in other patients.

Breathlessness at the end of life

For many patients who have been breathless on exertion, becoming chair- or bed-bound can reduce the problems of breathlessness. A few patients, however, become more breathless and hypoxic despite their reduced mobility. This causes distress and fear, sometimes with gasping respiration that has been described as 'air hunger'.[81] Lorazepam or midazolam can be helpful.[82] The aim is not sedation, but to allow the patient to be more relaxed and comfortable. Doses should start small, but are repeated until the patient is settled and relaxed, but not necessarily sedated. Lorazepam can be given q8–12h (half-life is 12–15 hours), while midazolam can be given as a continuous subcutaneous infusion. While such events can be distressing, helping the patient to be settled and comfortable creates an important opportunity to further discuss the reasons for the deterioration with the patient if they are able, or with their partner or relatives.

References

B = book; C = comment; Ch = chapter; CS-n = case study-number of cases; CT-n = controlled trial-number of cases; E = editorial; GC = group consensus; I = interviews; Let = letter; LS = laboratory study; MC = multi-center; OS-n = open study-number of cases; R = review; RCT-n = randomized controlled trial-number of cases; RS-n = retrospective survey-number of cases; SA = systematic or meta analysis.

1 Anderson H, Ward C, Eardley A *et al.* (2001) The concerns of patients under palliative care and a heart failure clinic are not being met. *Palliative Medicine.* **15**(4): 279–86. (OS-279)

2 Reuben DB, Mor V, Hiris J (1988) Clinical symptoms and length of survival in patients with terminal cancer. *Archives of Internal Medicine.* **148**(7): 1586–91. (RS)

3 Lloyd-Williams M (1996) An audit of palliative care in dementia. *European Journal of Cancer Care.* **5**(1): 53–5. (RS-17)

4 Neudert C, Oliver D, Wasner M, Borasio GD (2001) The course of the terminal phase in patients with amyotrophic lateral sclerosis. *Journal of Neurology.* **248**(7): 612–16. (I-121)

5 McCarthy M, Lay M, Addington-Hall J (1996) Dying from heart disease. *Journal of the Royal College of Physicians of London.* **30**(4): 325–8. (I-600)

6 Shee CD (1995) Palliation in chronic respiratory disease. *Palliative Medicine.* **9**(1): 3–12. (R, 51 refs)

7 Gibbs LME, Ellershaw JE, Williams MD (1997) Caring for patients with HIV disease: the experience of a generic hospice. *AIDS Care.* **9**(5): 601–7. (OS-24)

8 Edmonds P, Karlsen S, Khan S, Addington-Hall J (2001) A comparison of the palliative care needs of patients dying from chronic respiratory diseases and lung cancer. *Palliative Medicine.* **15**(4): 287–95. (I-636)

9 Heyse-Moore L, Beynon T, Ross V (2000) Does spirometry predict dyspnea in advanced cancer? *Palliative Medicine.* **14**(3): 189–95. (OS-155)

10 Plant H, Bredin M, Krishnasamy M, Corner J (2000) Working with resistance, tension and objectivity: conducting a randomised controlled trial of a nursing intervention for breathlessness including commentary by S. Bond. *Nt Research.* **5**(6): 426–36. (R)

11 Mancini I, Body JJ (1999) Assessment of dyspnea in advanced cancer patients. *Supportive Care in Cancer.* **7**(4): 229–32. (R, 15 refs)

12 Wilcock A, Crosby V, Clarke D, Tattersfield A (1999) Repeatability of breathlessness measurements in cancer patients. *Thorax.* **54**(4): 375. (OS-31)

13 O'Driscoll M, Corner J, Bailey C (1999) The experience of breathlessness in lung cancer. *European Journal of Cancer Care.* **8**(1): 37–43. (I-52)

14 Wilcock A, Crosby V, Hughes A *et al.* (2002) Descriptors of breathlessness in patients with cancer and other cardiorespiratory diseases. *Journal of Pain and Symptom Management.* **23**(3): 182–9. (OS-261)

15 Cox C (2002) Non-pharmacological treatment of breathlessness. *Nursing Standard.* **16**(24): 33–6. (R, 35 refs)

16 Davis C (1997) ABC of palliative care: breathlessness, cough, and other respiratory problems. *BMJ.* **315**: 931–4. (R)

17 Bailey C (1996) Breathe a little easier. *Nursing Times.* **92**: 55–8. (R)

18 Bredin M, Corner J, Krishnasamy M *et al.* (1999) Multicentre randomised controlled trial of nursing intervention for breathlessness in patients with lung cancer. *BMJ.* **318**: 901–4. (RCT-119)

19 Spence DP, Graham DR, Ahmed J *et al.* (1993) Does cold air affect exercise capacity and dyspnea in stable chronic obstructive pulmonary disease? *Chest.* **103**(3): 693–6. (RCT-16)

20 Kratzing CC, Cross RB (1984) Effects of facial cooling during exercise at high temperature. *European Journal of Applied Physiology & Occupational Physiology.* **53**(2): 118–20.

21 Armour W, Clark AL, McCann GP, Hillis WS (1998) Effects of exercise position on the ventilatory responses to exercise in chronic heart failure. *International Journal of Cardiology.* **66**(1): 59–63. (RCT-9)

22 Yap JC, Moore DM, Cleland JG, Pride NB (2000) Effect of supine posture on respiratory mechanics in chronic left ventricular failure. *American Journal of Respiratory & Critical Care Medicine.* **162**(4 Pt 1): 1285–91. (CT-20)

23 Collins JV, Clark TJ, Brown DJ (1975) Airway function in healthy subjects and patients with left heart disease. *Clinical Science & Molecular Medicine.* **49**(3): 217–28. (OS-112)

24 Hanning CD, Alexander-Williams JM (1995) Pulse oximetry: a practical review. *BMJ.* **311**: 367–70.

25 Ahmedzai S (1997) Palliation of respiratory symptoms. In: D Doyle, GWC Hanks, N MacDonald (eds) *The Oxford Textbook of Palliative Medicine* (2e). Oxford Medical Publications, Oxford. pp. 583–616. (Ch)

26 Tai NR, Atwal AS, Hamilton G (1999) Modern management of pulmonary embolism. *British Journal of Surgery.* **86**(7): 853–68. (R, 145 refs)

27 Johnson MJ (1997) Problems of anticoagulation within a palliative care setting: an audit of hospice inpatients taking warfarin. *Palliative Medicine.* **11**: 306–12.

28 Nazario R, Delorenzo LJ, Maguire AG (2002) Treatment of venous thromboembolism. *Cardiology in Review*. **10**(4): 249–59. (R, 66 refs)

29 Girard P, Stern JB, Parent F (2002) Medical literature and vena cava filters: so far so weak. *Chest*. **122**(3): 963–7. (SA, 32 refs)

30 Kelly GS (1998) Clinical applications of N-acetylcysteine. *Alternative Medicine Review*. **3**(2): 114–27. (R, 96 refs)

31 Robinson PJ (2002) Dornase alpha in early cystic fibrosis lung disease. *Pediatric Pulmonology*. **34**(3): 237–41. (R)

32 Wildiers H, Menten J (2002) Death rattle: prevalence, prevention and treatment. *Journal of Pain and Symptom Management*. **23**(4): 310–17. (RS-107).

33 Watts T, Jenkins K (1999) Palliative care nurses' feelings about death rattle. *Journal of Clinical Nursing*. **8**(5): 615–16. (OS-33)

34 Bennett MI (1996) Death rattle: an audit of hyoscine (scopolamine) use and review of management. *Journal of Pain and Symptom Management*. **12**(4): 229–33. (CT-100)

35 Hughes A, Wilcock A, Corcoran R, Lucas V, King A (2000) Audit of three antimuscarinic drugs for managing retained secretions. *Palliative Medicine*. **14**(3): 221–2. (OS)

36 Back IN, Jenkins K, Blower A, Beckhelling J (2001) A study comparing hyoscine hydrobromide and glycopyrrolate in the treatment of death rattle. *Palliative Medicine*. **15**(4): 329–36. (OS)

37 Mutagh FEM, Thorns A, Oliver DJ (2002) Hyoscine and glycopyrrolate for death rattle. *Palliative Medicine*. **16**: 449–50.

38 Clayton J, Fardell B, Hutton-Potts J, Webb D, Chye R (2003) Parenteral antibiotics in a palliative care unit: prospective analysis of current practice. *Palliative Medicine*. **17**(1): 44–8. (OS-41)

39 Spruyt O, Kausae A (1998) Antibiotic use for infective terminal respiratory secretions. *Journal of Pain and Symptom Management*. **15**: 263–4. (Let, CS-11)

40 Bricaire F, Castaing JL, Pocidalo JJ, Vilde JL (1988) Pharmacokinetics and tolerance of ceftriaxone after subcutaneous administration. [French] *Pathologie et Biologie*. **36**(5 Pt 2): 702–5. (CS-8)

41 Borner K, Lode H, Hampel B *et al*. (1985) Comparative pharmacokinetics of ceftriaxone after subcutaneous and intravenous administration. *Chemotherapy*. **31**(4): 237–45. (RCT-8)

42 Sutton PP, Gemmell HG, Innes N *et al*. (1988) Use of nebulised saline and nebulised terbutaline as an adjunct to chest physiotherapy. *Thorax*. **43**: 57–60.

43 Tamaoki J, Kohri K, Isono K, Nagai A (2000) Inhaled indomethacin in bronchorrhea in bronchioloalveolar carcinoma: role of cyclooxygenase. *Chest*. **117**(4): 1213–14. (Let)

44 Ahmedzai S, Regnard C (1995) Dyspnea. In: *Flow Diagrams in Advanced Cancer and Other Diseases*. Edward Arnold, London. pp. 48–53.

45 Tattersall MHN, Boyer MJ (1990) Management of malignant pleural effusions. *Thorax*. **45**: 81–2.

46 Schulze M, Boehle AS, Kurdow R *et al*. (2001) Effective treatment of malignant pleural effusion by minimal invasive thoracic surgery: thoracoscopic talc pleurodesis and pleuroperitoneal shunts in 101 patients. *Annals of Thoracic Surgery*. **71**(6): 1809–12. (RS-101)

47 Genc O, Petrou M, Ladas G, Goldstraw P (2000) The long-term morbidity of pleuroperitoneal shunts in the management of recurrent malignant effusions. *European Journal of Cardio-Thoracic Surgery*. **18**(2): 143–6. (RS-160)

48 Ramirez AJ, Towlson KE, Leaning MS *et al*. (1998) Do patients with advanced breast cancer benefit from chemotherapy? *British Journal of Cancer*. **78**(11): 1488–94. (OS-160)

49 Plataniotis GA, Kouvaris JR, Dardoufas C *et al*. (2002) A short radiotherapy course for locally advanced non-small cell lung cancer (NSCLC): effective palliation and patients' convenience. *Lung Cancer*. **35**(2): 203–7.

50 Davis CL, Lewith GT, Broomfield J, Prescott P (2001) A pilot project to assess the methodological issues involved in evaluating acupuncture as a treatment for disabling breathlessness. *Journal of Alternative & Complementary Medicine*. **7**(6): 633–9. (CT-16)

51 Filshie J, Penn K, Ashley S, Davis C (1996) Acupuncture for the relief of cancer-related breathlessness. *Palliative Medicine*. **10**: 145–50.

52 Nagy-Agren S, Haley HB (2002) Management of infections in palliative care patients with advanced cancer. *Journal of Pain and Symptom Management*. **24**: 64–70. (R, 11 refs)

53 Chen LK, Chou YC, Hsu PS *et al*. (2002) Antibiotic prescription for fever episodes in hospice patients. *Supportive Care in Cancer*. **10**(7): 538–41. (RS-535)

54 Oneschuk D, Fainsinger R, Demoissac D (2002) Antibiotic use in the last week of life in three different palliative care settings. *Journal of Palliative Care*. **18**(1): 25–8. (OS-150)

55 Vitetta L, Kenner D, Sali A (2000) Bacterial infections in terminally ill hospice patients. *Journal of Pain and Symptom Management*. **20**(5): 326–34. (OS-102)

56 Chan R, Hemeryck L, O'Regan M, Clancy L, Feely J (1995) Oral versus intravenous antibiotics for community acquired lower respiratory tract infection in a general hospital: open, randomised controlled trial. *BMJ*. **310**: 1360–2. (RCT-541)

57 Beringer P (2001) The clinical use of colistin in patients with cystic fibrosis. *Current Opinion in Pulmonary Medicine*. **7**(6): 434–40. (R, 30 refs)

58 Lin HC, Cheng HF, Wang CH *et al*. (1997) Inhaled gentamicin reduces airway neutrophil activity and mucus secretion in bronchiectasis. *American Journal of Respiratory & Critical Care Medicine*. **155**(6): 2024–9. (RCT-28)

59 Friedman NL (1996) Hiccups: a treatment review. *Pharmacotherapy*. **16**(6): 986–95. (R, 78 refs)

60 Rousseau P (2003) Hiccups in patients with advanced cancer: a brief review. *Progress in Palliative Care*. **11**(1): 10–12. (R, 27 refs)

61 Twycross RG, Wilcock A (2001) Respiratory symptoms. In: *Symptom Management in Advanced Cancer* (3e). Radcliffe Medical Press, Oxford. pp. 141–79.

62 Ahmedzai S, Davis C (1997) Nebulised drugs in palliative care. *Thorax.* 52(Suppl 2): S75–77.

63 Udezue E (2001) Lidocaine inhalation for cough suppression. *American Journal of Emergency Medicine.* 19(3): 206–7. (OS)

64 Davis CL (1994) The therapeutics of dyspnea. *Cancer Surveys.* 21: 85–98. (R, 78)

65 Walsh TD (1984) Opiates and respiratory function in advanced cancer. *Recent Results in Cancer Research.* 89: 115–17.

66 Boyd KJ, Kelly M (1997) Oral morphine as symptomatic treatment of dyspnea in patients with advanced cancer. *Palliative Medicine.* 11(4): 277–81. (OS-15)

67 Ward C (2002) The need for palliative care in the management of heart failure. *Heart.* 87: 294–8. (R, 37 refs)

68 Flowers B (2003) Palliative care for patients with end-stage heart failure. *Nursing Times.* 99: 30–2. (R, 14 refs)

69 Vercovitch M, Waller A, Adunsky A (1999) High dose morphine use in the hospice setting. *Cancer.* 86(5): 871–7. (RS-651)

70 Jennings AL, Davies AN, Higgins JP et al. (2002) A systematic review of the use of opioids in the management of dyspnea. *Thorax.* 57(11): 939–44. (SA-18)

71 Prandota J (2002) Furosemide: progress in understanding its diuretic, anti-inflammatory, and bronchodilating mechanism of action, and use in the treatment of respiratory tract diseases. *American Journal of Therapeutics.* 9(4): 317–28. (R, 123 refs)

72 Shimoyama N, Shimoyama M (2002) Nebulized furosemide as a novel treatment for dyspnea in terminal cancer patients. *Journal of Pain and Symptom Management.* 23(1): 73–6. (CS-3)

73 Stone P, Rix E (2002) Nebulized furosemide for dyspnea in terminal cancer patients. *Journal of Pain and Symptom Management.* 23(3): 274–5. (Let)

74 Nebulized furosemide for dyspnea in terminal cancer patients: author's response (2002) *Journal of Pain and Symptom Management.* 23(3): 275–6. (Let)

75 Bailey C (1995) Nursing as therapy in the management of breathlessness in lung cancer. *European Journal of Cancer Care.* 4: 184–90. (R, 24 refs)

76 Corner J, Plant H, A'Hern R et al. (1996) Non-pharmacological intervention for breathlessness in lung cancer. *Palliative Medicine.* 10: 299–305. (RCT-20)

77 Branthwaite MA (1989) Mechanical ventilation at home. *BMJ.* 298: 1409.

78 Branthwaite MA (1991) Non-invasive and domiciliary ventilation: positive pressure techniques. *Thorax.* 46: 208–12.

79 Polkey MI, Lyall RA, Davidson AC et al. (1999) Ethical and clinical issues in the use of home non-invasive mechanical ventilation for the palliation of breathlessness in motor neurone disease. *Thorax.* 54(4): 367–71. (R, 43 refs)

80 Shee CD, Green M (2003) Non-invasive ventilation and palliation: experience in a district general hospital and a review. *Palliative Medicine.* 17(1): 21–6. (CS-10)

81 Tarzian AJ (2000) Caring for dying patients who have air hunger. *Journal of Nursing Scholarship.* 32(2): 137–43. (OS-10)

82 Fainsinger RL, Waller A, Bercovici M et al. (2000) A multicentre international study of sedation for uncontrolled symptoms in terminally ill patients. *Palliative Medicine.* 14(4): 257–65. (OS-287)

83 Launois S, Bizec JL et al. (1993) Hiccup in adults: an overview. *European Respiratory Journal.* 6: 563–75.

84 Guelaud C, Similowski T et al. (1995) Baclofen therapy for chronic hiccup. *European Respiratory Journal.* 8: 235–7.

85 Wilcock A, Twycross R (1996) Midazolam for intractable hiccup. *Journal of Pain and Symptom Management.* 12: 59–61. (CS)

86 Gleeson C, Spencer D (1995) Blood transfusion and its benefits in palliative care. *Palliative Medicine.* 9: 307–13. (OS-97)

87 Monti M, Castelleni L, Berlusconi A, Cunietti E (1996) Use of red blood cell transfusions in terminally ill cancer patients admitted to a palliative care unit. *Journal of Pain and Symptom Management.* 12: 18–22. (OS-31)

88 Davies A, Wang S (1997) Blood transfusions in patients with advanced cancer. *Journal of Pain and Symptom Management.* 13: 318. (Let)

89 Irwin RS, Curley FJ, Bennett FM (1993) Appropriate use of antitussives and protussives. A practical review. *Drugs.* 46(1): 80–91. (R, 88 refs)

90 Dicpinigaitis PV, Dobkin JB (1997) Antitussive effect of the GABA-agonist baclofen. *Chest.* 111(4): 996–9. (RCT-12)

91 Ahmedzai S, Carter R, Mills RJ, Moram F (1985) Effects of nabilone on pulmonary function. *Proceedings of the Oxford Symposium on Cannabis.* IRL Press, Oxford. pp. 371–8.

92 Newall AR, Orser R, Hunt M (1996) The control of oral secretions in bulbar ALS/MND. *Journal of Neurological Sciences.* 139(Suppl): 43–4. (OS-16)

93 Nedefors T (1996) Xerostomia: prevalence and pharmacotherapy. With special reference to beta-adrenoreceptor antagonists. *Swedish Dental Journal.* 116(Suppl): 1–70. (Q-n3311, OS-12)

94 Abernethy AP, Currow DC, Frith P, Fazekas S, McHugh A, Bui C (2003) Randomised, double-blind, placebo controlled crossover trial of sustained release morphine for the management of refractory dyspnoea. *BMJ.* 327: 523–6. (RCT-48)

95 Hately J, Laurence V, Scott A et al. (2003) Breathlessness clinics within specialist care settings can improve the quality of life and functional capacity of patients with lung cancer. *Palliative Medicine.* 17: 410–17. (OS-30)

Skin problems

Clinical decision and action checklist

1 Is the skin healthy?
2 Is the skin dry?
3 Is the skin wet?
4 Is the skin broken?
5 Is the skin itchy?

Key points

- Preventing pressure damage starts with identifying patients at risk.
- Healing of pressure damage is not realistic if the prognosis is short.
- Dry skin is common and uncomfortable.

Introduction

A number of skin problems can occur in advanced disease, particularly dry skin, sweating, pressure ulcers and itch. Malignant ulcers are described in Malignant ulcers and fistulae (p. 109).

Maintaining a healthy skin

A healthy skin is supple, intact and a good color, but the skin is easily compromised in advanced disease. Assessing the risk of pressure damage is important and a number of pressure sore prediction scores are available, such as the Waterlow, Norton, or Braden risk scores.[1,2] For those at moderate or high risk of pressure damage special mattresses, seat cushions and careful handling will reduce the risk of tissue breakdown. Even using good quality static mattresses can significantly reduce the incidence and severity of pressure sores.[3] Adequate nutrition and hydration are important and it is possible that stress plays a part by delaying healing.[4]

Diagnosing skin problems

Diagnosing a skin problem is mainly visual:

Character	Possible cause
Dry	Dehydration, drugs, air conditioning
Wet	Sweating (anxiety, drugs, eczema, fever, hormonal deficiency, hyperthyroidism, infection), body fluids (urine, stool, exudate)
Bluish, purple	Venous congestion, local malignancy, cyanosis, bruising
Grey or black	Recent bruising, necrosis due to local pressure damage or arterial insufficiency
Pale or white	Acute arterial occlusion, anemia or hypotension
Redness	Rash (e.g. drugs, skin irritant or systemic infection), recent trauma (e.g. scratch or injury), vasodilatation (e.g. fever or infection)
Yellow or green	Old bruising, jaundice

Managing skin problems

Dry skin: Simple measures can prevent and treat a dry skin (*see* cd-2 opposite).

Broken skin: Early damage can be difficult to identify, although one suggestion is that the skin in early damage feels warmer than surrounding skin.[5] For a deep ulcer, cleansing and healing will take several months. Patients with a short prognosis (day by day deterioration) are unlikely to heal, and even debridement may be incomplete, but odor and pain can be controlled. Slower deterioration (week by week) may allow some healing of shallow ulcers if nutrition is adequate, but only cleansing in deeper ulcers.

Moist dressings for pressure ulcers: The ideal dressing maintains high humidity, removes exudate and toxins, provides thermal insulation, is impermeable to bacteria, free from particles and toxins, and capable of removal without further damage or pain.[6] Traditional gauzes, antiseptics and hypochlorites do not fulfil these needs.[7] Few trials have shown any one dressing to have an advantage, and choice will depend not only on the type of wound, but also on availability, experience of the carer, the site of the wound and patient preference or tolerance.[8] Hydrogels (e.g. Intrasite gel) are useful where slough and infection are present. Conformable polyurethane foam dressings (e.g. Allevyn, Lyofoam Extra) are useful for heavy exudates. Hydrocolloids (e.g. Comfeel, Duoderm) maintain a moist environment useful for debridement and healing.

Debridement of pressure ulcers: Necrotic tissue delays healing, produces odor and masks the extent of damage. Dressings that maintain a moist environment remove necrotic tissue without further damage.[9] A hard, dark eschar of dead skin can occasionally prevent access to the ulcer, but the eschar can be softened with moist dressings.

Other dressings: Semipermeable adhesive film dressings (e.g. Opsite, Tegaderm) are useful in maintaining humidity in shallow ulcers ($< 0.5\,cm$) or in protecting very early damage.

Itch: A wide range of skin disorders and systemic conditions are known to cause itching and an equally wide range of underlying mechanisms and treatments have been suggested.[10,45] Most treatments are based on small numbers or case studies.

Sweating: Some patients suffer profuse sweating, particularly at night. It may be due to fear or anxiety. Occasionally malignancy will produce a fever with sweating – measures such as cooling with a fan or sponge are effective. If the cause cannot be treated then systemic drugs can be tried, but their use is based on small numbers or case studies.

Clinical decision	If YES ⇒ Action
1 Is the skin healthy? (supple, intact, good colour)	• Check the skin and calculate a pressure risk score weekly (daily if the risk is moderate or high). • Ensure good hydration and nutrition (especially vitamin C and zinc).[11,12] • Ensure the skin is kept supple and prevent contact with urine or feces. • *If there is a moderate to high risk of pressure damage:* distribute pressure using special surfaces or mattresses. Keep the patient's upper body at no more than a 30° tilt and take care with positioning. Prevent trauma to pressure areas by ensuring careful moving and positioning. If the skin is dry *see* cd-2 below.
2 Is the skin dry?	• When bathing, use tepid water and hypoallergenic soaps.[13] Use an emollient cream or ointment within 5 mins of washing, then pat dry (do not rub).[10] Avoid lotions. • Increase ambient humidity, if necessary with a room humidifier.[10]
3 Is the skin wet?	• *If due to exposure to body fluids:* use a barrier preparation (e.g. zinc ointments or simethicone cream) or a barrier application (e.g. Sween cream, Cavilon solution (Canada only), Secura cream (US only), Baza Pro (US – differs from Canadian Baza Protect in containing an antifungal)).[14] • *If due to sweating:* treat causes such as anxiety, drugs, eczema, hormonal deficiency, hyperthyroidism or infection. Use fans and reduce the temperature in the room. For persistent fever: use acetaminophen PO or PR 1 g q4h or diclofenac PO 50 mg q8h.[15] For hormone deficiency in women try megestrol acetate 20–40 mg PO daily;[16] for men after prostate cancer treatment try cyproterone acetate 50 mg PO twice daily.[17] If sweating persists, try amitriptyline 10–50 mg at bedtime, propantheline 15–30 mg at bedtime,[18] or thalidomide 50–100 mg PO daily.[19,20] Check precautions for thalidomide.[46] (Special access status in North America.)
4 Is the skin broken?	• *Exclude these causes:* infection, arterial insufficiency, venous ulceration, or trauma due to sensory loss. • *If the prognosis is too short to allow healing* (e.g. day by day deterioration): choose dressings for comfort such as non-adherent, soft silicone net dressings (e.g. Mepitel).[21,22] • *If odor is present: see* cd-4 in Malignant ulcers and fistulae (p. 111). • *If pain is present: see* cd-6 in Malignant ulcers and fistulae (p. 111). • *If this is a malignant ulcer: see* Malignant ulcers and fistulae (p. 109). • *If the skin surface is intact but damaged:* Superficial damage: if pressure care is fully implemented, a dressing is not usually required for discoloration of skin. A blister or abrasion may need a light dressing for protection. Deep damage: this is likely to develop into an ulcer. If a hard eschar is present this needs moistening with hydrocolloid or hydrogel dressing for one week followed by debridement under sedation and/or analgesia. • *If this is an ulcer due to pressure damage:* Avoid harmful chemicals: e.g. chlorinated solutions or hydrogen peroxide. Superficial ulcer: provide an environment for re-epithelialization: moisture-retaining dressings (e.g. Allevyn, Lyofoam Extra, hydrocolloid dressings, Op-Site). Reassess as needed. Deep ulcer: provide an environment for granulation using moist cavity dressing (e.g. cavity foam dressing, calcium alginate or hydrogel). For heavy exudate *see* cd-5 in Malignant ulcers and fistulae (p. 111). If debris is present use 0.9% saline for irrigation.[23] Antiseptics such as iodine-based derivatives (e.g. povidone iodine fabric dressing) can reduce infection.[24] Surgical debridement in the OR may be appropriate in some patients.[25] Reassess the ulcer at each dressing change.
5 Is the skin itchy?	• Correct simple causes, such as stopping or changing a drug causing an itchy rash. Avoid lotions. • Treat any dry skin: *see* cd-2 above. • *If the itch is localized:* try local cooling with a cold compress.[26] Alternatives are topical clobetasol 0.05% ointment daily if inflammation is present,[27] capsaicin cream[28] or doxepin 5% cream q8h (not commercially available in Canada),[29] but all topical applications may themselves cause local sensitivity reactions. • *If the itch is generalized:* Systemic options: doxepin 75 mg PO at bedtime, ondansetron 4–8 mg PO or SC q8h,[30] paroxetine 10–20 mg PO on waking,[31] naltrexone 25–50 mg PO daily,[32] cimetidine 800 mg PO at bedtime[33,34] or thalidomide 50–100 mg PO daily.[35,36] (Special access status in North America.) NSAIDs help if there is inflammation.[37] UVB phototherapy has been used for itch due to uremia and cholestasis.[38–41] Massage has been used for itching due to scarring,[42] and TENS for malignant ulcers.[43]

Adapted from Bale and Regnard[44]
cd = clinical decision

References

B = book; C = comment; Ch = chapter; CS-n = case study-number of cases; CT-n = controlled trial-number of cases; E = editorial; GC = group consensus; I = interviews; Let = letter; LS = laboratory study; MC = multicenter; OS-n = open study-number of cases; R = review; RCT-n = randomized controlled trial-number of cases; RS-n = retrospective survey-number of cases; SA = systematic or meta analysis.

1 Birchall L (1993) Making sense of pressure sore calculators. *Nursing Times*. **89**: 34–7.

2 Galvin J (2002) An audit of pressure ulcer incidence in a palliative care setting. *International Journal of Palliative Nursing*. **8**(5): 214, 216, 218–21. (OS-542)

3 Hofman A, Geelkerken RH, Wille J, Hamming JJ, Hermans J, Breslau PJ (1994) Pressure sores and pressure-decreasing mattresses: controlled clinical trial. *The Lancet*. **343**: 568–71. (RCT-44)

4 Kiecolt-Glaser JK, Marucha PT, Malarkey WB, Mercado AM, Glaser R (1995) Slowing of healing by psychological stress. *The Lancet*. **346**: 1194–6. (CT-26)

5 Lowthian P (1994) Pressure sores: a search for definition. *Nursing Standard*. **9**: 30–2.

6 Turner TD (1985) Semiocclusive and occlusive dressings. In: T Ryan (ed) An environment for healing: the role of occlusion. *Royal Society of Medicine Congress and Symposium Series*. **88**: 5–14. (Ch)

7 Bale S (1987) Dressing leg ulcers. *Journal of District Nursing*. **5**: 9–13.

8 Anonymous (2002) Wound management products and elastic hosiery. In: *British National Formulary No 45 (March 2003)*. British Medical Association and the Royal Pharmaceutical Society of Great Britain, London.

9 Miller M (1994) The ideal healing environment. *Nursing Times*. **90**: 62–8. (Ch)

10 Bueller HA, Bernhard JD (1998) Review of pruritus therapy. *Dermatology Nursing*. **10**(2): 101–7. (R, 66 refs)

11 Goode HF, Burns E, Walker BE (1992) Vitamin C depletion and pressure sores in elderly patients with femoral neck fracture. *BMJ*. **305**: 925–7. (OS-21)

12 Dickerson JWT (1993) Ascorbic acid, zinc and wound healing. *Journal of Wound Care*. **2**: 350–3.

13 Bernhard JD (1994) General principles, overview, and miscellaneous treatments of itching. In: *Itch: mechanisms and management of pruritus*. McGraw-Hill, Inc, New York. pp. 367–81. (Ch)

14 Grocott P (1999) The management of fungating wounds. *Journal of Wound Care*. **8**(5): 232–4. (R, 24 refs)

15 Obořilová A, Jiří M, Pospíšil Z, Kořístek Z (2002) Symptomatic intravenous antipyretic therapy: efficacy of metamizol, diclofenac and propacetamol. *Journal of Pain and Symptom Management*. **24**(6): 608–15. (OS-254)

16 Wymenga AN, Sleijfer DT (2002) Management of hot flushes in breast cancer patients. *Acta Oncologica*. **41**(3): 269–75. (R, 56 refs)

17 Cervenakov I, Kopecny M, Jancar M, Chovan D, Mal'a M (2000) 'Hot flush', an unpleasant symptom accompanying antiandrogen therapy of prostatic cancer and its treatment by cyproterone acetate. *International Urology & Nephrology*. **32**(1): 77–9. (OS-31)

18 Canaday BR, Stanford RH (1995) Propantheline bromide in the management of hyperhidrosis associated with spinal cord injury. *Annals of Pharmacotherapy*. **29**(5): 489–92. (CS-2)

19 Peuckmann V, Fisch M, Bruera E (2000) Potential novel uses of thalidomide: focus on palliative care. *Drugs*. **60**(2): 273–92. (R, 120 refs)

20 Deaner PB (2000) The use of thalidomide in the management of severe sweating in patients with advanced malignancy: trial report. *Palliative Medicine*. **14**: 429–31. (OS-10).

21 Gotschall CS, Morrison MI, Eichelberger MR (1998) Prospective randomized study of the efficacy of Mepitel on partial thickness scalds in children. *Journal of Burn Care Rehabilitation*. **19**: 279–83. (RCT)

22 Taylor R (1999) Use of a silicone net dressing in severe mycosis fungoides. *Journal of Wound Care*. **8**(9): 429–30. (CS-1)

23 Glide S (1997) Cleaning choices. *Nursing Times*. **88**: 74–8.

24 Gilchrist B on behalf of the European Tissue Repair Society (1997) Should iodine be recognised in wound management? *Journal of Wound Care*. **6**: 148–50.

25 Bale S (1997) A guide to wound debridement. *Journal of Wound Care*. **6**: 179–82. (R)

26 Fruhstorfer H, Hermanns M, Latzke L (1986) The effects of thermal stimulation on clinical and experimental itch. *Pain*. **24**: 259–69. (OS-18)

27 Lorenz B, Kaufman RH, Kutzner SK (1998) Lichen sclerosus. Therapy with clobetasol propionate. *Journal of Reproductive Medicine*. **43**(9): 790–4. (RS-81)

28 Weisshaar E, Heyer G, Forster C, Handwerker HO (1998) Effect of topical capsaicin on the cutaneous reactions and itching to histamine in atopic eczema compared to healthy skin.

Archives of Dermatological Research. **290**(6): 306–11. (RCT)

29 Richelson E (1979) Tricyclic antidepressants and histamine H1 receptors. *Mayo Clinic Proceedings.* **54**: 669–74. (R)

30 Muller C, Pongratz S, Pidlich J, Penner E, Kaider A, Schemper M, Raderer M, Scheithauer W, Ferenci P (1998) Treatment of pruritus in chronic liver disease with the 5-hydroxytryptamine receptor type 3 antagonist ondansetron: a randomized, placebo-controlled, double-blind cross-over trial. *European Journal of Gastroenterology & Hepatology.* **10**(10): 865–70. (RCT)

31 Zylicz Z, Smits C, Krajnik M (1998) Paroxetine for pruritus in advanced cancer. *Journal of Pain and Symptom Management.* **16**(2): 121–4. (CS-5)

32 Peer G, Kivity S, Agami O, Fireman E, Silverberg D, Blum M, Iaina A (1996) Randomised cross-over trial of naltrexone in uraemic patients. *Lancet.* **348**: 1552–4. (RCT-15)

33 Harrison AR, Littenberg G, Goldstein L, Kaplowitz N (1979) Pruritis, cimetidine and polycythaemia. *New England Journal of Medicine.* **300**: 433–4. (Let)

34 Aymard JP, Lederlin P, Witz F *et al.* (1980) Cimetidine for pruritus in Hodgkin's disease. *BMJ.* **280**: 151–2.

35 Moraes M, Russo G (2001) Thalidomide and its dermatologic uses. *American Journal of the Medical Sciences.* **321**(5): 321–6. (R, 44 refs)

36 Daly BM, Shuster S (2000) Antipruritic action of thalidomide. *Acta Dermato-Venereologica.* **80**(1): 24–5. (OS-11)

37 Twycross RG (1981) Pruritus and pain in *en cuirass* breast cancer. *Lancet.* **ii**: 696. (Let)

38 Gilchrest BA, Rowe JW, Brown RS, Steinman TI, Arndt KA (1979) Ultraviolet phototherapy of uremic pruritus: long-term results and possible mechanism of action. *Annals of Internal Medicine.* **91**: 17–21. (OS-7)

39 Hanid MA, Levi AJ (1980) Phototherapy for pruritus in primary biliary cirrhosis. *Lancet.* **2**: 530. (Let)

40 Lim HW, Vallurupalli S, Meola T, Soter NA (1997) UVB phototherapy is an effective treatment for pruritus in patients infected with HIV. *Journal of the American Academy of Dermatology.* **37**(3 Pt 1): 414–17. (OS-21)

41 Jeanmougin M, Rain JD, Najean Y (1996) Efficacy of photochemotherapy on severe pruritus in polycythemia vera. *Annals of Hematology.* **73**(2): 91–3. (CS-11)

42 Patino O, Novick C, Merlo A, Benaim F (1999) Massage in hypertrophic scars. *Journal of Burn Care & Rehabilitation.* **20**(3): 268–71; discussion 267. (RCT-30)

43 Grocott P (1999) The management of fungating wounds. *Journal of Wound Care.* **8**(5): 232–4. (R, 24 refs)

44 Bale S, Regnard C (1995) Pressure sores. In: *Flow Diagrams in Advanced Cancer and Other Diseases.* Edward Arnold, London. pp. 54–6. (Ch)

45 Twycross R, Greaves MW, Handwerker H, Jones EA, Libretto SE, Szepietowski JC, Zylicz Z (2003) Itch: scratching more than the surface. *Quarterly Journal of Medicine.* **96**: 7–26. (R, 211 refs)

46 Twycross R, Wilcock A, Charlesworth S, Dickman A (2003) Thalidomide. In: *PCF2: Palliative Care Formulary.* Radcliffe Medical Press, Oxford. pp. 237–9 (also on www.palliativedrugs.com).

Terminal phase (the last hours and days)

Clinical decision and action checklist

1 Does the medication need reviewing?
2 Are symptoms present or anticipated?
3 Are interventions continuing?
4 Is communication difficult?
5 Is insight uncertain?
6 Are religious and spiritual needs uncertain?
7 Is there uncertainty about informing others?
8 Is there uncertainty that the plan of care has been discussed?

Key points

- The last hours and days are a time of adjustments for the patient and carers.
- Most patients die peacefully without distress.
- If distress does occur, sedation is not first-line treatment.

Introduction

This advice refers to patients who are dying. A steady deterioration is common in cancer, so that a day-by-day or hour-by-hour deterioration is likely to indicate the terminal phase. However, in some patients with cancer, and in many patients with neurological or cardiac disease, several life-threatening episodes may precede the terminal phase. Patients in the terminal phase have several common features:

> **The signs and symptoms of a dying patient**
> - Deteriorating day by day or faster because of their underlying condition, or an irreversible complication of their disease.
> - Patient expresses a realization that they are dying.
> - Reduced cognition, drowsy or comatose.
> - Bed-bound.
> - Taking little food or fluid and having difficulty with oral medication.
> - Altered breathing pattern.
> - Peripherally cyanosed and cold.

Exacerbations of pain or breathlessness are unusual in patients whose symptoms have been well controlled until this point.[1] This final phase starts a median of 23 hours before death, varying from a few hours to several days.[2] Many patients are awake and rational until this terminal phase.

A time of adjustments

The terminal phase is a crucial time of adjustments for all:

- *Stopping unnecessary drugs:* It is often possible to simplify drug regimes as a patient deteriorates.
- *Continuing with other drugs by an appropriate route:* The subcutaneous and buccal routes are useful and kind alternatives.
- *Ensure PRN medication is available or prescribed:* metoclopramide, hydromorphone or morphine injection, hyoscine/scopolamine patch, or glycopyrrolate and midazolam should be available in the patient's home or on the ward.
- *Controlling physical symptoms:* Adjustments (psychological or social) are impossible if there is troublesome pain, nausea or breathlessness.
- *Giving explanations:* Lack of information is a common cause of problems. Like drugs, information must be titrated to the individual. *See* Breaking difficult news (p. 25) and Helping the person with the effects of difficult news (p. 29).
- *Anticipating changes:* Although it is not possible to anticipate every crisis, planning ahead is essential. For example, many patients suffer from bronchial secretions at the end of life – having hyoscine/hyoscyamine/scopolamine patch, or glycopyrrolate available is sensible.
- *Giving and accepting adequate support:* Duty demands we provide support, but clinical governance insists we also accept help, advice and support when we are unsure of the situation.
- *Setting realistic goals:* Goals change as a patient deteriorates, but one can still foster hope even if that is now about comfort. Resuscitation issues may need to be discussed – *see* Issues around resuscitation (p. 193).
- *Ensuring that religious and spiritual care is offered:* Ask the patient, partner or family if they would like to talk to a chaplain/spiritual advisor or other professional.
- *Explaining changes to the partner, family and carers:* They should be given as much (or as little) information as they need (with the patient's consent).
- *Helping the patient, partner, family and carers understand the changes:* Although changes are frightening, it can be comforting for some patients, partners or relatives to have the natural and gentle course of a death explained.
- *Informing other team members:* The family physician and/or hospital consultant will need to know what is happening.
- *Ensuring the environment is appropriate:* Comfortable and as quiet (or noisy) as they want.
- *Anticipating the death:* For some patients, families and carers this can be a valuable time to consider issues such as funeral arrangements and organ donation.

Managing symptoms

These are discussed in detail elsewhere in the Guide. A key issue is that when helping a distressed patient **sedation is *not* first line treatment**. Other approaches are tried first, and even if drugs with sedative actions are used, low doses are chosen and then titrated to the individual. Opioids are never used to 'settle' a patient.

Noisy or moist breathing: Positional change may be enough to reduce the airway secretions, otherwise hyoscine/hyoscyamine/scopolamine patch, or glycopyrrolate help at least half of such patients.

Urinary incontinence: This will probably subside as the patient's renal function reduces. Consider the use of pads or catheter (indwelling or intermittent), or use sheaths for male patients.

Pain: Consider causes such as urinary retention, constipation, uncomfortable position, infection, and pressure sore pain in addition to known disease-related pain.

Restlessness/agitation/confusion: If other measures are inappropriate, consider a benzodiazepine.

Clinical decision	If YES ⇒ Action
Patient is deteriorating day by day because of their underlying condition, or because of an irreversible complication of their disease.	
1 Does the medication need reviewing?	**Care Pathway for the Dying Patient (CPDP)** **CPDP Goal 1: Current medication assessed and non-essentials discontinued.** *See* table overleaf for review of medication. • Stop all non-essential medication. • If unable to swallow, convert to SC route either as intermittent dosing or as continuous SC infusion.
2 Are symptoms present or anticipated?	**CPDP Goal 2: As required subcutaneous medication written up as per CPDP protocol** A *Pain* (also *see* Diagnosing and treating pain (p. 39)): *If not on oral opioid:* If the patient is in pain: give parenteral opioid SC. If the pain is controlled: prescribe parenteral opioid SC q4h PRN. *If already on morphine:* If the patient is in pain: give one tenth to one sixth of the 24-hour dose. If the pain is controlled: convert to parenteral opioid SC infusion. – conversion: generally, the SC dose is 50% of the PO dose (hydromorphone, morphine) – prescribe PRN dose of opioid as one tenth to one sixth of 24 hr dose of SC infusion. *If uncertain about conversions:* contact a palliative care physician or nurse for advice. B *Nausea and vomiting* (also *see* Nausea and vomiting (p. 113)): If present: give metoclopramide 10 mg q6h SC. If absent: prescribe metoclopramide 10 mg SC q6h PRN. C *Respiratory tract secretions* (also *see* Respiratory problems (p. 131)): If present: give hyoscine hydrobromide/scopolamine 400 mcg SC (0.4 mg), hyoscyamine (0.125–0.25 mg PO/SL q4h PRN – max 1.5 mg/d), glycopyrrolate 400 microgram SC q4h PRN, or scopolamine patch (US) q72h. If absent: prescribe hyoscine hydrobromide 400 microgram or glycopyrrolate 400 microgram SC q4h PRN. D *Terminal restlessness and agitation* (also *see* cd-4 in Emergencies (p. 207)): If present: give midazolam 5–10 mg SC. If absent: prescribe midazolam 5–10 mg SC q4h PRN. E *After 24 hours:* Review the medication and if two or more PRN doses have been needed then either consider a regular regime (including an SC infusion) for 24 hours, or increase the present dose. *If problems are still present after 24 hours:* contact the palliative care team for advice.
3 Are interventions continuing?	**CPDP Goal 3: Discontinue inappropriate interventions** • Discontinue interventions such as regular blood tests, turning regimes, vital signs. • Ensure that a DNR – Do Not Resuscitate decision – has been documented. *See* Issues around resuscitation (p. 193).
4 Is communication difficult?	**CPDP Goal 4: Ability to communicate in English assessed as adequate** • Assess the ability to communicate in English. • For patients who are unconscious or have severe communication problems *see* Identifying distress in the person with severe communication difficulty (p. 33).
5 Is insight uncertain?	**CPDP Goal 5: Insight into condition assessed** • Assess the insight of the patient, partner and family about the situation.
6 Are religious and spiritual needs uncertain?	**CPDP Goal 6: Religious/spiritual needs assessed with patient and family** • Assess the religious and spiritual needs with the patient, partner and family. • Ask if the patient, partner or family wish to see a spiritual advisor, priest or chaplain.
7 Is there uncertainty about informing others?	**CPDP Goal 7: Identify how the family and others are to be informed of the patient's impending death.** **CPDP Goal 8: Family and other people involved are given relevant hospital information.** **CPDP Goal 9: All key people are aware of the patient's condition.** • If the patient agrees, give the partner, family and others relevant information. • Ensure the key professionals are aware of the patient's condition.
8 Is there uncertainty that the plan of care has been discussed?	**CPDP Goal 10: Plan of care explained and discussed with the patient and family.** **CPDP Goal 11: Family and other people involved express an understanding of the plan of care.** • Explain the plan with the patient, partner and family. • Make sure the partner, family and others express an understanding of the plan of care.

Adapted with permission from the Liverpool Care Pathway for the Dying Patient[3]
cd = clinical decision

Table continued overleaf

Reviewing drugs in the last hours and days

Drug	Suggested action	Alternative action
Analgesics		
acetaminophen	stop	acetaminophen 500 mg PR
weak opioids	hydromorphone SC 0.5–1.0 mg q1h PRN	hydromorphone SC infusion
strong opioids	give SC at equivalent doses	transdermal fentanyl (will need at least 12 hours for effect, and a strong opioid as breakthrough)
ketamine	continue by SC infusion (or intermittent SC)	–
NSAIDs	stop	diclofenac 100 mg PR once daily or ketoralac 30 mg SC
Antiemetics		
dimenhydrinate	continue by SC injection	dimenhydrinate PR q8h
haloperidol	continue by SC injection once at night	methotrimeprazine SC once at night (Canada only)
hyoscine/scopolamine	continue by SC injection or infusion	transdermal hyoscine hydrobromide/scopolamine patch
methotrimeprazine (Canada only)	continue by SC injection once at night	chlorpromazine PR once at night
metoclopramide	continue by SC injection or infusion	domperidone PR q8h (in US only available from compounding pharmacies)
Antiepileptics		
gabapentin for neuropathic pain	sodium valproate PR	SC ketamine or opioid
valproate, phenytoin, carbamazepine for seizures	phenobarbital 60–80 mg q8 or 12h SC (injection not currently available in Canada) or sodium valproate PR	midazolam SC infusion for prevention midazolam buccally for status
Antimicrobial agents		
chest infections	hyoscine/hyoscyamine/scopolamine, or glycopyrrolate for excess bronchial secretions	single dose of 500 mg ceftrioxone IM or SC
fungal infections	stop systemic anti-fungal	topical miconazole
Gram –ve infections	stop oral antibiotic	metronidazole 400 mg PR q8h
Cardiovascular		
antiarrhythmics	stop	–
antihypertensives	stop	–
ACE inhibitor	stop	furosemide SC as needed
furosemide	stop	furosemide SC as needed
Corticosteroids		
e.g. dexamethasone	stop if condition deteriorates rapidly (but beware of agitation on stopping corticosteroids)	If used as co-analgesic give as single SC injection
Endocrine and metabolic drugs		
bisphosphonates	stop	–
hypoglycemics	stop	–
octreotide	stop	–
Gastrointestinal drugs		
antacids	stop	–
laxatives	stop	Bisacodyl suppository
PPI, H$_2$ antagonists	stop	ranitidine SC infusion[5]
Hematological drugs		
erythropoietin	stop	–
iron, B$_{12}$	stop	–
Psychotropic drugs		
antidepressants for depression	stop (but beware of agitation on stopping SSRI and SNRI drugs)	clomipramine 10–50 mg IM once at night
amitriptyline for neuropathic pain	carbamazepine PR once daily	clomipramine 10–50 mg IM once at night
benzodiazepines	midazolam SC	diazepam PR once at night
haloperidol	continue by SC injection	methotrimeprazine SC (Canada only)
methotrimeprazine	continue by SC injection	chlorpromazine PR
Miscellaneous		
baclofen	diazepam PR once at night	midazolam SC infusion
dantrolene	diazepam PR once at night	midazolam SC infusion
bronchodilators	stop	nebulized salbutamol
enteral nutrition	stop	SC fluids only (review needed daily)
wound management	minimize dressing changes	–

Breathlessness: Consider changing the patient's position, increasing air movement (fan, open windows), oxygen, relaxation, and explanation. Consider a benzodiazepine to reduce any fear and/or an opioid to relieve the feeling of breathlessness.

Nausea/vomiting: Continue anti-emetics by the most appropriate route.

Sweating: Keep the patient cool, regularly change the bed linen, and use cotton nightwear. Involve the family in sponging the patient if they wish.

Jerking/twitching/plucking: This can be myoclonic jerks due to excessive opioid, in which case reduce the dose or change opioid. Other causes are uremia or an altered neurological state. Low dose midazolam may help.

The death

How it seems for the patient: What is observed for most patients with advanced illness is a gentle 'winding down' of the body's systems. Even in cardiac and respiratory failure, sudden, dramatic deaths are uncommon. At the end it is more a gentle absence of life than a sudden presence of death. Peaceful silence is the most obvious feature.

How it seems for the carers:[4] Some find it easy to cry, others feel as though they have dried up. Some feel the urge to speak, often to express relief. Others feel it's an anticlimax because, in a sense, the patient left hours or days before. Many are so numbed with grief that they feel helpless and useless, but may not admit to this. Others cannot remember names, addresses and telephone numbers. This needs to be understood and information may have to be given to another member of the family.

Occasionally a relative or partner has been unable to adjust to the deterioration of the patient and reacts with shock or anger to what is obvious to everyone else. It is rare for such people to be truly ignorant of the facts, it is just that they have not been able to face the terrible reality. Experienced help and support from a palliative care specialist (doctor, nurse, chaplain/spiritual advisor or social worker) may be needed.

How it is for the professional carer: It often feels awkward. There is an overwhelming urge to do something such as checking the pulse or breathing, moving a pillow, making tea. There are no rules, but there are some principles:

- Take your cue from the family or partner – enable them to do it their way.
- Silence is awkward, but is right in the right place (there's nothing you can say that will make it better).
- If those present want to talk, then talk; if they're silent, then let them be silent.

- Someone *will* need to check the patient has died. Don't pronounce death until at least several minutes have elapsed from the last breath. Some patients take an occasional breath for several minutes.
- After the death, ask those present if they want to stay, and if so, whether they want to be alone.

The arrangements

The carer now has a number of responsibilities:

- helping the family contact friends and relatives
- asking them whether it is to be a burial or a cremation
- helping them choose an undertaker
- if a post mortem is needed, obtaining consent and explaining the arrangements
- explaining how to register a death.

The death certificate: The death certificate should be filled out by the doctor who saw the patient within the last few days. The cause of death is, for example, 'Carcinoma of stomach', not the mode of death such as 'respiratory arrest' or 'coma'. Because the next of kin do not receive a copy of the death certificate, or any notification of the cause of death, they may wish to question the attending physician about the cause of death. Such questions should be answered honestly, but considerately.

Post mortems: In many provinces in Canada and most states in the US, when death is due to industrial disease (e.g. asbestosis), injury, neglect, suspicious circumstances, or within the normal recovery time of an operation, referral to the medical examiner (ME) is mandated. The ME may demand a post mortem, so the relative's permission is not needed, but they should be informed. For all other deaths a post mortem can be a valuable way of finding out why a disease behaved the way it did. In this case, a relative's permission is essential and usually it is not difficult to ask if this is done sensitively (e.g. 'It would help us to examine Michael to find out why he had so much pain'), and it is made clear that the relative or partner can refuse. For some families, it can be helpful to discuss this ahead of the death. The funeral may be delayed by up to a day by a post mortem.

Organ donation: Many patients, families and carers are willing to consider this and see it as something good coming out of a tragedy. Which organs can be used, and how soon they should be removed will depend on local policy, and the local transplant co-ordinator should be contacted for advice. Corneas and heart valves can often be used. The transplant team can remove organs rapidly and discreetly.

References

B = book; C = comment; Ch = chapter; CS-n = case study-number of cases; CT-n = controlled trial-number of cases; E = editorial; GC = group consensus; I = interviews; LS = laboratory study; MC = multi-center; OS-n = open study-number of cases; PC = personal communication; R = review; RCT-n = randomized controlled trial-number of cases; RS-n = retrospective survey-number of cases; SA = systematic or meta analysis.

1 Henriksen H, Riis J, Christophersen B, Moe C (1997) Distress symptoms in hospice patients. *Ugeskrift for Laeger.* **159**(47): 6992–6. (OS-117)
2 Morita T, Ichiki T, Tsunoda J, Inoue S, Chihara S (1998) A prospective study on the dying process in terminally ill cancer patients. *American Journal of Hospice & Palliative Care.* **15**(4): 217–22. (OS-100)
3 Ellershaw J, Ward C (2003) Care of the dying patient: the last hours and days of life. *BMJ.* **326**: 30–4. (R, 24 refs)
4 Doyle D (1994) *Caring for a Dying Relative: a guide for families.* Oxford University Press, Oxford.
5 Dickman A (2003) SC ranitidine or omeprazole. Bulletin board on www.palliativedrugs.com, 11 Feb. (PC)

Urinary and sexual problems

Clinical decision and action checklist

1 Is a UTI symptom present?
2 Has the urine changed colour?
3 Is pain present?
4 Are sexual difficulties present?
5 Is urinary incontinence present?
6 Has urinary output changed?
7 Has urinary frequency changed?

Key points

- Urinary problems are common in advanced disease.
- Urinary tract infection symptoms may be non-specific in the elderly and neurologically impaired.
- Intermittent self-catheterization is an underused but effective technique for several urinary problems.
- Sexual problems are often not discussed nor explored by professionals.

Introduction

A wide range of urinary problems can be caused by local cancer, or by any condition that impairs mobility or pelvic neurological function. Consequently urinary problems are common in advanced disease and have a major impact on self-esteem and quality of life.[1]

Infections

In adults, a crystal clear urine of normal color that is negative for nitrites and leukocyte esterase is likely to be free of infection.[2–4] There are four key symptoms of infection: dysuria, frequency, back pain and hematuria.[5] Women with two of these symptoms have a 90% chance of a UTI.[5] In the elderly or in neurologically impaired patients, symptoms may be non-specific, e.g. confusion, myoclonic jerks, increased seizures. When a patient first presents with an infection single dose antibiotics are adequate. Culture is unnecessary for most women,[6,7] but in children, a normal dipstick does not exclude infection and culture is needed.[8,9] Culture and 7-day courses of antibiotics are necessary for recurrent infection, in the elderly or if the genitourinary tract is abnormal. Patients with urethral catheters invariably have urine that contains bacteria and treatment is only required in the presence of local or systemic symptoms.

Bleeding

It is unusual for blood loss to be severe, so oral iron supplements may be sufficient to prevent symptomatic anemia. Often it is the patient's anxiety that is uppermost and reassurance may be the most effective treatment. Infection should always be excluded. Palliative radiotherapy can reduce hematuria arising from a bleeding cancer in the urinary tract. Bladder irrigation with a 1% alum solution can reduce severe bleeding from the bladder.[10] Embolization of the internal iliac artery has also been used.[11] Aminocaproic or tranexamic acid* may help but can produce hard clots that can cause obstruction and are difficult to remove.[12]

Pain

Trigone pain: The trigone is at the base of the bladder, surrounding the urethral opening. Irritation of this area can cause pain that radiates to the tip of the distal urethra. Catheter balloons are a common cause and reducing the balloon volume can help as well as avoiding tension on the catheter itself. Intermittent catheterization is an alternative (*see* p. 155).

Bladder pain due to tumor or persistent infection can be eased with local anesthetic instilled into the bladder. Lidocaine can be used on a once daily basis when mixed with bicarbonate to reduce systemic absorption.[13,14] Bupivacaine may be simpler and more effective.[15] Intravesical opioid may also be effective.[16] Instillation of drugs into the bladder can be done using intermittent catheterization (*see* p. 155).

Ureteric pain ('renal colic') can be severe. Hyoscine butylbromide (Canada) or hyoscyamine/scopolamine (US) will provide immediate relief. Strong opioids are as effective as NSAIDs,[17] and the potential renal adverse effects of NSAIDs make them a third-line treatment.[18] As an alternative, acupuncture has been used successfully in ureteric pain.[19]

Persistent pain from the renal tract may require ketamine or spinal analgesia.

Other urinary problems

Urinary retention: Constipation is a common cause of retention in the elderly, debilitated or neurologically impaired. Morphine is an unusual cause of retention and more common causes are tricyclic antidepressants and drugs with antimuscarinic actions. Urethral obstruction is more common in older men due to an enlarged prostate. Other causes of urethral and ureteric obstructions are uncommon.

Incontinence: This is a distressing symptom with effects on self-esteem, personal hygiene and social interaction, although many patients manage to cope if the problem is mild.[20,21] Permanent catheterization should be a last resort since there are many causes which can be treated (see clinical decision table). Desmopressin is a synthetic analog of vasopressin (antidiuretic hormone) which reduces urinary output overnight and is occasionally helpful in otherwise intractable nocturnal incontinence.[22,23] A fluid intake/output chart is started, and no fluids given after 6 pm. It is important that the patient produces a daytime output of at least 500 ml, otherwise water intoxication can occur. An intranasal or oral dose is given at bedtime.

Catheter problems: Blockage is the commonest problem and is usually related to infection.[27] There is no evidence that regular bladder washouts reduce the risk of catheter blockage.[28,29] Bypassing of urine around a catheter may be due to:

---

*Aminocaproic acid is not available in Canada. In the US topical preparations can be obtained from a compounding pharmacy.

Clinical decision	If YES ⇒ Action

1 Is a UTI symptom present? (dysuria, frequency, back pain, or hematuria)	• Test the urine for nitrites, leukocyte esterase and protein.
	• *If the urine test is positive for nitrites, or leukocytes:*
	  – in women with a normal GU tract: give trimethoprim 200 mg q12h for 3 days.
	  – in all other patients: culture the urine. Start trimethoprim 200 mg q12h (1–2 mg/kg q12h for children) for 3 days.
	  If the infection persists: culture the urine and give a 7-day course of a cephalosporin (continue for 2 weeks if pyelonephritis is present).
	• *If an enterovesical fistula is present* (mixed enterococci on culture): treat only if the symptoms are troublesome since eradication of infection is impossible.
	• *If the urine dipstick test is negative:* consider candida if local symptoms are present.[24]

2 Has the urine changed colour?	• **If the urine is positive for blood on testing:** Exclude and treat a urinary tract infection (*see* cd-1 above). *If the bleeding is severe:* insert a 18–24Ch gauge catheter and irrigate with 0.9% saline to remove clots. Instil with 1% alum solution 50 ml for 30 minutes. If this is insufficient, instil 1% alum at a rate of 5 ml/hour for 24–72 hours. *See* also Bleeding (p. 67). *If the source of bleeding is unclear:* refer to a urologist to consider a pyelogram or cystoscopy. *If a tumor is the source of bleeding:* consider aminocaproic or tranexamic acid 1–1.5 g PO q8–12h but there is a risk of producing hard clots that can cause obstruction. Refer to an oncologist to consider radiotherapy or embolization. • **If this is not blood:** Reassure the patient. Consider other causes of colour change: orange-red (senna, bile, rifampicin, rhubarb), red-brown (adriamycin, bile, beetroot, food dyes), green-black (mitoxantrone, bile).

3 Is pain present?	• **Pain in the midline**
	If the pain is in the penis or urethra: test the urine to exclude a UTI.
	If the trigone (base of bladder) is being irritated (produces pain felt at the tip of the urethra):
	  – irritation by catheter: reduce the volume of balloon, try a smaller size catheter or consider intermittent catheterization. Avoid tension on the catheter.
	  – irritation due to tumor or persistent cystitis: try a bladder instillation of bupivacaine 50 mg (e.g. 20 ml 0.25% solution) for 15 mins q12h. For a once daily regimen, try instilling lidocaine 200 mg (e.g. 10 ml 2% solution) with 10 ml of 8.4% sodium bicarbonate.[13]
	If the pain is felt in the lower abdomen: this may be bladder irritability or spasm due to:
	  – catheter: reduce the balloon volume. Consider intermittent catheterization.
	  – cystitis (persistent infection, NSAIDs, some cytotoxics[25]): treat the cause if possible, otherwise try instilling bupivacaine or lidocaine as above.
	  – unstable bladder: *see* incontinence (neuropathic bladder) (*see* cd-5 overleaf).
	  – urinary retention: *see* decreased urine output (*see* cd-6 overleaf).
	• **Unilateral pain**
	If the pain is in the groin: this may be colic due to irritation or obstruction of the ureter. Treat the cause. For pain relief give hyoscine butylbromide (Canada only) 20 mg IV or SC. Consider starting a strong opioid (or giving a breakthrough dose of an existing opioid). An NSAID can be tried if the renal function is good. For ureteric obstruction due to tumor, try dexamethasone 16 mg daily.
	If the pain is felt in the loin: this may be renal capsule distension or irritation.
	  – infection: exclude TB or pyelonephritis.
	  – hemorrhage: hydromorphone 2 mg or morphine 10 mg SC if not on an opioid, otherwise use equivalent of current analgesia. Consider ketamine.
	  – tumor: start opioid or increase existing opioid by 50% if needed. If renal function is poor, avoid NSAIDs.
	  – bilateral ureteric obstruction: *see* cd-6 overleaf.

4 Are sexual difficulties present?	• Has the couple's usual physical intimacy changed? Is this a problem for them? If the answer is yes to both questions, consider the following (*see* also the notes on p. 155): *Erectile impotence:* exclude reversible causes such as anxiety, depression, and drugs (antihypertensives, antidepressants, beta-blockers, lipid lowering drugs, thiazides, spironolactone). Consider a trial of sildenafil 25–50 mg 1 hour before sexual activity (contraindicated if hypotensive, on nitrates, recent CVA, or recent myocardial infarction). *Vaginal pain on intercourse:* exclude hormonal deficiency causing dryness or vaginitis. *Intercourse physically impossible* (e.g. local tumor): explore other ways to stimulate the partner or express physical closeness. • Enable open discussion of sexuality and body image.

Table continued overleaf

5	Is urinary incontinence present?	• **If a fistula is present (vesicovaginal or vesicorectal):** Plan regular voiding through the urethra, using water-absorbent pads the rest of the time. Regular intermittent catheterization may help by keeping the bladder empty. • **In the absence of a fistula** Exclude overflow due to urethral or catheter obstruction (urge to micturate, full bladder on examination): *see* decreased urine output (*see* cd-6 below). *Confusional state causing inappropriate micturition: see* Confusional states (delirium and dementia) (p. 171). *Total urinary incontinence* (i.e. no control present, usually due to local tumor): catheterization with long-term indwelling catheter. *Stress incontinence* (incontinence on straining): exclude a hypotonic bladder (*see* below). Consider oxybutynin 3–5 mg q8h or tolterodine 1–2 mg q12h.[51] Other options are external pads, support prostheses and urethral inserts.[52] *Neurological* (caused by damage to neurological control of bladder): – *Hypotonic (neuropathic) bladder* (symptoms are difficulty in initiating micturition, intermittent stream, incomplete emptying, recurrent infections, stress incontinence; caused by damage to the sacral plexus or due to spinal cord compression below T11): teach intermittent catheterization. – *Unstable bladder* (causes frequency, nocturia, and urgency; caused by damage to suprasacral pathways): oxybutynin 3–5 mg q8h or tolterodine 1–2 mg q12h.[51] – *Unsustained bladder* (features same as unstable bladder, but symptoms are worsened by oxybutynin or other antimuscarinic drugs; caused by spinal cord damage or multiple sclerosis): teach intermittent catheterization. *Bypassing catheter:* reduce balloon volume or change to smaller size catheter. *Poor mobility:* refer to physiotherapist. Consider sheath catheter or intermittent catheterization. • **If nights are disturbed by incontinence** (and only if renal function is normal): give desmopressin 10–40 microgram intranasally or 100–400 microgram PO at night to stop overnight renal production of urine. • **Manage the consequences of incontinence:** use barrier preparations to protect skin. Personal hygiene: provide encouragement and help to wash regularly and change clothes if needed. Consider the sexual and psychological consequences.
6	Has urinary output changed?	• **Increased urine output**: consider these causes and treat if possible: cardiac failure with nocturia, chronic renal failure, diabetes mellitus, diabetes insipidus (pituitary or nephrogenic), diuretics, hypercalcemia. • **Decreased urine output** *Dehydration:* may require correction: *see* Nutrition and hydration problems (p. 119). *Obstruction of both ureters:* start dexamethasone 8 mg in the morning. Consider referral to the urologists for insertion of a ureteric stent.[53] *Obstruction of urethra:* distortion caused by fecal impaction (*see* Constipation (p. 75)); blockage by tumor (a suprapubic catheter may be needed); increased sphincter tone caused by antimuscarinic drugs (reduce dose or stop drugs). Obstruction of catheter: washout or replace. *Endocrine:* syndrome of inappropriate antidiuretic hormone (SIADH) causing fluid overload. Demeclocycline blocks the effect of ADH and is given PO 300–600 mg q12h. *See* cd-7e in Emergencies (p. 213). *Neurological:* exclude cord compression (*see* cd-9a in Emergencies (p. 213))
7	Has urinary frequency changed?	• **Increased frequency** Causes of increased urine output: *see* cd-6 above. Bladder irritability: – infection: *see* cd-1 on previous page. – unstable bladder: *see* cd-5 above. – anxiety: *see* Anxiety (p. 165). – obstruction with overflow: *see* decreased urine output (cd-5 above). *Small capacity bladder* (due to tumor): ensure regular voiding or try intermittent catheterization. • **Decreased frequency** *Causes of decreased urinary output: see* cd-6 above. *Antimuscarinic drugs* (e.g. hyoscine, tricyclic antidepressants) causing increased sphincter tone: reduce dose or stop drug. *Neurological problems: see* cd-5 above.

Adapted from Regnard and Mannix[26]
cd = clinical decision

1   a large balloon causing bladder irritability
2   a large catheter that is stretching and reducing the seal provided by the bladder sphincter or
3   obstruction of the catheter.

Choosing the correct catheter gauge is important: size 12–16Ch catheters will drain clear and dilute urine, 16–18Ch will drain urine containing debris, and 18Ch or larger are needed to drain clots.[28] Catheters with balloon sizes greater than 10 ml are best avoided.[28]

Intermittent self-catheterization

This is an underused procedure that is safe, effective and is suitable for both men and women.[30,31] It is the treatment of choice in neuropathic bladder,[32,33] but can be used in many other situations.[34–36] Because the bladder is emptied completely, the risk of infection is reduced in those with residual urine.[37] The following technique should be used at least four times a day by patients or carers.[38,39] Sterility is *not* necessary during the procedure:

1   Wash the hands.
2   Wash the skin around urethra with warm water.
3   Cover a 10Ch reusable catheter with KY lubricant jelly.
4   Insert the catheter until urine flows.
5   Once urine has stopped flowing slowly withdraw the catheter, gently rotating the catheter until no further urine flows.
6   Rinse the catheter in tap water and leave immersed in a 0.016% sodium hypochlorite solution (Hygeol in 300 ml water) for at least 30 minutes.
7   Allow the catheter to dry, and cover with clean paper tissue until the next time.

Sexual problems

Despite the many ways in which advanced disease can cause sexual dysfunction, it is uncommon for sexual problems to be discussed or explored.[40–45] In reality, many couples find it helpful that the subject has been openly discussed, whether or not it is a problem in their relationship.[46] They have often assumed it was an inevitable part of treatment or the illness and suffered in silence.[47]

Erectile impotence: Some causes can be solved simply, such as stopping a drug that is causing erectile impotence. If erectile impotence persists, a trial of sildenafil is worthwhile, as many patients with advanced disease do not have the inclination or time to wait for a full impotence assessment.

Hormonal deficiency: In women this can cause painful intercourse because of dryness and vaginitis that may be helped by lubrication or estrogen creams.

Altered body image: This can impair a patient's perception of their sexuality. While open discussion will help, some patients will need cognitive behavioral therapy or skilled psychosexual counseling.

Urinary incontinence and discharge: Incontinence has only a modest effect on sexual satisfaction,[48] but the distress of incontinence may result in reduced sexual interest. Vaginal discharge or bleeding due to tumor will often result in a cessation of intercourse.

Sex and the catheter: Some patients with catheters and their partners are still able and willing to consider intercourse, but they are afraid of the catheter. Women can have intercourse with an indwelling catheter, but the catheter can reduce satisfaction.[49] Intermittent self-catheterization is a better alternative.[28] Men who are able to achieve an erection can do so with a catheter present. Gentle intercourse is possible for men with a disconnected catheter (after draining the bladder), and placing a condom over the penis and catheter.[50] If the ejaculatory mechanism is undamaged this can still occur with a catheter, but may be painful. Alternatives are self-recatheterization or intermittent catheterization if there is no urethral obstruction, or a condom catheter if incontinence was the original reason for a catheter.[28]

Problems preventing intercourse: Local cancer, painful infection, severe incontinence, fistulae or previous surgery may prevent penetrative intercourse. Patients and their partners may wish to explore other ways of achieving sexual satisfaction. The help of a psychosexual counselor can be invaluable.

References

B = book; C = comment; Ch = chapter; CS-n = case study-number of cases; CT-n = controlled trial-number of cases; E = editorial; GC = group consensus; I = interviews; Let = letter; LS = laboratory study; MC = multi-center; OS-n = open study-number of cases; Q-n = questionnaire-number completed; R = review; RCT-n = randomized controlled trial-number of cases; RS-n = retrospective survey-number of cases; SA = systematic or meta analysis.

1 Smith DB (1999) Urinary continence issues in oncology. *Clinical Journal of Oncology Nursing.* **3**(4): 161–7. (R, 25 refs)

2 Flanagan PG, Rooney PG, Davies EA, Stout RW (1989) Evaluation of four screening tests for bacteriuria in elderly people. *Lancet.* **1**(8647): 1117–19. (CT-418)

3 Tremblay S, Labbé J (1994) Crystal clear urine and infection. *Lancet.* **343**: 479–80. (Let)

4 Clague JE, Horan MA (1994) Urine culture in the elderly: author's reply. *Lancet.* **344**: 1779–80.

5 Bent S, Nallamothu BK, Simel DL, Fihn SD, Saint S (2002) Does this woman have an acute uncomplicated urinary tract infection? *JAMA.* **287**(20): 2701–10. (SA, 52 refs)

6 Anon (1995) Urinary tract infection. *MeReC Bulletin.* **6**: 29–32.

7 Wagenlehner FM, Naber KG (2001) Uncomplicated urinary tract infections in women. *Current Opinion in Urology.* **11**(1): 49–53. (R, 31 refs)

8 Gorelick MH, Shaw KN (1999) Screening tests for urinary tract infection in children: a meta-analysis. *Pediatrics.* **104**: e54. (SA, 32 refs)

9 Thayyil-Sudhan S, Gupta S (2000) Dipstick examination for urinary tract infections. *Archives of Disease in Children.* **82**: 271–2. (Let)

10 Bullock N, Whitaker RH (1985) Massive bladder haemorrhage. *BMJ.* **291**: 1522–3. (E)

11 Gujral S, Bell R, Kabala J, Persad R (1999) Internal iliac artery embolisation for intractable bladder haemorrhage in the peri-operative phase. *Postgraduate Medical Journal.* **75**(881): 167–8. (CS-1)

12 Schultz M, van der Lelie H (1995) Microscopic haematuria as a relative contraindication for tranexamic acid. *British Journal of Haematology.* **89**(3): 663–4. (CS-3)

13 Henry R, Patterson L, Avery N, Tanzola R, Tod D, Hunter D, Nickel JC, Morales A (2001) Absorption of alkalized intravesical lidocaine in normal and inflamed bladders: a simple method for improving bladder anesthesia. *Journal of Urology.* **165**(6 Pt 1): 1900–3. (OS-24)

14 Birch BR, Miller RA (1994) Absorption characteristics of lignocaine following intravesical instillation. *Scandinavian Journal of Urology & Nephrology.* **28**(4): 359–64. (CT-11)

15 McInerney PD, Grant A, Chawla J, Stephenson TP (1992) The effect of intravesical Marcain instillation on hyperreflexic detrusor contractions. *Paraplegia.* **30**(2): 127–30. (OS-36)

16 McCoubrie R, Jeffrey D (2003) Intravesical diamorphine for bladder spasm. *Journal of Pain and Symptom Management.* **25**(1): 1–2. (Let, CS-1)

17 Cordell WH, Larson TA, Lingeman JE, Nelson DR, Woods JR, Burns LB, Klee LW (1994) Indomethacin suppositories versus intravenous titrated morphine for the treatment of ureteral colic. *Annals of Emergency Medicine.* **23**: 262–9. (RCT-75)

18 Shokeir AA (2002) Renal colic: new concepts related to pathophysiology, diagnosis and treatment. *Current Opinion in Urology.* **12**(4): 263–9. (R, 57).

19 Lee Y, Lee W, Chen M, Huang JK, Chung C, Chang LS (1992) Acupuncture in the treatment of renal colic. *Journal of Urology.* **147**: 16–18. (RCT)

20 Bogner HR, Gallo JJ, Sammel MD, Ford DE, Armenian HK, Eaton WW (2002) Urinary incontinence and psychological distress in community-dwelling older adults. *Journal of the American Geriatrics Society.* **50**(3): 489–95. (I-781)

21 Fultz NH, Herzog AR (2001) Self-reported social and emotional impact of urinary incontinence. *Journal of the American Geriatrics Society.* **49**(7): 892–9. (I-1326)

22 Rittig S, Knusden B, Sorensen S *et al.* (1989) Longterm double-blind crossover study of desmopressin intranasal spray in the management of nocturnal enuresis. In: SR Medow (ed) *Desmopressin in Nocturnal Enuresis.* Horus Medical, Sutton Coldfield. pp. 43–55. (Ch)

23 Miller M (2000) Nocturnal polyuria in older people: pathophysiology and clinical implications. *Journal of the American Geriatrics Society.* **48**(10): 1321–9. (R, 104 refs)

24 Anon (1988) Urinary tract candidosis. *Lancet.* **ii**: 1000–2.

25 Bramble FJ, Morley R (1997) Drug-induced cystitis: the need for vigilance. *British Journal of Urology.* **79**(1): 3–7. (R, 18 refs)

26 Regnard C, Mannix K (1995) Urinary problems. In: *Flow Diagrams in Advanced Cancer and Other*

Diseases. Edward Arnold, London. pp. 39–43. (Ch)

27 Getliffe K (1996) Bladder instillations and bladder washouts in the management of catheterised patients. *Journal of Advanced Nursing.* **23**(3): 548–54. (R, 49 refs).

28 Pomfret I (2000) Catheter care in the community. *Nursing Standard.* **14**(27): 46–51. (R, 23 refs)

29 Winn C (1998) Complications with urinary catheters. *Professional Nurse (Study Supplement).* **13**(5): S7–10. (R)

30 Doherty W (2000) Intermittent catheterisation: draining the bladder. *Nursing Times.* **96**(31 NTplus): 13. (R, 2 refs)

31 Hunt GM, Oakeshott P, Whitaker RH (1996) Intermittent catheterisation: simple, safe, and effective but underused. *BMJ.* **312**(7023): 103–7. (R, 35 refs)

32 Wyndaele JJ, Madersbacher H, Kovindha A (2001) Conservative treatment of the neuropathic bladder in spinal cord injured patients. *Spinal Cord.* **39**(6): 294–300. (R, 44 refs)

33 Yavuzer G, Gök H, Tuncer S, Soygür T, Arikan N, Arasil T (2000) Compliance with bladder management in spinal cord injury patients. *Spinal Cord.* **38**(12): 762–5. (OS-50)

34 Winn C, Thompson J (1999) Urinary catheters for intermittent use. *Professional Nurse.* **14**(12): 859–62, 864–5. (R, 32 refs)

35 Duffin H (2000) Intermittent self-catheterisation. *Journal of Community Nursing.* **14**(10): 29–30, 32. (CS-1)

36 Jolley S (1997) Intermittent catheterisation for post-operative urine retention. *Nursing Times.* **93**(33): 46–7. (OS)

37 Biering-Sorensen F, Bagi P, Hoiby N (2001) Urinary tract infections in patients with spinal cord lesions: treatment and prevention. *Drugs.* **61**(9): 1275–87. (R, 73 refs)

38 Anonymous (1991) Underused: intermittent self catheterisation. *Drug and Therapeutics Bulletin.* **29**: 37–9.

39 Hunt G, Whitaker R, Oakeshott P (1993) *The User's Guide to Intermittent Catheterisation.* Family Publications Ltd (in association with the British Medical Association), London. (B)

40 Schover LR (1999) Counseling cancer patients about changes in sexual function. *Oncology (Huntington).* **13**(11): 1585–91; discussion 1591–2, 1595–6. (R)

41 Shell JA (2002) Evidence-based practice for symptom management in adults with cancer: sexual dysfunction. *Oncology Nursing Forum.* **29**(1): 53–66. (SA, 104 refs)

42 Penson RT, Gallagher J, Gioiella ME, Wallace M, Borden K, Duska LA, Talcott JA, McGovern FJ, Appleman LJ, Chabner BA, Lynch TJ Jr (2000) Sexuality and cancer: conversation comfort zone. *Oncologist.* **5**(4): 336–44. (R)

43 Ofman US (1995) Preservation of function in genitourinary cancers: psychosexual and psychosocial issues. *Cancer Investigation.* **13**(1): 125–31. (R, 47 refs)

44 Andersen BL (1990) How cancer affects sexual functioning. *Oncology (Huntington).* **4**(6): 81–8; discussion 92–4. (R, 30 refs)

45 Cort E (1998) Nurses' attitudes to sexuality in caring for cancer patients. *Nursing Times.* **94**(42): 54–6. (OS)

46 Ananth H, Jones L, King M, Tookman A (2003) The impact of cancer on sexual function: a controlled study. *Palliative Medicine.* **17**: 202–5. (Q-120)

47 Hughes MK (2000) Sexuality and the cancer survivor: a silent coexistence. *Cancer Nursing.* **23**(6): 477–82. (R, 55 refs)

48 Lalos O, Berglund A, Lalos A (2001) Impact of urinary and climacteric symptoms on social and sexual life after surgical treatment of stress urinary incontinence in women: a long-term outcome. *Journal of Advanced Nursing.* **33**(3): 316–27. (OS-45)

49 Watanabe T, Rivas DA, Smith R, Staas WE Jr, Chancellor MB (1996) The effect of urinary tract reconstruction on neurologically impaired women previously treated with an indwelling urethral catheter. *Journal of Urology.* **156**(6): 1926–8. (OS-18)

50 Rigby D (1998) Long-term catheter care. *Professional Nurse (Study Supplement).* **13**(5S): 14–15.

51 Anonymous (2001) Managing incontinence due to detrusor instability. *Drug and Therapeutics Bulletin.* **39**: 59–64.

52 Sasso KC (1998) New treatment options for stress incontinence. *RN.* **61**(9): 36–9. (R, 6 refs)

53 Smith P, Bruera E (1995) Management of malignant ureteral obstruction in the palliative care setting. *Journal of Pain and Symptom Management.* **10**: 481–6.

Psychological symptoms

- Anger

- Anxiety

- Confusional states (delirium and dementia)

- Withdrawal and depression

Anger

Clinical decision and action checklist

1 Acknowledge what anger does to you.
2 Acknowledge the person's anger.
3 Are several family members angry?
4 Is the person controlled and contained?
5 Is the anger appropriate?
6 Is the anger inappropriate?
7 Is the anger escalating?
8 Is the person depressed?
9 Is the anger causing isolation?
10 Is the anger persisting?

Key points

- Many situations in advanced disease can cause anger.
- Be aware of what anger does to you.
- Apologize if you are at fault, never apologize for others.
- Anger should defuse rapidly. If it does not, be prepared to stop the interview and leave.

Introduction

Advanced illness produces many reasons to be angry, such as unrealized ambitions, loss of control, feelings of hopelessness, depression, persistent symptoms and spiritual conflicts. Anger can be an accompanying feature of pain,[1] anticipatory grief[2] or depression.[3,4] It is more common in adult children and in care-givers not living with the patient.[2] Anger can present in different ways:

Expression	Level of anger	Target of anger
Active	Proportionate	Correctly directed
Passive	Out of proportion	Misdirected

Anger that is actively expressed, proportionate or correctly directed is easier to help than anger that is passive, out of proportion or misdirected. No assumptions should be made about the anger until it has been assessed.

161

Getting started

Be aware of what anger does to you: It is common to be emotionally affected when confronted by an angry person. Some professionals feel irritated, in which case they need to suppress this irritation to avoid escalating the anger. Other professionals become withdrawn at the anger being directed at them, and need to be more assertive in order to be believed and help the angry person effectively. The key is to be calm but clear.[5] If your reaction makes it difficult for you to help an angry person it would be best to ask someone else to see the angry person, and to consider getting advice or teaching on helping an angry person.

Acknowledge the anger: e.g. 'I can see this has made you angry. How can I help?' While this may seem unnecessary, it gives the person a clear message that you have noticed their anger and that you are taking it seriously. Most people want to know that the professional is prepared to listen and help.

The setting: With an angry person it is usually impossible to choose the right setting. If the setting seems particularly awkward (e.g. a busy corridor) then as the discussion progresses it is reasonable to suggest an alternative, more private venue.

The appropriateness of anger: The cause can be elicited by asking, 'What's happened to make you feel like this?' The extent of the anger can be clarified by asking, 'On a scale of 0 to 10, how angry have you been?' Most anger is understandable in that (a) its reasons can be understood, and (b) some people in distressing situations become angry.

Apologizing: When the anger is correctly directed at the professional, and that anger is proportionate to the situation, it is best to apologize. For example: 'I'm sorry you were kept waiting for so long – it would make me angry too.' However, when the anger is about the behavior of another health professional, avoid the temptation to defend that person since (a) it is not your place to defend others, and (b) trying to defend the other person will fail to defuse the anger and will only result in the accusation that 'You lot all stick together!' You can still show your concern without being defensive, for example: 'I can see why you're angry.' Then suggest that they speak or write to the individual to express their concerns.

Escalating anger

The steps so far should have defused most people's anger *within a few minutes*. At the very least, it should be no worse. Occasionally, however, the anger escalates. If this happens:

- Position yourself by the nearest exit.
- Acknowledge the escalating anger, e.g. 'I can see you're having difficulty controlling your anger.'
- Set limits. Admitting to them that their anger is making you feel uncomfortable should switch the focus from anger to the underlying emotion such as fear or sadness. If they cannot switch, they are unlikely to calm down.
- If the person cannot accept the limits, end the interview and leave immediately to avoid the risk of being assaulted.

Persisting anger

There are several reasons for persisting anger:

1 this is a person's normal behaviour
2 a clinical depression
3 unrealized ambitions, e.g. not seeing children grow up
4 loss of control because of weakness or immobility, or
5 spiritual anger.

The last four may need additional or specialist help.[6–8]

Clinical decision	If YES ⇒ Action
1 Acknowledge what anger does to you (if such situations always make you very angry or very passive, ask someone else to conduct the interview).	
2 Acknowledge the person's anger, e.g. 'I can see you're angry, how can I help?'	
3 Are several family members angry?	• Take someone with you from a different discipline, e.g. if you are a doctor ask a nurse or social worker to join you.
4 Is the person controlled and contained?	• *If the person is passively angry:* Acknowledge the anger (e.g. 'Am I right that this has made you angry?'). Negotiate to discuss the cause (e.g. 'Can you explain why you're feeling like this?'). Encourage the expression of anger (e.g. 'Just how angry have you been?'). • *If you (the professional) are the only person who is angry:* you should withdraw and seek support.
5 Is the anger appropriate?	• *If it is correctly directed and proportionate to the situation* (e.g. appointments are running (very) late): Identify the level of anger. Show understanding without being defensive (e.g. 'I'd be angry too'). Enable them to express their anger. Apologize if you have made an error (do not apologize for others).
6 Is the anger inappropriate?	• *If it is misdirected* (e.g. anger at a family physician that chemotherapy failed): Check this (e.g. 'I can see that you're angry that the treatment didn't work, but could you tell me why your anger is directed at me?'). Explore the causes of anger that may be uncovered. • *If the setting is difficult:* suggest moving to a quiet room. • If the level is out of proportion to the situation: Go to cd-7 below.
7 Is the anger escalating?	• Position yourself near the room exit with the door open. • Set limits (e.g. 'I can see that this has made you very angry. I want to help, but your anger is beginning to make me feel uncomfortable. If you don't feel you can control your anger, I wouldn't feel comfortable continuing.'). • **If the person cannot accept limits this is likely to be pathological anger.** **Stop the interview and leave the room immediately.** (e.g. 'In that case I have to stop this discussion now.')
8 Is the person depressed?	e.g. apathetic or expressing feelings of hopelessness. • *See* Withdrawal and depression (p. 177).
9 Is the anger causing isolation?	• Acknowledge their isolation (e.g. 'Your anger seems to have left you isolated'). • Explore the effects of the isolation on relationships.
10 Is the anger persisting?	• *If this is normal behavior:* usually no action is needed. Most naturally angry people recognize this and acknowledge its presence. Occasionally limits have to be set as in cd-7 above. • *If this is unusual behavior for the person:* Are there causes unconnected to the illness? Ask for specialist advice and help for the person (e.g. cognitive therapy).

Adapted from Faulkner, Maguire and Regnard[9]
cd = clinical decision

References

B = book; C = comment; Ch = chapter; CS-n = case study-number of cases; CT-n = controlled trial-number of cases; E = editorial; GC = group consensus; I = interviews; LS = laboratory study; MC = multi-center; OS-n = open study-number of cases; R = review; RCT-n = randomized controlled trial-number of cases; RS-n = retrospective survey-number of cases; SA = systematic or meta analysis.

1   Sela RA, Bruera E, Conner-Spady B, Cumming C, Walker C (2002) Sensory and affective dimensions of advanced cancer pain. *Psycho-Oncology.* **11**(1): 23–34. (OS-111)

2   Chapman KJ, Pepler C (1998) Coping, hope, and anticipatory grief in family members in palliative home care. *Cancer Nursing.* **21**(4): 226–34. (I-61)

3   Robbins PR, Tanck RH (1997) Anger and depressed affect: interindividual and intra-individual perspectives. *Journal of Psychology.* **131**(5): 489–500. (OS-78)

4   Koh KB, Kim CH, Park JK (2002) Predominance of anger in depressive disorders compared with anxiety disorders and somatoform disorders. *Journal of Clinical Psychiatry.* **63**(6): 486–92. (OS-402)

5   Garnham P (2001) Understanding and dealing with anger, aggression and violence. *Nursing Standard.* **16**(6): 37–42. (R, 11 refs)

6   Brittlebank A, Regnard C (1990) Terror or depression? A case report. *Palliative Medicine.* **4**: 317–19. (CS-1)

7   Ramsay N (1992) Referral to a liaison psychiatrist from a palliative care unit. *Palliative Medicine.* **6**: 54–60.

8   Moorey S, Greer S (2002) Cognitive techniques II: applications of cognitive techniques to common problems. In: *Cognitive Behaviour Therapy for People with Cancer.* Oxford University Press, Oxford. pp. 126–31. (Ch)

9   Faulkner A, Maguire P, Regnard C (1995) The angry person. In: *Flow Diagrams in Advanced Cancer and Other Diseases.* Edward Arnold, London. pp. 81–5. (Ch)

Anxiety

1 Does the person feel apprehensive, tense or on edge?
2 Can an anxiety state be excluded?
3 Is an anxiety state present?
4 Is the person functioning poorly?
5 Are somatic symptoms distressing?
6 Do sudden panics or phobic episodes occur?
7 Is the anxiety persisting?

Key points

- Anxiety is common in advanced disease, but not inevitable or untreatable.
- Much anxiety can be eased with clear communication and simple measures.
- Anxiety and depression often coexist.
- Specialist help is needed for persistent, severe anxiety.

Introduction

Life-threatening illness creates an uncertain future that causes anxiety that may increase as the illness progresses. Anxiety in turn makes it more difficult for the patient to cope with suffering. Anxiety is common in advanced disease,[1] but is missed in more than half of patients,[2] or not recorded in medical notes.[3] It is associated with symptoms such as anorexia,[4] depression,[5] is commoner in younger adults,[6] and when information is inadequate.[7] It is also common in partners and relatives.[8]

Identifying anxiety

Features of anxiety are *apprehensive expectation* (e.g. fear, rumination, tendency to perceive situations in a threatening way), *vigilance and scanning* (e.g. irritability, poor concentration, difficulty getting to sleep, tendency to perceive bodily sensations in a threatening way), *motor tension* (e.g. trembling, tension, restlessness) and *autonomic hyperactivity* (e.g. sweating, dry mouth, cold hands, tachycardia, diarrhea). In advanced disease, anxiety is often associated with depression. The Hospital Anxiety and Depression (HAD) scale is a simple screening tool that is more useful for anxiety than depression,[9] but may not be sufficiently sensitive for use in palliative care.[10]

Anxiety state: This has a persistent, dominating and intrusive quality accompanied by at least four anxiety-related symptoms for at least two weeks. If severe, it can cause disorganized functioning (*see* later on this page).

Drug-induced restlessness (akathisia): This can mimic the motor tension aspects of anxiety, but patients may deny any severe anxiety. Examples of drugs that may cause this are haloperidol, hyoscine, methotrimeprazine, metoclopramide and the tricyclic antidepressants (e.g. amitriptyline).

Helping the anxious person

Supportive measures: Enabling a person to express their feelings and giving the information they need can do much to ease anxiety. Helping the individual to look for links between thoughts and feelings can generate more realistic interpretations. For example, feeling 'out of control with all that machinery' can be changed into, 'It's good to think all that technology is there to help.' Similar approaches have been used with visualization and guided imagery.[11–14] Simple anxiety management techniques can be helpful, such as distraction or relaxation. Muscle relaxation techniques are best avoided as it can worsen the anxiety of some people who are excessively vigilant of their bodily sensations. Autogenic relaxation (deep relaxation and self-hypnosis) is a better alternative,[15] but there is equivocal evidence for its success in anxiety.[16] The evidence for reflexology in treating anxiety is conflicting.[17,18] Other approaches include hypnosis,[19] music therapy[20] and aromatherapy.[21,22]

Disorganized functioning: As anxiety worsens, the individual becomes increasingly distracted from daily activities. As it becomes more severe, it begins to intrude on everyday decisions such as what to wear or whether to get washed. Decisions become increasingly erratic and are made on the spur of the moment. Moderate disorganization will ease with anxiety suppressants such as the benzodiazepines. Severe disorganization will require antipsychotics. Although haloperidol, olanzepine and methotrimeprazine are effective in severe anxiety,[23–25] risperidone is more effective.[26–28]

Panic: This occurs suddenly without an obvious cause, is intense and can last 5–20 minutes. A fear of dying and loss of control are often provoked by the episodes. Although there is no obvious warning, individuals can be taught to identify triggers or specific thoughts that precede a panic. These thoughts may give some clue as to the cause, but also provide a means of instituting self-taught controls that with practice can prevent panic-triggering thoughts initiating a panic episode. Intranasal or buccal midazolam can help reduce isolated panics related to procedures.[29]

Phobias: Situations or objects are interpreted as occasions when help is impossible, difficult or embarrassing. If individuals feel humiliated by these feelings they will find it hard to disclose their phobia. Treatment often needs specialist help, requiring a combination of cognitive behavioral therapy and antidepressants.[30,31]

When problems persist

Specialist help will be needed to unravel mixed disorders (e.g. mixed anxiety and depression), to diagnose unusual presentations, deal with a persistent anxiety state or provide further therapy.[32,33] This help may be from a psychiatrist, psychologist, counselor or social worker.[34] Cognitive behavioral therapy can be particularly helpful.[35] In reality, however, which specialist is enlisted is more likely to depend on what is available locally.

Clinical decision	If YES ⇒ Action
1 Does the person feel apprehensive, tense or on edge?	• Exclude: Drug-induced motor restlessness (akathisia). The patient appears restless but may deny any anxiety (*see* notes opposite for list of drugs). Stop the drug causing the reaction. *Confusional state: see* Confusional states (delirium and dementia) (p. 171). • *Start supportive measures:* Supportive communication. Offer information if patient wishes this (if the information is likely to be difficult news, *see* Breaking difficult news (p. 25)). Explore causes of anxiety by encouragement to disclose concerns (*see* Helping the person with the effects of difficult news (p. 29)). Look for links between thoughts and feelings. Explore possible solutions, e.g. by helping the person to form more realistic interpretations or visualize more positive images. Look at how to change procedures that are causing anxiety. Consider relaxation, massage, aromatherapy or music therapy.
2 Can an anxiety state be excluded?	• *If this is moderate anxiety:* Teach relaxation exercises (distraction, autogenic relaxation). Enable access to aromatherapy and massage, if available.
3 Is an anxiety state present?	• Characteristics: Persistent apprehension for more than 2 weeks and for more than 50% of the time. This is different to their usual mood. Four or more features of anxiety are present • Follow the clinical decisions below.
4 Is the person functioning poorly?	• *If disorganization is moderate* (poor concentration, but able to care for themselves): Start a benzodiazepine: for minimal sedation use lorazepam 0.5–1 mg PO or sublingually.[36] If insomnia is the problem use temazepam 10–40 mg at bedtime. • *If disorganization is severe* (tormented, unable to care for themselves or make a decision): Start an antipsychotic: for minimal sedation use risperidone 2–4 mg (0.5–1 mg in elderly) PO once daily. If sedation is needed use olanzepine 5–10 mg PO once daily or methotrimeprazine (Canada only) 25–50 mg q8h PO or SC. • *If the disorganization persists:* refer for specialist help and advice.
5 Are somatic symptoms distressing?	i.e. autonomic hyperactivity (e.g. tremor, tachycardia, sweating, diarrhea). • Consider a β-blocker, e.g. propranolol 10–40 mg q8h (NB: risk of hypotension if used with lorazepam, temazepam or methotrimeprazine).
6 Do sudden panics or phobic episodes occur?	• Seek out triggers and explore thoughts. • *For panic:* provide explanation and company. – single episodes (e.g. during MRI scan): 2–4 mg midazolam spray intranasally[29] or midazolam solution sublingually. – repeated episodes: clomipramine 25 mg at night (10 mg if > 70 years), or an SSRI antidepressant such as paroxetine 10–40 mg PO once in the morning.[37] • *For phobias:* consider lorazepam 0.5–1 mg sublingually 1–2 hours before exposure to precipitating event. If persistent, consider clomipramine or an SSRI as above for panic. • Refer for cognitive behavioral therapy if available.[38]
7 Is the anxiety persisting?	• Consider: – the concurrent presence of depression (*see* Withdrawal and depression (p. 177)). – referral for specialist advice and help.

Adapted from Maguire, Faulkner and Regnard[39]
cd = clinical decision

References

B = book; C = comment; Ch = chapter; CS-n = case study-number of cases; CT-n = controlled trial-number of cases; E = editorial; GC = group consensus; I = interviews; LS = laboratory study; MC = multi-center; OS-n = open study-number of cases; Q-n = questionnaire-number of respondents; R = review; RCT-n = randomized controlled trial-number of cases; RS-n = retrospective survey-number of cases; SA = systematic or meta analysis.

1 Tremblay A, Breitbart W (2001) Psychiatric dimensions of palliative care. *Neurologic Clinics.* **19**(4): 949–67. (R, 63 refs)

2 Krishnasamy M, Wilkie E, Haviland J (2001) Lung cancer health care needs assessment: patients' and informal carers' responses to a national mail questionnaire survey. *Palliative Medicine.* **15**(3): 213–27. (Q-279)

3 Strömgren AS, Groenvold M, Pedersen L, Olsen AK, Spile M, Sjøgren P (2001) Does the medical record cover the symptoms experienced by cancer patients receiving palliative care? A comparison of the record and patient self-rating. *Journal of Pain and Symptom Management.* **21**(3): 189–96. (OS-58)

4 Hawkins C (2000) Anorexia and anxiety in advanced malignancy: the relative problem. *Journal of Human Nutrition & Dietetics.* **13**(2): 113–17. (Q-147)

5 Devanand DP (2002) Comorbid psychiatric disorders in late life depression. *Biological Psychiatry.* **52**(3): 236–42. (R, 51)

6 Walsh D, Donnelly S, Rybicki L (2000) The symptoms of advanced cancer: relationship to age, gender, and performance status in 1000 patients. *Supportive Care in Cancer.* **8**(3): 175–9. (OS-100)

7 Fallowfield LJ, Jenkins VA, Beveridge HA (2002) Truth may hurt but deceit hurts more: communication in palliative care. *Palliative Medicine.* **16**(4): 297–303. (R)

8 Aranda SK, Hayman-White K (2001) Home caregivers of the person with advanced cancer: an Australian perspective. *Cancer Nursing.* **24**(4): 300–7. (I-42)

9 Le Fevre P, Devereux J, Smith S, Lawrie SM, Cornbleet M (1999) Screening for psychiatric illness in the palliative care inpatient setting: a comparison between the Hospital Anxiety and Depression Scale and the General Health Questionnaire-12. *Palliative Medicine.* **13**(5): 399–407. (OS-79)

10 Lloyd-Williams M, Friedman T, Rudd N (2001) An analysis of the validity of the Hospital Anxiety and Depression Scale as a screening tool in patients with advanced metastatic cancer. *Journal of Pain and Symptom Management.* **22**(6): 990–6. (OS-100)

11 Green L (1994) Touch and visualisation to facilitate a therapeutic relationship in an intensive care unit – a personal experience. *Intensive & Critical Care Nursing.* **10**(1): 51–7. (R, 30 refs)

12 Thompson MB, Coppens NM (1994) The effects of guided imagery on anxiety levels and movement of clients undergoing magnetic resonance imaging. *Holistic Nursing Practice.* **8**(2): 59–69. (RCT-41)

13 Hattan J, King L, Griffiths P (2002) The impact of foot massage and guided relaxation following cardiac surgery: a randomized controlled trial. *Journal of Advanced Nursing.* **37**(2): 199–207. (RCT-25)

14 Van Fleet S (2000) Relaxation and imagery for symptom management: improving patient assessment and individualizing treatment. *Oncology Nursing Forum.* **27**(3): 501–10. (R, 77 refs)

15 Wright S, Courtney U, Crowther D (2002) A quantitative and qualitative pilot study of the perceived benefits of autogenic training for a group of people with cancer. *European Journal of Cancer Care.* **11**(2): 122–30. (R)

16 Ernst E, Kanji N (2000) Autogenic training for stress and anxiety: a systematic review. *Complementary Therapies in Medicine.* **8**(2): 106–10. (SA, 11 refs)

17 Williamson J, White A, Hart A, Ernst E (2002) Randomised controlled trial of reflexology for menopausal symptoms. *BJOG: an International Journal of Obstetrics & Gynaecology.* **109**(9): 1050–5. (RCT-75)

18 Stephenson NL, Weinrich SP, Tavakoli AS (2000) The effects of foot reflexology on anxiety and pain in patients with breast and lung cancer. *Oncology Nursing Forum.* **27**(1): 67–72. (RCT-23)

19 Liossi C, White P (2001) Efficacy of clinical hypnosis in the enhancement of quality of life of terminally ill cancer patients. *Contemporary Hypnosis.* **18**(3): 145–60. (RCT-50)

20 Hilliard RE (2001) The use of music therapy in meeting the multidimensional needs of hospice patients and families. *Journal of Palliative Care.* **17**(3): 161–6. (CS-4)

21 Hadfield N (2001) The role of aromatherapy massage in reducing anxiety in patients with

malignant brain tumours. *International Journal of Palliative Nursing.* **7**(6): 279–85. (CS-8)

22 Wilkinson S, Aldridge J, Salmon I, Cain E, Wilson B (1999) An evaluation of aromatherapy massage in palliative care. *Palliative Medicine.* **13**(5): 409–17. (RCT-103)

23 Currier GW, Trenton A (2002) Pharmacological treatment of psychotic agitation. *CNS Drugs.* **16**(4): 219–28. (R, 63 refs)

24 Khojainova N, Santiago-Palma J, Kornick C, Breitbart W, Gonzales GR (2002) Olanzapine in the management of cancer pain. *Journal of Pain and Symptom Management.* **23**(4): 346–50. (OS-8)

25 Mintzer J, Faison W, Street JS, Sutton VK, Breier A (2001) Olanzapine in the treatment of anxiety symptoms due to Alzheimer's disease: a post hoc analysis. *International Journal of Geriatric Psychiatry.* **16**(Suppl 1): S71–7. (RCT)

26 Blin O, Azorin JM, Bouhours P (1996) Antipsychotic and anxiolytic properties of risperidone, haloperidol, and methotrimeprazine in schizophrenic patients. *Journal of Clinical Psychopharmacology.* **16**(1): 38–44. (RCT-63)

27 Chouinard G, Jones B, Remington G, Bloom D, Addington D, MacEwan GW, Labelle A, Beauclair L, Arnott W (1993) A Canadian multicenter placebo-controlled study of fixed doses of risperidone and haloperidol in the treatment of chronic schizophrenic patients. *Journal of Clinical Psychopharmacology.* **13**: 25–40. (RCT-135)

28 Conley RR, Mahmoud R (2001) A randomized double-blind study of risperidone and olanzapine in the treatment of schizophrenia or schizoaffective disorder. *American Journal of Psychiatry.* **158**(5): 765–74. (RCT-377)

29 Hollenhorst J, Munte S, Friedrich L, Heine J, Leuwer M, Becker H, Piepenbrock S (2001) Using intranasal midazolam spray to prevent claustrophobia induced by MR imaging. *American Journal of Roentgenology.* **176**(4): 865–8. (RCT-54)

30 Rogers P, Gournay K (2001) Phobias: nature, assessment and treatment. *Nursing Standard.* **15**(30): 37–43. (R, 29 refs)

31 Blomhoff S, Haug TT, Hellstrom K, Holme I, Humble M, Madsbu HP, Wold JE (2001) Randomised controlled general practice trial of sertraline, exposure therapy and combined treatment in generalised social phobia. *British Journal of Psychiatry.* **179**: 23–30. (RCT-387)

32 Brittlebank A, Regnard C (1990) Terror or depression? A case report. *Palliative Medicine.* **4**: 317–19.

33 Ramsay N (1992) Referral to a liaison psychiatrist from a palliative care unit. *Palliative Medicine.* **6**: 54–60.

34 Sheldon FM (2000) Dimensions of the role of the social worker in palliative care. *Palliative Medicine.* **14**(6): 491–8. (R, 14 refs)

35 Moorey S, Greer S (2002) Cognitive techniques II: applications of cognitive techniques to common problems. In: *Cognitive Behaviour Therapy for People with Cancer.* Oxford University Press, Oxford. pp. 121–6. (Ch)

36 Barraclough J (1997) ABC of palliative care: Depression, anxiety, and confusion. *BMJ.* **315**: 1365–8. (R)

37 Wagstaff AJ, Cheer SM, Matheson AJ, Ormrod D, Goa KL (2002) Paroxetine: an update of its use in psychiatric disorders in adults. *Drugs.* **62**(4): 655–703. (R, 179 refs)

38 Cosgrave E, McGorry P, Allen N, Jackson H (2000) Depression in young people: a growing challenge for primary care. *Australian Family Physician.* **29**(2): 123–7, 145–6. (R, 21 refs)

39 Maguire P, Faulkner A, Regnard C (1995) The anxious person. In: *Flow Diagrams in Advanced Cancer and Other Diseases.* Edward Arnold, London. pp. 73–6. (Ch)

Confusional states (delirium and dementia)

Clinical decision and action checklist

1 Is memory failure present?
2 Has alertness changed?
3 Is concentration impaired?
4 Is the patient experiencing unusual sights or sounds?
5 Has behavior altered?
6 Explain the cause and treatment.
7 Is urgent control of disturbance necessary?

Key points

- Provide company, a constant routine and a light, quiet environment.
- Always assume a patient understands.

Introduction

Confusion is common in the terminal stages of advanced disease and is associated with a short prognosis.[1–6]

Symptoms of confusion

Acute confusional states (delirium): Six features are highly specific: acute onset, fluctuating course, disorganized thinking, inattention, memory impairment and disorientation. Four are less specific: altered sleep-awake cycle, abnormal psychomotor activity, perceptual disturbance and altered alertness (an alternating pattern of hypo-alertness and hyper-alertness is commonest).[7] Acute confusion is likely if there are four or more features.[8] Simple rating tools can be useful,[9–11] but disordered writing skills may be a simple and sensitive sign.[12]

Chronic confusional states (dementia) can appear similar to acute states, but with a history of years or months, symptoms that fluctuate less, and the patient's alertness is unlikely to have changed. Dementia related to some diseases can develop rapidly over a few months (e.g. Down's syndrome, AIDS, Batten's disease) and can be associated with other problems such as epilepsy.

Memory failure: This is common and often due to a failure to take in information. In the dementias there is a failure to retain information because of irreversible cortical damage.

Alteration in alertness: This can be an increase or decrease in alertness.[7] Drugs and infection are the commonest causes. Hypercalcemia should always be suspected in patients with malignancy who have unexplained confusion. In the dementias, alertness is unchanged.

Impaired concentration: This can occur independently of any change in alertness. An extreme form is seen in 'frozen terror', where severe anxiety produces a state of immobile withdrawal.[13]

Abnormal experiences: Misperceptions have an external stimulus and occur with reduced alertness or concentration. For example, a patient may think they see someone to one side, only to turn and find no one is there. Hallucinations are much less common and have no outside stimulus, e.g. seeing a green cat climb up a wall. While misperceptions and hallucinations may be two ends of a spectrum, their differentiation is important,[14] e.g. with morphine, misperceptions will usually disappear as tolerance to drowsiness occurs, whereas hallucinations require a change in dose or opioid. It is also important to understand that some misperceptions and hallucinations are not frightening to the patient and may even be comforting, such as seeing a long-lost relative or seeing a friendly pet.

Altered behavior: This can cause the most difficulties in managing a confused patient. When due to a reversible, acute confusional state, treating the cause of the confusion will return the behavior to normal. If the behavior is distressing to the patient, behavior modification or medication may be needed.

Helping the confused patient

Find the cause: The commonest causes of delirium are drugs, organ failure, hypoxia, infection and hypercalcemia, many of which can be treated.[15] Dehydration may contribute to acute confusion but the evidence that rehydration alone is helpful is equivocal.[16–21]

Working together: Confusional states can be frightening for patients, family and staff. An informed, interdisciplinary approach is essential.[22] Confused patients can understand explanations, although if their concentration is impaired this explanation may have to be repeated several times. It is also important to provide the partner and relatives with information.[23] Families can help to identify if a patient is distressed.

Urgent control of disturbance: Confusion is not always distressing to the patient, but occasionally the behavior risks harm to the confused patient or others, or there is a clear consensus that the patient is distressed by the experience. Because escape and paranoia are two common features it may take a great deal of explanation and a calm, well-lit environment. Drugs should be a last resort.[24] If needed, they should be chosen on the basis of the symptoms.[25] In the absence of abnormal behavior, and in the presence of anxiety, benzodiazepines will help suppress the anxiety to a level that is manageable for the patient. However, benzodiazepines can worsen confusion,[26] and when abnormal behavior or severe anxiety is present then antipsychotic medication is needed. A few patients need both. It is unusual to need to sedate a confused patient,[2] but irreversible confusion causing persistent suffering in the last hours and days of a patient's life may need drugs in doses that cause sedation (*see* also Emergencies: severe agitation (cd-4, p. 207)).[27–31] For dose equivalents, *see* p. 174.

Clinical decision	If YES ⇒ Action
1 Is memory failure present?	• Orient frequently in time, place and person. • Ensure that there is a constant environment and encourage activity. • *If a cerebral tumor is present:* start high-dose dexamethasone and consider cranial irradiation. • *If the history suggests dementia* (*see* notes opposite): plan for longer-term care.
2 Has alertness changed?	• Consider the following: Drugs recently started: many drugs can cause confusion. Stop all except absolutely essential drugs. Reduce the dose of essential drugs or change to alternatives. If opioid toxicity signs are present (myoclonus, pinpoint pupils) reduce the dose or change the opioid.[32–35] Beware of drugs with long half lives that may cause problems a week or more after starting (e.g. amitriptyline, diazepam or methadone). Drug, alcohol or nicotine withdrawal: this tends to cause increased alertness. Restart the missing drug, alcohol or nicotine (e.g. nicotine patch). • Exclude the following: Infection: reduce pyrexia, examine the chest, test urine. Treat if possible. Biochemical cause: (hypercalcemia, uremia, inappropriate ADH secretion). Treat if possible. Cardiac or respiratory disease: (ventricular failure, pleural effusion, pulmonary metastases). Treat if possible. Recent trauma: (long bone fracture, subdural hematoma). • *If dehydrated: see* Nutrition and hydration problems (p. 119). Rehydration may improve some patients with acute confusion, but is only one of several approaches.[5] • *If alertness is severely reduced,* try methylphenidate 2.5–5 mg in the morning, increasing if necessary to 10–15 mg.[36–40] Anxiety, nervousness and insomnia are common adverse effects.
3 Is concentration impaired?	• *Exclude an anxiety state:* – *anxiety is present:* consider worries that may be distracting the patient such as ignorance about the diagnosis, communication problems, or social problems. – *in the absence of anxiety:* consider causes of distraction such as pain. – exclude psychiatric illness such as clinical depression.
4 Is the patient experiencing unusual sights or sounds?	• Ensure a well-lit, quiet and consistent environment. • *If patient is misinterpreting an external stimulus:* review the causes of altered alertness above. • *If patient is hallucinating (no external stimulus):* – exclude drugs, or chemical withdrawal. – if these are distressing the patient *see* cd-7 below. – consider a psychotic illness and refer as appropriate.
5 Has the behavior altered?	(e.g. wandering, paranoid, euphoric, manic, depressed) • Exclude the causes of memory failure in cd-1 above. • Consider drugs as in cd-2 above. • Consider psychiatric illness and refer as appropriate.
6 **Explain** the cause of confusion, possible treatment and management to patient (and to family and staff).	
7 Is urgent control of disturbance necessary?	• Ensure that the environment is well-lit and quiet with a minimum of staff changes. • *In the absence of abnormal experiences or altered behavior:* To reduce anxiety with minimal sedation: lorazepam 0.5–1 mg PO or sublingually. If sedation is required: midazolam 2–10 mg SC or sublingual q1h PRN (or 20–120 mg SC infusion per 24 hours). • *In the presence of aggression:* haloperidol 2.5–10 mg hs PO or SC[41] or risperidone PO 0.5–2 mg at bedtime.[46] • *In the presence of abnormal experiences or altered behavior:* – if sedation needs to be kept to a minimum: haloperidol 2.5–10 mg hs PO or SC[42] or risperidone PO 0.5–2 mg at bedtime.[43–46] – if sedation is required: olanzapine PO 5–10 mg daily[47–50] or methotrimeprazine (Canada only) 12.5–100 mg q8h PO or SC (or as SC infusion 25–300 mg per 24 hours). • *If the patient is suffering from persistent agitation: see* cd-4 Emergencies (p. 207).

Adapted from Stedeford and Regnard[51]
cd = clinical decision

The following columns show approximate dose equivalents:[52]

Benzodiazepines	Antipsychotics
diazepam 5 mg	chlorpromazine 100 mg
midazolam 2.5 mg	methotrimeprazine 50 mg
lorazepam 0.5 mg	haloperidol 2.5 mg
clonazepam 0.25 mg	risperidone 0.5 mg

References

B = book; C = comment; Ch = chapter; CS-n = case study-number of cases; CT-n = controlled trial-number of cases; E = editorial; GC = group consensus; I = interviews; Let = letter; LS = laboratory study; MC = multi-center; OS-n = open study-number of cases; R = review; RCT-n = randomized controlled trial-number of cases; RS-n = retrospective survey-number of cases; SA = systematic or meta analysis.

1 Caraceni A, Nanni O, Maltoni M, Piva L, Indelli M, Arnoldi E, Monti M, Montanari L, Amadori D, De Conno F (2000) Impact of delirium on the short term prognosis of advanced cancer patients. Italian Multicenter Study Group on Palliative Care. *Cancer.* **89**(5): 1145–9. (OS-393)

2 Fainsinger RL, De Moissac D, Mancini I, Oneschuk D (2000) Sedation for delirium and other symptoms in terminally ill patients in Edmonton. *Journal of Palliative Care.* **16**(2): 5–10. (OS-150)

3 Morita T, Tsunoda J, Inoue S, Chihara S (1999) Survival prediction of terminally ill cancer patients by clinical symptoms: development of a simple indicator. *Japanese Journal of Clinical Oncology.* **29**(3): 156–9. (OS-245)

4 Hall P, Schroder C, Weaver L (2002) The last 48 hours of life in long-term care: a focused chart audit. *Journal of the American Geriatrics Society.* **50**(3): 501–6. (RS-185)

5 Lawlor PG, Gagnon B, Mancini IL, Pereira JL, Hanson J, Suarez-Almazor ME, Bruera ED (2000) Occurrence, causes, and outcome of delirium in patients with advanced cancer: a prospective study. *Archives of Internal Medicine.* **160**(6): 786–94. (OS-113)

6 Pereira J, Hanson J, Bruera E (1997) The frequency and clinical course of cognitive impairment in patients with terminal cancer. *Cancer.* **79**(4): 835–42. (RS-321)

7 O'Keeffe ST, Lavan JN (1999) Clinical significance of delirium subtypes in older people. *Age & Ageing.* **28**(2): 115–19. (OS-94)

8 Inouye SK, van Dyck CH, Alessi CA, Balkin S, Siegal AP, Horwitz RI (1990) Clarifying confusion: the confusion assessment method – a new method for detection of delerium. *Annals of Internal Medicine.* **113**: 941–8. (OS-56)

9 Smith MJ, Breitbart WS, Platt MM (1995) A critique of instruments and methods to detect, diagnose and rate delirium. *Journal of Pain and Symptom Management.* **10**: 35–77. (SA, 237 refs).

10 Brietbart W, Sparrow B (1998) Management of delirium in the terminally ill. *Progress in Palliative Care.* **6**: 107–13. (R, 82 refs)

11 Morita T, Tsunoda J, Inoue S, Chihara S, Oka K (2001) Communication capacity scale and agitation distress scale to measure the severity of delirium in terminally ill cancer patients: a validation study. *Palliative Medicine.* **15**(3): 197–206. (OS-30)

12 Macleod AD, Whitehead LE (1997) Dysgraphia and terminal delirium. *Palliative Medicine.* **11**(2): 127–32. (CT-10)

13 Brittlebank A, Regnard C (1990) Terror or depression? A case report. *Palliative Medicine.* **4**: 317–19. (CS-1)

14 Stedeford A (1994) Confusion. In: *Facing Death: patients, families and professionals* (2e). Sobell Publications, Oxford. pp. 149–63. (Ch)

15 Morita T, Tei Y, Tsunoda J, Inoue S, Chihara S (2001) Underlying pathologies and their associations with clinical features in terminal delirium of cancer patients. *Journal of Pain and Symptom Management.* **22**(6): 997–1006. (OS-237)

16 Cerchietti L, Navigante A, Sauri A, Palazzo F (2000) Clinical trial. Hypodermoclysis for control of dehydration in terminal-stage cancer. *International Journal of Palliative Nursing.* **6**(8): 370–4. (RCT-42)

17 Soden K, Hoy A, Hoy W, Clelland S (2002) Artificial hydration in patients dying in a district general hospital. *Palliative Medicine.* **16**(6): 542–3. (OS-111)

18 Fainsinger RL, Bruera E (1997) When to treat dehydration in a terminally ill patient? *Supportive Care in Cancer.* **5**(3): 205–11. (R, 54 refs)

19 Bruera E, Franco JJ, Maltoni M, Watanabe S, Suarez-Almazor M (1995) Changing pattern of agitated impaired mental status in patients with advanced cancer: association with cognitive monitoring, hydration, and opioid rotation. *Journal of Pain and Symptom Management.* **10**(4): 287–91. (RS-279)

20 Dunphy K, Finlay I, Rathbone G, Gilbert J, Hicks F (1995) Rehydration in palliative and terminal care:

if not – why not? *Palliative Medicine.* **9**(3): 221–8. (R, 32 refs)

21 Dunlop RJ, Ellershaw JE, Baines MJ, Sykes N, Saunders CM (1995) On withholding nutrition and hydration in the terminally ill: has palliative medicine gone too far? A reply. *Journal of Medical Ethics.* **21**(3): 141–3.

22 McAndrew C, Vandivort M (2001) The six principles of excellent clinical care for dementia: nurse practitioners and physicians working together. *Nurse Practitioner Forum.* **12**(1): 12–22. (R, 29 refs)

23 Gagnon P, Charbonneau C, Allard P, Soulard C, Dumont S, Fillon L (2002) Delirium in advanced cancer: a psychoeducational intervention for family caregivers. *Journal of Palliative Care.* **18**(4): 253–61. (CT-124)

24 Anon (2003) Drugs for disruptive features in dementia. *Drug and Therapeutics Bulletin.* **41**(1): 1–4. (R, 39 refs)

25 Conn DK, Lieff S (2001) Diagnosing and managing delirium in the elderly. *Canadian Family Physician.* **47**: 101–8. (R, 44 refs)

26 Breitbart W, Marotta R, Platt MM, Weisman H, Derevenco M, Grau C, Corbera K, Raymond S, Lund S, Jacobson P (1996) A double-blind trial of haloperidol, chlorpromazine, and lorazepam in the treatment of delirium in hospitalized AIDS patients. *American Journal of Psychiatry.* **153**(2): 231–7. (RCT-244)

27 Morita T, Tsunoda J, Inoue S, Chihara S (2000) Pain and symptom management. Terminal sedation for existential distress. *American Journal of Hospice & Palliative Care.* **17**(3): 189–95. (RS-248)

28 Cheng C, Roemer-Becuwe C, Pereira J (2002) Clinical note. When midazolam fails. *Journal of Pain and Symptom Management.* **23**(3): 256–65. (CS-2)

29 Chiu T, Hu W, Lue B, Cheng S, Chen C (2001) Sedation for refractory symptoms of terminal cancer patients in Taiwan. *Journal of Pain and Symptom Management.* **21**(6): 467–72. (OS-276)

30 Fainsinger RL, Waller A, Bercovici M, Bengtson K, Landman W, Hosking M, Nunez-Olarte JM, deMoissac D (2000) A multicentre international study of sedation for uncontrolled symptoms in terminally ill patients. *Palliative Medicine.* **14**(4): 257–65. (OS-387)

31 Fainsinger RL, Landman W, Hoskings M, Bruera E (1998) Sedation for uncontrolled symptoms in a South African hospice. *Journal of Pain and Symptom Management.* **16**(3): 145–52. (OS-23)

32 Morita T, Tei Y, Tsunoda J, Inoue S, Chihara S (2002) Increased plasma morphine metabolites in terminally ill cancer patients with delirium: an intra-individual comparison. *Journal of Pain and Symptom Management.* **23**(2): 107–13. (OS-131)

33 Davis MP, Horvitz HR (2002) Increased plasma morphine metabolites and delirium. *Journal of Pain and Symptom Management.* **24**(3): 273. (Let)

34 Morita T, Tei Y, Inoue S (2002) Increased plasma morphine metabolites and delirium: author's response. *Journal of Pain and Symptom Management.* **24**(3): 273–4. (Let)

35 Lawlor PG (2002) The panorama of opioid-related cognitive dysfunction in patients with cancer: a critical literature appraisal. *Cancer.* **94**(6): 1836–53. (SA, 164 refs)

36 Homsi J, Walsh D, Nelson K (2000) Psychostimulants in supportive care. *Supportive Care in Cancer.* **8**: 385–97. (R, 141 refs)

37 Sugawara Y, Akechi T, Shima Y, Okuyama T, Akizuki N, Nakano T, Uchitomi Y (2002) Efficacy of methylphenidate for fatigue in advanced cancer patients: a preliminary study. *Palliative Medicine.* **16**: 261–3. (OS)

38 Breitbart W, Rosenfeld B, Kaim M, Funesti-Esch J (2001) A randomized, double-blind, placebo-controlled trial of psychostimulants for the treatment of fatigue in ambulatory patients with human immunodeficiency virus disease. *Archives of Internal Medicine.* **161**(3): 411–20. (RCT-144)

39 Dein S, George R (2002) A place for psychostimulants in palliative care? *Journal of Palliative Care.* **18**(3): 196–9. (R, 27 refs)

40 Morita T, Otani H, Tsunoda J, Inoue S, Chihara S (2000) Successful palliation of hypoactive delirium due to multi-organ failure by oral methylphenidate. *Supportive Care in Cancer.* **8**(2): 134–7. (CS-1)

41 Lonergan E, Luxenberg J, Colford J (2000) Haloperidol for agitation in dementia (Cochrane Review). *The Cochrane Library, 2002; Issue 2.* Update Software Ltd, Oxford. (www.cochrane.org)

42 Breitbart W, Strout D (2000) Delirium in the terminally ill. *Clinics in Geriatric Medicine.* **16**(2): 357–72. (R, 90 refs)

43 Lee MA, Leng ME, Tiernan EJ (2001) Risperidone: a useful adjunct for behavioural disturbance in primary cerebral tumours. *Palliative Medicine.* **15**(3): 255–6.

44 Lodge P, Tanner M, McKeogh MM (1998) Risperidone in the management of agitation in HIV dementia. *Palliative Medicine.* **12**(3): 206–7. (Let)

45 Katz IR, Jeste DV, Mintzer JE, Clyde C, Napolitano J, Brecher M (1999) Comparison of risperidone and placebo for psychosis and behavioral disturbances associated with dementia: a randomized, double-blind trial. Risperidone Study Group. *Journal of Clinical Psychiatry.* **60**(2): 107–15. (RCT-625)

46 De Deyn PP, Rabheru K, Rasmussen A, Bocksberger JP, Dautzenberg PL, Eriksson S, Lawlor BA (1999) A randomized trial of risperidone, placebo, and haloperidol for behavioral symptoms of dementia. *Neurology.* **53**(5): 946–55. (RCT-344)

47 Breitbart W, Tremblay A, Gibson C (2002) An open trial of olanzapine for the treatment of delirium in hospitalized cancer patients. *Psychosomatics.* **43**(3): 175–82. (OS-79)

48 Khojainova N, Santiago-Palma J, Kornick C, Breitbart W, Gonzales GR (2002) Olanzapine in

the management of cancer pain. *Journal of Pain and Symptom Management.* **23**(4): 346–50. (CS-8)

49 Sipahimalani A, Masand PS (1998) Olanzapine in the treatment of delirium. *Psychosomatics.* **39**(5): 422–30. (CS-8)

50 Street JS, Clark WS, Gannon KS, Cummings JL, Bymaster FP, Tamura RN, Mitan SJ, Kadam DL, Sanger TM, Feldman PD, Tollefson GD, Breier A (2000) Olanzapine treatment of psychotic and behavioral symptoms in patients with Alzheimer disease in nursing care facilities: a double-blind, randomized, placebo-controlled trial. The HGEU Study Group. *Archives of General Psychiatry.* **57**(10): 968–76. (RCT-206)

51 Stedeford A, Regnard C (1995) Confusional states. In: *Flow Diagrams in Advanced Cancer and Other Diseases.* Edward Arnold, London. pp. 68–72. (Ch)

52 Lloyd-Williams M (2003) *Delirium and dementia in palliative care.* Lecture given at Advanced Course in Pain and Symptom Management, 19 June 2003.

Withdrawal and depression

Clinical decision and action checklist

1 Acknowledge the withdrawal.
2 Is this the patient's usual behavior?
3 Is the patient unwilling to continue talking?
4 Does the patient feel everything is meaningless?
5 Is anger present?
6 Are fears, guilt or shame present?
7 Is the patient feeling depressed?
8 Is the withdrawal persisting?

Key points

- Withdrawal can occur for many reasons, but depression is often missed.
- Depression may respond within two weeks of starting an antidepressant.

Introduction

Withdrawal has many possible causes and these should be excluded before assuming a depression is present. The proportion of patients with advanced disease who have a clinical depression varies between studies and depends partly on the assessment tools used. It has been suggested that a median of 15% of cancer patients and up to 25% of AIDS patients suffer from depression.[1,2]

Getting started

Acknowledge what is happening: Although this may seem unnecessary, it gives the person a clear message that you have noticed their withdrawal and that you are taking it seriously.

Causes of withdrawal: This may be the person's usual behavior, but other causes include depression, distraction due to pain, a confusional state, drowsiness (caused by drugs, infection or a biochemical disturbance), exhaustion, severe anxiety or fear, collusion preventing the person from talking for fear of upsetting a partner or relative, or reduced facial expression due to drugs (e.g. haloperidol, metoclopramide) or neurological disease (e.g. Parkinson's, motor neuron disease).

Depression

Depression can be missed since it is easily misinterpreted as sadness or masked by anxiety.[3–7] Recognizing depression depends on the patient's manner, identifying clues in interviews and the use of screening tools.[8] Screening tools increase the likelihood of diagnosis and treatment,[9–11] but none are ideal.[12] The Hospital Anxiety and Depression (HAD) scale needs to have a higher cut-off threshold to be useful.[2,6] The Edinburgh postnatal depression scale may be a more useful screening tool.[3,6,13] A simple screening tool may be to ask, 'Have you had a depressed mood most of the day nearly every day?'.[6,14,15] The diagnosis of depression is made on the following characteristics.

---

1   A persistent feeling of a depressed mood ($>$ 2 weeks for $>$ 50% of the time) in the absence of a psychosis.
2   This is a change to their usual mood.
3   There is a loss of interest and enjoyment.
4   Three or more of the following depressive-related symptoms are present: diurnal variation in mood, repeated or early morning wakening, impaired concentration, loss of interest or enjoyment, feelings of hopelessness, guilt, shame or feeling a burden to others, thoughts of self-harm, desire for hastened death (loss of energy, appetite and sex drive are less useful).

The four diagnostic criteria of depression (adapted from DSM IV[16,17])

Loss of energy, appetite and sex drive are more likely to be due to the disease itself and cannot be used as diagnostic indicators. In contrast, thoughts of self-harm and a desire for a hastened death are strong indicators of depression.[6,18–20] Suicidal thoughts are not always an indicator of depression since some patients will express a realistic wish that they would prefer to be dead rather than be in pain, a burden, or immobile. This may be interpreted as a request for euthanasia, but feelings of hopelessness are more likely to indicate genuine suicidal thoughts and sustained suicidal thoughts require closer assessment and screening for depression.[21,22] Suicides are rare in palliative care patients,[23,24] but are associated with a fear of losing autonomy and independence.[25]

Helping the withdrawn patient

Causes of withdrawal should be treated if possible, but the most helpful approach is developing trust between the carer and the withdrawn person. Continuing to show kindness, despite the person's perception of hopelessness, demonstrates to the person that they are worthwhile.

Depression should be treated if present,[26] but there is little research on treating depression in advanced disease and it is necessary to use evidence from other depressed patients.[2,27] Antidepressants are still the quickest way to achieve a response and if the depression started recently the response may occur in less than 2 weeks. SSRI antidepressants do not have fewer adverse effects than tricyclic antidepressants and may also be less effective than tricyclics, although SNRIs may be more effective than SSRIs.[8,28,29] Nausea and vomiting are common on the first dose of SSRIs and SNRIs and a withdrawal reaction (headache, nausea, paresthesiae, dizziness and anxiety) can occur on abrupt withdrawal.[30] Low dose tricyclics (below 100mg/day) may be as effective as higher doses.[31] If adverse effects are a problem and the depression is mild to moderate, the herb St John's Wort (*Hypericum perforatum*) is effective.[32] Venlafaxine can reduce neuropathic pain and may be helpful in patients with coexisting depression.[33] Treatment with antidepressants should continue for 4–6 months.[8]

Persisting withdrawal

Methylphenidate has a role if a rapid response is needed, especially in a very withdrawn patient.[34,35] Cognitive behavioral therapy (CBT) is also helpful in suitable patients, particularly in preventing relapse.[36–39] CBT is as effective as antidepressants but takes longer to be effective.[40] If the depression persists or has complicating features (e.g. agitation, paranoia) it is essential to ask for advice and help from psychiatry colleagues.[41]

Clinical decision	If YES ⇒ Action
1 **Acknowledge the withdrawal:** e.g. 'You seem quiet and withdrawn today, can I help?'	
2 **Is this the patient's usual behavior?**	• Normally introverted or quiet personality: offer time to establish trust.
3 **Is the patient unwilling to continue talking?**	• Establish a dialogue: acknowledge the difficulties and negotiate further discussion (e.g. 'Can you bear to tell me why you find it so difficult to talk to me just now?'). • Exclude the following: Confusional state: *see* Confusional states (delirium and dementia) (p. 171). Distraction by a persistent symptom such as pain. Drugs causing akinesia (e.g. haloperidol, metoclopramide, methotrimeprazine). Neurological causes: motor neurone disease, Parkinson's disease, Parkinsonism due to brain damage (e.g. encephalitis, dementia, tumor). Fatigue and weakness related to the illness, or causes of drowsiness: *see* Fatigue, drowsiness, lethargy and weakness (p. 101). Collusion with a partner or relative that prevents the person from talking openly: see the patient alone. Guilt or shame: explore the reasons, although this may be due to an underlying depression. Severe anxiety or fear ('frozen terror'): *see* Anxiety (p. 165). • If no cause can be found, acknowledge the patient's refusal to continue and express a willingness to help in the future if needed.
4 **Does the patient feel everything is meaningless?**	• Explore what it was that previously gave their life meaning. • Ask whether they would like to contact a spiritual advisor, priest or chaplain. • Exclude a clinical depression (*see* cd-7 below).
5 **Is anger present?**	• *See* Anger (p. 161).
6 **Are fears, guilt or shame present?**	• Identify, clarify and specify the concerns: *see* Helping the person with the effects of difficult news (p. 29). • *If the patient is apprehensive, tense or on edge: see* Anxiety (p. 165). • *If guilt or shame is present:* If this is unrealistic, help a patient to reframe thoughts about the emotion. If this is realistic, check if patient could accept self-forgiveness. Exclude a clinical depression since guilt and shame are common in depression.
7 **Is the patient feeling depressed?**	• *A depressive illness is present if there is:* 1 Persistent low mood (> 2 weeks for > 50% of time). 2 A change to their usual mood. 3 A loss of interest and enjoyment. 4 Four other depressive-related symptoms (*see* notes opposite). • Start an anti-depressant (use lower doses in the elderly) If neuropathic pain is present, consider using venlafaxine 37.5–75 mg daily. If adverse effects are a problem, and the depression is of mild to moderate severity, consider St John's Wort 170 mg daily.
8 **Is the withdrawal persisting?**	• Refer for specialist advice and help, including cognitive behavioral therapy. • If a rapid response is needed, consider methylphenidate 5 mg in the morning, titrated up to 20 mg if necessary.[42]

Adapted from Maguire, Faulkner and Regnard[43]
cd = clinical decision

References

B = book; C = comment; Ch = chapter; CS-n = case study-number of cases; CT-n = controlled trial-number of cases; E = editorial; GC = group consensus; I = interviews; Let = letter; LS = laboratory study; MC = multi-center; OS-n = open study-number of cases; Q = questionnaire; R = review; RCT-n = randomized controlled trial-number of cases; RS-n = retrospective survey-number of cases; SA = systematic or meta analysis.

1 Breibart W, Chochinov HV, Passik S (1997) Psychiatric aspects of palliative care. In: D Doyle, GWC Hanks, N MacDonald (eds) *The Oxford Textbook of Palliative Medicine* (2e). Oxford Medical Publications, Oxford. pp. 933–54. (Ch)

2 Hotopf M, Chidgey J, Addington-Hall J, Lan Ly K (2002) Depression in advanced disease: a systematic review. Part 1. Prevalence and case finding. *Palliative Medicine.* **16**: 81–97. (SA, 77 refs)

3 Lloyd-Williams M (2002) Is it appropriate to screen palliative care patients for depression? *American Journal of Hospice & Palliative Care.* **19**(2): 112–14. (OS)

4 Stiefel R, Die Trill M, Berney A, Olarte JM, Razavi A (2001) Depression in palliative care: a pragmatic report from the Expert Working Group of the European Association for Palliative Care. *Supportive Care in Cancer.* **9**(7): 477–88. (R, 113 refs)

5 Lloyd-Williams M, Friedman T, Rudd N (1999) A survey of antidepressant prescribing in the terminally ill. *Palliative Medicine.* **13**(3): 243–8. (OS-1046)

6 Lloyd-Williams M, Spiller J, Ward J (2003) Which depression screening tools should be used in palliative care? *Palliative Medicine.* **17**(1): 40–3. (SA, 15 refs)

7 Kessler D, Bennewith O, Lewis G, Sharp D (2002) Detection of depression and anxiety in primary care: follow up study. *BMJ.* **325**: 1016–17. (OS-179)

8 Peveler R, Carson A, Rodin G (2002) ABC of psychological medicine: depression in medical patients. *BMJ.* **323**: 149–52. (R)

9 Passik SD, Kirsh KL, Theobald D, Donaghy K, Holtsclaw E, Edgerton S, Dugan W (2002) Use of a depression screening tool and a fluoxetine-based algorithm to improve the recognition and treatment of depression in cancer patients: a demonstration project. *Journal of Pain and Symptom Management.* **24**(3): 318–27. (OS-35)

10 Lloyd-Williams M (2001) Screening for depression in palliative care patients: a review. *European Journal of Cancer Care.* **10**(1): 31–5. (R, 40 refs)

11 Lloyd-Williams M (2002) The stability of depression scores in patients who are receiving palliative care. *Journal of Pain and Symptom Management.* **24**(6): 593–7. (OS-72)

12 Urch CE, Chamberlain J, Field G (1998) The drawback of the hospital anxiety and depression scale in the assessment of depression in hospice inpatients. *Palliative Medicine.* **12**: 395–6. (OS-52)

13 Lloyd-Williams M, Friedman T, Rudd N (2000) Criterion validation of the Edinburgh postnatal depression scale as a screening tool for depression in patients with advanced metastatic cancer. *Journal of Pain and Symptom Management.* **20**(4): 259–65. (OS-100)

14 Chochinov HM, Wilson KG, Enns M, Lander S (1994) Prevalence of depression in the terminally ill: effects of diagnostic criteria and symptom threshold judgements. *American Journal of Psychiatry.* **154**: 674–6. (I-134)

15 Whooley MA, Avins AL, Miranda J, Browner WS (1997) Case-finding instruments for depression. Two questions are as good as many. *Journal of General Internal Medicine.* **12**(7): 439–45. (OS-536)

16 American Psychiatric Association (1994) *Diagnostic and Statistical Manual of Mental Disorders – Fourth Edition (DSM-IV).* American Psychiatric Association, Washington. (B)

17 Lloyd-Williams M (2002) Diagnosis and treatment of depression in palliative care. *European Journal of Palliative Care.* **9**(5): 186–8. (R, 21 refs)

18 Lloyd-Williams M (2002) How common are thoughts of self-harm in a UK palliative care population? *Supportive Care in Cancer.* **10**(5): 422–4. (OS-248)

19 Breitbart W, Rosenfeld B, Pessin H, Kaim M, Funesti-Esch J, Galietta M, Nelson CJ, Brescia R (2000) Depression, hopelessness, and desire for hastened death in terminally ill patients with cancer. *JAMA.* **284**(22): 2907–11. (OS-92)

20 Chochinov HM, Wilson KG, Enns M, Mowchun N, Lander S, Levitt M, Clinch JJ (1995) Desire for death in the terminally ill. *American Journal of Psychiatry.* **152**(8): 1185–91. (I-200)

21 Chochinov HM, Wilson KG, Enns M, Lander S (1998) Depression, hopelessness, and suicidal ideation in the terminally ill. *Psychosomatics.* **39**(4): 366–70. (OS-196)

22 Block SD (2000) Assessing and managing depression in the terminally ill patient. ACP-ASIM End-of-Life Care Consensus Panel. American

College of Physicians – American Society of Internal Medicine. *Annals of Internal Medicine.* **132**(3): 209–18. (R)

23 Ripamonti C, Filiberti A, Totis A, De Conno F, Tamburini M (1999) Suicide among patients with cancer cared for at home by palliative-care teams. *Lancet.* **354**(9193): 1877–8. (Let, CS-5)

24 Grzybowska P, Finlay I (1997) The incidence of suicide in palliative care patients. *Palliative Medicine.* **11**(4): 313–16. (Q)

25 Filiberti A, Ripamonti C, Totis A, Ventafridda V, De Conno F, Contiero P, Tamburini M (2001) Characteristics of terminal cancer patients who committed suicide during a home palliative care program. *Journal of Pain and Symptom Management.* **22**(1): 544–53. (I, CS-5)

26 Block SD for the ACP-ASIM End-of-Life Care Consensus Panel (2000) Assessing and managing depression in the terminally ill patient. *Annals of Internal Medicine.* **132**(3): 209–18. (R, 95 refs)

27 Lan Ly K, Chidgey J, Addington-Hall J, Hotopf M (2002) Depression in advanced disease: a systematic review. Part 2. Treatment. *Palliative Medicine.* **16**: 279–84. (SA, 23 refs)

28 Anderson IM (2001) Meta-analytical studies on new antidepressants. *British Medical Bulletin.* **57**: 161–78. (SA, 32 refs)

29 Moon CA, Vince M (1996) Treatment of major depression in general practice: a double-blind comparison of paroxetine and lofepramine. *British Journal of Clinical Practice.* **50**(5): 240–4. (RCT-138)

30 Edwards JG, Anderson I (1999) Systematic review and guide to selection of selective serotonin reuptake inhibitors. *Drugs.* **57**(4): 507–33. (R, 118 refs)

31 Furukawa TA, McGuire H, Barbui C (2002) Meta analysis of effects and side effects of low dosage tricyclic antidepressants in depression: systematic review. *BMJ.* **325**: 991–5. (SA-141)

32 van Gurp G, Meterissian GB, Haiek LN, McCusker J, Bellavance F (2002) St John's wort or sertraline? Randomized controlled trial in primary care. *Canadian Family Physician.* **48**: 905–12. (RCT-87)

33 Tasmuth T, Hartel B, Kalso E (2002) Venlafaxine in neuropathic pain following treatment of

breast cancer. *European Journal of Pain: Ejp.* **6**(1): 17–24. (RCT)

34 Rozans M, Dreisbach A, Lertora JJ, Kahn MJ (2002) Palliative uses of methylphenidate in patients with cancer: a review. *Journal of Clinical Oncology.* **20**(1): 335–9. (R, 49 refs)

35 Pereira J, Bruera E (2001) Depression with psychomotor retardation: diagnostic challenges and the use of psychostimulants. *Journal of Palliative Medicine.* **4**(1): 15–21. (CS-1)

36 Maguire P, Hopwood P, Tarrier N, Howell T (1985) Treatment of depression in cancer patients. *Acta Psychiatrica Scandanavica.* **72**: 81–4.

37 Blanch J, Rousaud A, Hautzinger M, Martinez E, Peri JM, Andres S, Cirera E, Gatell JM, Gasto C (2002) Assessment of the efficacy of a cognitive-behavioural group psychotherapy programme for HIV-infected patients referred to a consultation-liaison psychiatry department. *Psychotherapy & Psychosomatics.* **71**(2): 77–84. (CT-39)

38 Scott J (2001) Cognitive therapy for depression. *British Medical Bulletin.* **57**: 101–13. (SA)

39 Teasdale JD, Scott J, Moore RG, Hayhurst H, Pope M, Paykel ES (2001) How does cognitive therapy prevent relapse in residual depression? Evidence from a controlled trial. *Journal of Consulting & Clinical Psychology.* **69**(3): 347–57. (CT-158)

40 Thompson LW, Coon DW, Gallagher-Thompson D, Sommer BR, Koin D (2001) Comparison of desipramine and cognitive/behavioral therapy in the treatment of elderly outpatients with mild-to-moderate depression. *American Journal of Geriatric Psychiatry.* **9**(3): 225–40. (RCT-102)

41 Ramsay N (1992) Referral to a liaison psychiatrist from a palliative care unit. *Palliative Medicine.* **6**: 54–60. (RS)

42 Homsi J, Walsh D, Nelson KA, LeGrand S, Davis M (2000) Methylphenidate for depression in hospice practice: a case series. *American Journal of Hospice & Palliative Care.* **17**(6): 393–8. (CS-10)

43 Maguire P, Faulkner A, Regnard C (1995) The withdrawn patient. In: *Flow Diagrams in Advanced Cancer and Other Diseases.* Edward Arnold, London. pp. 77–80. (Ch)

Difficult decisions

- Making ethical choices
  (written jointly with Bryan Vernon[1])

- Decisions around competency
  (written jointly with Dorothy Matthews,
  Lynn Gibson and Justin Amery)

- Issues around resuscitation[2]

Making ethical choices

Clinical decision and action checklist

1 Is an alternative course of action available?
2 Could something color your judgment?
3 Whose interests are best served?
4 What values are involved?
5 What consequences could there be?
6 What professional issues are there?
7 Is a decision still unclear?

Key points

- Most clinical decisions have ethical aspects, but only some decisions need extensive ethical reviews.
- Asking for advice from team members and other professionals is essential.

Introduction

Difficult decisions in clinical care often involve ethical issues.[3–5] This does not mean that every difficult clinical decision must include an extensive review of the ethical issues involved, but it can be helpful to screen for ethical issues.

Issues about the decision

There is rarely no choice: A common starting point is the belief that there is no choice. In reality it is rare that no choices exist. Invariably there may be solutions that were rejected as undesirable, but which advice or investigation indicate are feasible. An example might be the rejection of major surgery for bowel obstruction, when surgical advice indicates that a simple loop colostomy can be easily and quickly performed. It is also possible that advice and investigation uncover solutions that had not been considered. For example, advice from a pain specialist could indicate the possibility of regional blocking procedures for an apparently intractable pain. The key here is to ask for advice.

What is influencing the decision?

Prejudice: It is difficult to believe that discrimination exists in health care. In reality, there is good evidence that some people find it harder than others to get access to health care.[6–11]

Whose interests? Different solutions will have the interests of different groups at their center. Deciding whose interest links with which decision can make the best decision clearer.

Which values? Different solutions have different values. It can help to identify the best option if issues are considered such as the use of resources, whether an action is caring, or if an action breaks established rules.

Consequences of a decision

It is important to consider the effects of a course of action with regard to benefit, rights and professional issues. Additional advice can be invaluable, if only to expand the discussion.

When a decision is still unclear

Even after checking through the issues and the consequences of different solutions, a clear solution can be elusive. It is essential to ensure that all necessary advice has been sought. If time is short, then waiting to see developments can make a decision clearer (*see* cd-7 in table). If the situation is less urgent, then a meeting bringing together the patient, partner or relative, advisors and the multidisciplinary team may find a solution. In the US, the Joint Commission on Accreditation of Health Care Organizations (JCAHO) mandates health care institutions to have a mechanism to resolve ethical issues. As a result, most institutions will have an ethics consultation team or ethics committee which is familiar with end-of-life decision making. Most institutions in Canada also have a clinical ethics consultation team or committee. They are very helpful for providing appropriate recommendations in difficult situations. Courts are a last resort but can help to find a solution in rare cases where a solution is imperative. In the US, the ideal of patient autonomy is so powerful that the Patient Self-Determination Act[12] has been enacted to enhance and preserve patient autonomy. Advance directives are encouraged to honor the patient's wishes, but less than one-fifth of patients complete one.[13]

In the US, many important legal principles in end-of-life care are widely accepted among the states. It is important for health care providers to become familiar with their state's specific laws.

Clinical decision	If YES ⇒ Action

1 Do you wonder if an alternative course of action is available?	People may claim that they had no choice, but this is rarely true.
	• Consider if there are:
	  – undesirable courses of action that you have discounted implicitly
	  – desirable courses of action which you have yet to imagine.
	• Are you sure this is an ethical issue? Could it be a clinical issue for which there is insufficient information to make a clear decision?
	• Ask for advice from all the team or other specialists.

2 Is there any chance something could color your judgment?	• Review your prejudices on age, class, ethnicity, gender, intellectual ability, lifestyle or religion.

3 Is the decision in someone's interest?	• Consider which course of action is in:
	  – the patient's best interests (and promotes their autonomy)?
	  – the partner's or family's best interests (and if everyone's voice is being heard)?
	  – society's best interests?
	  – your best interest?

4 Are values part of this decision?	• Consider:
	  – Is this course of action caring?
	  – Is this a good use of resources?
	  – What values are being sacrificed?
	  – Does this involve breaking a rule I would normally follow?
	  – Is this decision equitable, i.e. can the healthcare system make the same decision for every eligible patient?

5 Will there be consequences to your action?	• Consider whether this course of action will:
	  – cause harm?
	  – result in benefit?
	  – violate anyone's rights or legitimate expectations?

6 Are there professional issues?	• Consider:
	  – How would you advise a colleague to act in similar circumstances?
	  – What would your colleagues think?
	  – Does professional guidance exist on this issue?
	  – Are you acting within the law?
	  – How would you justify your decision in the media?

7 Is a decision still unclear?	• Ensure that you have:
	  – involved the patient if they are able to contribute (if they cannot, ask the partner, relative or designated decision-maker about the patient's previously expressed views).
	  – shared the issues with your team and asked their views.
	  – asked other colleagues for advice.
	  If a decision is still not possible:
	• If time is short (rapid deterioration, terminal phase) use the 'rule of 3':
	  – If deterioration is hour by hour wait 3 hours, if day by day wait 3 days.
	  – After the wait, if the patient is worse this suggests that no intervention is appropriate, but if the patient is stable or better then further intervention may be appropriate.
	• If time is less urgent consider:
	  – a meeting with the team, patient, partner or relative and external advisor (e.g. palliative care specialist, ethicist, chaplain, spiritual advisor).
	The courts can be helpful in situations where agreement cannot be reached.

cd = clinical decision

Decisions around competency

Clinical decision and action checklist

1 Exclude reversible causes of reduced cognition.
2 Is an emergency a possibility?
3 Screening decisions.
4 Is the person competent for this decision?
5 Is the person not competent for this decision?
6 Is a clear decision difficult?
7 Document the decision.
8 Is the test/procedure likely to be distressing?

Key points

- Competency depends on the decision to be made.
- 'Best interests' and decisions using estimates of quality of life are prone to error.

Introduction

Preferences for care and consent for treatment emerge best from a process of discussion and feedback.[14] In young children, it is necessary to establish early on who has parental responsibility and who will be the health care proxy/proxy decision makers. This discussion is best left until a trusting relationship has developed with the care team, but this is not always possible. In situations where parental responsibility is shared (e.g. separated parents or a child under a care order), it is important to establish early on how difficult decisions will be addressed. This may involve a case conference at an early stage.

Assessing competency

Depression and reversible causes of reduced cognition should be excluded.

Competent adults and children are able to:[15]

1 remember and understand the reasons for, and details about, the test or treatment
2 believe this information
3 weigh the information in the balance and arrive at a choice.

These three tests of competency have important implications:

- *Competency does not apply to all decisions:* A patient may be competent for one decision, but not for another.[16] People with learning disabilities find the most difficult issues are participants' rights, options and the impact of their choices.[16]
- *A child can be competent:* Such children can give consent to treatment. They can probably also refuse a proposed treatment to which consent has been given by the parents,[17] but this is not a clear situation.
- *Parents must be competent too:* Occasionally parents have similar problems to a non-competent child. The parents' competence must be assessed before they can make decisions on their child's behalf.
- *Tests of cognition do not predict competency:* Even in patients with cognitive impairment, the capacity to make a decision can vary greatly and some are able to make valid advance directives if this is done with someone whom the person knows and trusts.[18,19] Consequently an abnormal cognition test does not exclude the possibility that an individual has the capacity to make a valid decision.[20,21] This parallels the issue in children, where competency is not determined by age, but by maturity and the ability to understand.[17,22] A young child may be able to communicate feelings through stories, play or art. An older child below 16 may be able to understand and discuss abstract and difficult issues.
- *Information must be understandable:* Clear information is crucial,[23] especially for a child or in the presence of cognitive impairment. Information may have to be presented in stages.[24] If verbal expression is limited, then any assessment should rely on other forms of expression.[24]

Decisions in the non-competent patient

Deciding on a patient's 'best interests' seems a pragmatic process that is particularly useful in emergencies,[25] but it is open to errors.[26] Estimates of quality of life by professionals are poor indicators of a patient's best interests.[27,28] A better approach is to consider two situations:

1 *Emergency treatment:* This is when the physician has the *option* of providing treatment to prevent death or a serious deterioration in physical or mental health.
2 *Necessary treatment:* Treatment must be necessary and realistic. In many cases, with open discussion, the decisions are clear to the clinical team and the partner, relatives or parents. Relatives and parents (or the designated decision-maker) can give invaluable information as to the current or previously expressed wishes of the patient. On occasions, consensus is difficult. This may be because more discussion is needed or the available information is incomplete. There may be a 'health care proxy/proxy decision maker' (in children this is usually the parents). It is rare to have to fall back on the courts for a decision. *See* also Making ethical choices (p. 185).

Carrying out the test/procedure

Regardless of competency, everything should be done to minimize discomfort and distress arising from tests or treatments. Examples are a pre-appointment visit or the use of topical anesthetic for venepuncture. Occasionally it is clear that a distressing test or procedure is needed in a non-competent patient. Titrated doses of sublingual midazolam[29–31] or lorazepam oral or sublingual can be used to minimize or eliminate any distress.[32,33] The sublingual and buccal routes are better tolerated in children than the intranasal route.[34]

Clinical decision	If YES ⇒ Action
1 **Exclude and treat depression and reversible causes of reduced cognition:** *see* Withdrawal and depression (p. 177) and Confusional states (delirium and dementia) (p. 171).	
2 **Is an emergency a possibility?**	• It is helpful at an early stage to plan what would happen in an emergency. For example, if a child is to be left in your care, you need to know the parents' wishes if an emergency arises. *See* also Issues around resuscitation (p. 193).
3 **Screening decisions** • Is the test/ procedure unlikely to influence care? • Is the care or treatment unrealistic or impractical?	• 'Yes' to either of these screening questions means that the test or procedure should not be done at present. • Review the position regularly. In the absence of new information, a guide would be to review: – daily in patients deteriorating day by day – weekly in patients deteriorating week by week – monthly in patients deteriorating month by month.
4 **Is the person competent for this decision?** • Can they remember and understand the information? • Do they believe the information? • Can they weigh the information in the balance and arrive at a choice?	• *For an adult who is competent:* explain the test/procedure, and ask the patient for permission to proceed. • *For a child who is competent:* – for proposed treatment: a competent child can give consent or may be able to refuse, even if this is different to the parent's wishes. – for current treatment: a competent child can give consent to continue treatment, but refusal of current treatment needs careful consideration if this is against either the parent's wishes or the clinician's advice. *See* cd-6 below.
5 **Is the patient not competent for this decision?** (NB: in the case of a child, parents need to be competent too)	• *For an emergency:* It is acceptable to use treatment that prevents death or a serious deterioration in physical or mental health (e.g. treat hypercalcemia). • *For any other necessary treatment:* Arrange a multidisciplinary team meeting and invite the partner or relatives to (1) explain the current situation, (2) enquire if the patient has previously expressed wishes about care, (3) explore the possibility of undue influence and (4) explain the reasons, advantages and disadvantages of the test or procedure.
6 **Is a clear decision difficult?**	• Review the tests in cd-3 and cd-4 above. • *If there is insufficient information:* obtain information. If this is unhelpful, agree an observation period (*see* cd-7 in Making ethical choices (p. 187)). • *If no consensus is possible:* agree to postpone the test/procedure and agree to a review time or date. If consensus is still difficult, arrange for a formal review by a senior clinician who is experienced in the patient's condition, but is not part of the clinical team. Involvement of an ethics consultant may be necessary if serious differences in opinions persist.

Table continued overleaf

7 Document the decision and the process leading to that decision.

8 Is the test/ procedure likely to be distressing for the patient?	• Explore simple approaches, such as topical local anesthetic for venepuncture, and ensuring the environment is comfortable and familiar. Give explanations at the patient's cognitive level (verbal, visual).
	
	• *For a hospital appointment or procedure in hospital:* consider a pre-appointment visit to assess the patient's level of acceptance and comfort with the environment. Pre-plan any visits to ensure the minimum waiting time and good access if the patient is disabled.
	
	• *If distress is still likely AND consensus has been reached to go ahead with the test/procedure:* continue as follows:
	  – have available flumazenil 200 microgram IV (a reversal agent for benzodiazepines) and basic resuscitation equipment (Ambu bag, oxygen, simple airway).
	  – three hours before test/procedure: reduce anxiety with lorazepam 0.5 mg PO or sublingual, repeated hourly up to maximum of 1.5 mg.
	  – if necessary, give midazolam 2.5 mg sublingually, repeated after 10 mins. If little or no effect, repeat with 2.5 mg (maximum 10 mg or 0.5 mg/kg for a child).
	  NB: Retain the eyelash reflex. The aim is not sedation, but to reduce anxiety.
	  – *If these doses have had no effect:* cancel the test/procedure for that day. Consider repeating on another day with higher starting doses, e.g. 1 mg lorazepam and 2.5–5 mg midazolam (or up to 0.75 mg/kg for a child).

cd = clinical decision

Issues around resuscitation

Clinical decision and action checklist

1 Is it impossible to anticipate the exact circumstances of the arrest?
2 Is the patient dying because of an irreversible condition?
3 Can the circumstances of the arrest be anticipated?
4 Regularly reassess the need for resuscitation.
5 Have the circumstances changed?

Key points

- An advance decision can only be made if the circumstances of the arrest can be anticipated.
- Patients and relatives should not be burdened with a decision when resuscitation is not an option.

Introduction

The American Medical Association (AMA) has endorsed the concept of Do-Not-Resuscitate (DNR) orders,[35] and most recently produced guidelines for the 'optimal use' of advance directives.[36] In Canada the Canadian Medical Association (CMA) and the Canadian Medical Protective Association (CMPA) have given advice on resuscitation decisions.[37,38] Several papers have commented on the application of resuscitation guidelines in clinical practice.[39–45]

Resuscitation: what it is and what it is not

These are resuscitation measures: Cardiac massage, artificial respiration (cardiopulmonary resuscitation – CPR). These CPR treatment measures will be instituted by local staff, but would precipitate calling emergency services and admission to an acute hospital.

These are comfort and palliative treatment measures: Analgesia, antibiotics, symptom control, feeding (any route), hydration (any route), oxygen and hospital admission for investigation, seizure control, and airways suction. These comfort and treatment measures are instituted after assessment, consultation with patient and family, and on the basis of clinical need.

Principles of resuscitation decisions

- At best, 60% of all resuscitations are successful, and up to half of these patients become well enough to return home,[46] but the discharge rate is lower in other series,[47] and reduces to 1% in non-witnessed arrests.[48] Some patients will choose CPR treatment even if the success rate is as low as 10%.[49] However, at the end of an irreversible terminal disease (e.g. cancer) CPR treatment will not succeed and is not a treatment option.
- Decisions made without knowing the exact circumstances of the arrest are of little help to the clinical team attending an arrest since a vague 'blanket' advance directive would make it difficult to know if it applies to the current situation. This should never prevent a discussion about CPR if the patient wants this.
- It is unethical to offer a treatment that will not work. In order to facilitate discussion with patients or relatives about CPR treatment at the natural end of life, establishing or reaffirming the patient's goals of care is important. If the clinical team is

'as certain as it can be' that resuscitation would fail,[37] CPR treatment should then not be offered as a realistic option when discussed with the patient and/or health care proxy/proxy decision maker/family. It will still be necessary to discuss this reality as openly as the patient or family wishes.

- In cases where the circumstances of an arrest can be anticipated, it is essential to obtain the patient's view. The only exceptions are if the patient is not competent or the patient does not want to discuss the matter. In these circumstances the view of the health care proxy/proxy decision maker or the next-of-kin should be obtained. Depression must be identified, as its treatment increases the likelihood of acceptance of CPR treatment.[50]
- The patient must be given as much information as they wish about their situation.[39]
- Medical decisions should be based on immediate health needs, and not on an opinion on quality of life.[27] This is because such opinions by health professionals are subjective and often at variance with the view of the patient.[28]
- 'Futility' is an unhelpful term with a tendency for subjective interpretation. Treatments should be decided in terms of acceptance to the patient, feasibility, likely success, risks and availability.[51]
- Since circumstances can arise which are not envisioned when the decision process is completed, the anticipated circumstances for the decision must be documented.
- Asking patients and relatives is uncomfortable but is easier if they have the information they want about the situation and they are allowed time for discussion and to make their decision.
- The principle of a 'default treatment' (e.g. doing CPR if no directive exists) is ethically suspect. No other treatments are offered by default. The reality is that clinical teams have to do what they always have done, make an assessment with the information they have at the time (including the advance directive and relatives' wishes) and act in the best interests of the patient.

Clinical decision	If YES ⇒ Action
1 **Is it impossible to anticipate the exact circumstances of the arrest?**	It is not possible to make a decision that would help a clinical team decide whether to attempt CPR in an unexpected arrest. This should never prevent a discussion about CPR if the patient or family or health care proxy/proxy decision maker wishes this. • In Canada a competent person should be involved in discussion about CPR, but in exceptional circumstances, e.g. imminently dying, such discussions may be inappropriate. In the US when discussing CPR treatment with the patient and/or health care proxy/proxy decision maker/next-of-kin, do it in the context of the overall goals of care rather than addressing it in isolation. It is important to not unnecessarily burden the patient and/or health care proxy/proxy decision maker/family with a CPR decision, but rather provide your valued input as a health care professional as to whether or not you feel that CPR is 'medically indicated' in the present circumstances. • Continue to communicate progress to the patient (and to the partner/family/health care proxy/proxy decision maker if the patient agrees). If the patient wishes, this may include information about the nature of CPR and its likely success in different clinical situations. • Continue to elicit and respond to the other concerns of the patient, partner, family and health care proxy/proxy decision maker. • Review the situation regularly to check if circumstances have changed. • In the event of an unexpected arrest, carry out CPR if there is a possibility of success.
2 **Is the patient dying because of an irreversible condition?**	CPR cannot be successful as the patient is dying naturally from their condition. • 'AND' = Allow a Natural Death. Effective palliative care should be in place to ensure a comfortable and peaceful time for the patient, and adequate support for the partner, family and health care proxy/proxy decision maker. *See* Terminal phase (the last hours and days) (p. 145). • In Canada a competent person should be involved in discussion about CPR, but in exceptional circumstances, e.g. imminently dying, such discussions may be inappropriate. In the US when discussing CPR treatment with the patient and/or health care proxy/proxy decision maker/next-of-kin, do it in the context of the overall goals of care rather than addressing it in isolation. It is important to not unnecessarily burden the patient and/or health care proxy/proxy decision maker/family with a CPR decision, but rather provide your valued input as a health care professional as to whether or not you feel that CPR is 'medically indicated' in the present circumstances. • Document the fact that CPR is not medically indicated. • Continue to communicate progress to the patient (and to the partner/family/health care proxy/proxy decision maker if the patient agrees). *See* Breaking difficult news (p. 25). • Continue to elicit the patient's, partner's, family's and health care proxy's/proxy decision maker's concerns. • Review regularly to check if circumstances have changed.
3 **Can the circumstances of the arrest be anticipated?**	e.g. previous life-threatening events or a condition where an arrest is likely. A fully informed advance directive on CPR is possible. • *Decide on the competency of the patient: see* Decisions around competency (p. 189). • *Consider the consequences of discussion of CPR with patient, family and health care proxy/proxy decision maker:* some will already have made clear their wish to discuss such issues. Others will have made clear that they do **not** want to discuss this, while some will be uncertain. • *If the patient is competent for this decision:* exclude and treat reversible causes (e.g. confusional state, depression). Discuss the options of CPR vs DNR with the patient. • *If the patient is not competent for this decision:* enquire about previous wishes from the partner, family or health care proxy/proxy decision maker to help the clinical team make the best decision (*see* Decisions around competency (p. 189)). • Document the decision *and* the anticipated circumstances of the arrest. • Continue to communicate progress to the patient (and to the partner, family and health care proxy/proxy decision maker if the patient agrees). • Continue to elicit the concerns of the patient, partner, family and health care proxy/proxy decision maker. • Review regularly to check if circumstances have changed. • In the event of the expected arrest, act according to the patient's wishes (or if the patient was not competent, follow the decision made by the health care proxy/proxy decision maker or surrogate decision maker).
4 **Regularly reassess the need for resuscitation** (while this does not mean burdening the patient and family with a CPR decision each time, it does require staff to be sensitive in picking up any change of views during discussions with the patient, partner, family or health care proxy/proxy decision maker).	
5 **Have the circumstances changed?**	• Start again at cd-1 above.

cd = clinical decision

References

B = book; C = comment; CC = Court case; Ch = chapter; CS-n = case study-number of cases; CT-n = controlled trial-number of cases; E = editorial; GC = group consensus; I = interviews; Let = letter; LS = laboratory study; MC = multi-center; OS-n = open study-number of cases; Q-n = questionnaire-number of respondents; R = review; RCT-n = randomized controlled trial-number of cases; RS-n = retrospective survey-number of cases; SA = systematic or meta analysis.

1 Vernon B (2003) Personal communication. Senior Lecturer, Department of Family Medicine, University of Newcastle on Tyne.

2 Regnard C, Matthews D, Gibson L (2003) *DNAR (Do Not Attempt Resuscitation) Policy.* Northgate and Prudhoe NHS Trust, Morpeth.

3 Quill TE, Lee BC, Nunn S (2000) Palliative treatments of last resort: choosing the least harmful alternative. University of Pennsylvania Center for Bioethics Assisted Suicide Consensus Panel. *Annals of Internal Medicine.* **132**(6): 488–93. (R)

4 Quill TE, Byock IR (2000) Responding to intractable terminal suffering: the role of terminal sedation and voluntary refusal of food and fluids. ACP-ASIM End-of-Life Care Consensus Panel. American College of Physicians-American Society of Internal Medicine. *Annals of Internal Medicine.* **132**(5): 408–14. (R, 65 refs)

5 Latimer EJ (1998) Ethical care at the end of life. *CMAJ (Canadian Medical Association Journal).* **158**(13): 1741–7. (R, 30 refs)

6 Dhruev N (2002) Not just skin-deep: how systems sustain racism. *Nursing Times.* **98**(23): 26–7. (R, 6 refs)

7 Taywaditep KJ (2001) Marginalization among the marginalized: gay men's anti-effeminacy attitudes. *Journal of Homosexuality.* **42**(1): 1–28. (R, 100 refs)

8 Ward D (2000) Ageism and the abuse of older people in health and social care. *British Journal of Nursing.* **9**(9): 560–3. (R, 30 refs)

9 Surlis S, Hyde A (2001) HIV-positive patients' experiences of stigma during hospitalization. *Journal of the Association of Nurses in AIDS Care.* **12**(6): 68–77. (R, 39 refs)

10 Garofalo R, Katz E (2001) Health care issues of gay and lesbian youth. *Current Opinion in Pediatrics.* **13**(4): 298–302. (R, 38 refs)

11 Bonham VL (2001) Race, ethnicity, and pain treatment: striving to understand the causes and solutions to the disparities in pain treatment. *Journal of Law, Medicine & Ethics.* **29**(1): 52–68. (R, 111 refs)

12 The Patient Self-Determination Act of 1990 (PSDA) (Sections 4206 and 4571 of the Omnibus Budget Reconciliation Act of 1990 PL 101–508). Effective 1 December 1991.

13 Meisel A, Snyder L, Quill T (2000) Seven legal barriers to end-of-life care: myths, realities, and grains of truth. *JAMA.* **284**: 2495–501.

14 Prendergast TJ (2001) Advance care planning: pitfalls, progress, promise. *Critical Care Medicine.* **29**(2): N34–9. (R, 49 refs)

15 Re C (1994) 1 *FLR* 31. (CC)

16 Arscott K, Dagnan D, Stenfert Kroese B (1999) Assessing the ability of people with a learning disability to give informed consent to treatment. *Psychological Medicine.* **29**(6): 1367–75. (OS-40)

17 Spencer GE (2000) Children's competency to consent: an ethical dilemma. *Journal of Child Health Care.* **4**(3): 117–22. (R, 46 refs)

18 Rempusheski VF, Hurley AC (2000) Advance directives and dementia. *Journal of Gerontological Nursing.* **26**(10): 27–34. (R, 34 refs)

19 Kim SY, Karlawish JH, Caine ED (2002) Current state of research on decision-making competence of cognitively impaired elderly persons. *American Journal of Geriatric Psychiatry.* **10**(2): 151–65. (R, 72 refs)

20 Barbas NR, Wilde EA (2001) Competency issues in dementia: medical decision making, driving, and independent living. *Journal of Geriatric Psychiatry & Neurology.* **14**(4): 199–212. (R, 79 refs)

21 Reid-Proctor GM, Galin K, Cummings MA (2001) Evaluation of legal competency in patients with frontal lobe injury. *Brain Injury.* **15**(5): 377–86. (R, 32 refs)

22 *Gillick v Wisbech Area Health Authority* (1986). (CC)

23 Taylor HA (1999) Barriers to informed consent. *Seminars in Oncology Nursing.* **15**(2): 89–95. (R, 35 refs)

24 Wong JG, Clare ICH, Holland AJ, Watson PC, Gunn M (2000) The capacity of people with a 'mental disability' to make a health care decision. *Psychological Medicine.* **30**(2): 295–306. (CT-61)

25 Larkin GL, Marco CA, Abbott JT (2001) Emergency determination of decision-making capacity: balancing autonomy and beneficence in the emergency department. *Academic Emergency Medicine.* **8**(3): 282–4. (R, 23 refs)

26 Donnelly M (2001) Decision-making for mentally incompetent people: the empty formula

of best interests? *Medicine & Law.* **20**(3): 405–16. (R, 44 refs)

27 Mencap (2001) *Considerations of 'quality of life' in cases of medical decision making for individuals with severe learning disabilities.* Mencap, London. (summary available on www.mencap.org.uk/ht ml/campaigns/health_pubs.htm) (B)

28 Costantini M, Mencaglia E *et al.* (2000) Cancer patients as 'experts' in defining quality of life domains. A multicentre survey by the Italian Group for the Evaluation of Outcomes in Oncology (IGEO). *Quality of Life Research.* **9**: 151–9.

29 Khalil S, Philbrook L, Rabb M, Wagner K, Jennings C, Chuang AZ, Lemak NA (1998) Sublingual midazolam premedication in children: a dose response study. *Paediatric Anaesthesia.* **8**(6): 461–5. (RCT-102)

30 Scott RC, Besag FM, Boyd SG, Berry D, Neville BG (1998) Buccal absorption of midazolam: pharmacokinetics and EEG pharmacodynamics. *Epilepsia.* **39**(3): 290–4. (CT-10)

31 Lim TW, Thomas E, Choo SM (1997) Premedication with midazolam is more effective by the sublingual than oral route. *Canadian Journal of Anaesthesia.* **44**(7): 723–6. (RCT-100)

32 Ghanchi FD, Khan MY (1997) Sublingual lorazepam as premedication in peribulbar anesthesia. *Journal of Cataract & Refractive Surgery.* **23**(10): 1581–4. (RCT)

33 Spenard J, Caille G, de Montigny C, Vezina M, Ouellette J, Lariviere L, Trudel F (1988) Placebo-controlled comparative study of the anxiolytic activity and of the pharmacokinetics of oral and sublingual lorazepam in generalized anxiety. *Biopharmaceutics & Drug Disposition.* **9**(5): 457–64. (RCT-12)

34 Karl HW, Rosenberger JL, Larach MG, Ruffle JM (1993) Transmucosal administration of midazolam for premedication of pediatric patients. Comparison of the nasal and sublingual routes. *Anesthesiology.* **78**(5): 885–91. (RCT-93).

35 American Medical Association Council on Ethical and Judicial Affairs (1987) *Do-not-resuscitate orders: Report B. Proceeding of the House of Delegates of the AMA.* Chicago: 170–1.

36 American Medical Association Council on Ethical and Judicial Affairs (1998) Optimal use or orders not to intervene and advance directives. *Psychology, Public Policy and Law.* **4**: 668–75.

37 CMA (1995) Policy Summary. Joint statement on resuscitative interventions (update). *Canadian Medical Association Journal.* **153**(11): 1652A–C.

38 Evans KG, Henderson GL (2002) *A Medico-Legal Handbook for Physicians in Canada.* Canadian Medical Protective Association, Ottawa.

39 Randall F (2002) Recent guidance on resuscitation: patients' choices and doctors' duties. *Palliative Medicine.* **15**: 449–50. (E)

40 Romano-Critchley G, Sommerville A (2001) Professional guidelines on decisions relating to cardiopulmonary resuscitation: introduction. *Journal of Medical Ethics.* **7**: 308–9. (Let)

41 Gill R (2001) Decisions relating to cardiopulmonary resuscitation: commentary 1 – CPR and the cost of autonomy. *Journal of Medical Ethics.* **27**: 317–18.

42 Luttrell S (2001) Decisions relating to cardiopulmonary resuscitation: commentary 2 – some concerns. *Journal of Medical Ethics.* **27**: 319–20.

43 Watt H (2001) Decisions relating to cardiopulmonary resuscitation: commentary 3 – degrading lives? *Journal of Medical Ethics.* **27**: 321–3.

44 Saunders J (2001) Perspectives on CPR: resuscitation or resurrection? *Clinical Medicine.* **1**(6): 457–60. (R)

45 Willard C (2000) Cardiopulmonary resuscitation for palliative care patients: a discussion of ethical issues. *Palliative Medicine.* **14**(4): 308–12. (R, 16 refs)

46 Zoch TW, Desbiens NA, DeStefano F, Stueland DT, Layde PM (2000) Short- and long-term survival after cardiopulmonary resuscitation. *Archives of Internal Medicine.* **160**(13): 1969–73. (RS-948)

47 Dumot JA, Burval DJ, Sprung J, Waters JH, Mraovic B, Karafa MT, Mascha EJ, Bourke DL (2001) Outcome of adult cardiopulmonary resuscitations at a tertiary referral center including results of 'limited' resuscitations. *Archives of Internal Medicine.* **161**(14): 1751–8. (RS-445)

48 Brindley PG, Markland DM, Mayers I, Kutsogiannis DJ (2002) Predictors of survival following in-hospital adult cardiopulmonary resuscitation. *CMAJ (Canadian Medical Association Journal).* **167**(4): 343–8. (RS-247)

49 Murphy DJ, Burrows D, Santilli S, Kemp AW, Tenner S, Kreling B, Teno J (1994) The influence of the probability of survival on patients' preferences regarding cardiopulmonary resuscitation. *New England Journal of Medicine.* **330**(8): 545–9. (I-287)

50 Eggar R, Spencer A, Anderson D, Hiller L (2002) Views of elderly patients on cardiopulmonary resuscitation before and after treatment for depression. *International Journal of Geriatric Psychiatry.* **17**(2): 170–4. (OS-50)

51 Waisel DB, Truog RD (1995) The cardiopulmonary resuscitation-not-indicated order: futility revisited. *Annals of Internal Medicine.* **122**(4): 304–8. (R)

Emergencies

Emergencies

Emergency	Clinical decision	Page		Emergency	Clinical decision	Page
Adrenocortical insufficiency	7a	(p. 211)		Hyperviscosity	8b	(p. 213)
Agitation	4	(p. 207)		Hypoglycemia	7d	(p. 213)
Air hunger	6b	(p. 209)		Hypotension	3c	(p. 205)
Anaphylaxis	3d	(p. 207)		Magnesium deficiency	7f	(p. 213)
Asthma	6e	(p. 209)		Neutropenia	8c	(p. 213)
Breathlessness	6	(p. 209)		Pain	5	(p. 207)
Bronchospasm	6e	(p. 209)		Pleural effusion	6f	(p. 211)
Cardiac arrest	2a	(p. 205)		Pleuritic pain	5e	(p. 209)
Chest pain	6c	(p. 209)		Peritonitis	5d	(p. 207)
Diabetes mellitus	7c & d	(pp. 211, 213)		Raised IC pressure	9b	(p. 214)
DIC	8a	(p. 213)		Respiratory arrest	3b	(p. 205)
Drug toxicity	3	(p. 205)		Seizures	2d	(p. 205)
Fracture	5c	(p. 207)		SIADH	7e	(p. 213)
Heart failure	6d	(p. 209)		Spinal cord compression	9a	(p. 213)
Hemorrhage	2c	(p. 205)		Stridor	6g	(p. 211)
Hypercalcemia	7b	(p. 211)		Tumor lysis syndrome	7g	(p. 213)
Hyperglycemia	7c	(p. 211)		Vena caval obstruction	9d	(p. 214)

Advice on children written by Renee McCulloch

Clinical decision and action checklist

1 Is comfort the only aim?
2 Is this a sudden collapse?
3 Are drugs the cause?
4 Is severe agitation present?
5 Is severe pain present?
6 Is the patient breathless?
7 Is there a metabolic cause ?
8 Is there a hematological cause?
9 Is a tumor causing local pressure problems?
10 Is the need for treatment uncertain?
11 Has the situation been explained?

Key points

- Several drugs and conditions can mimic the terminal phase of an illness, but are reversible.
- Treating emergencies can improve comfort and reduce distress even if the prognosis is unaltered.
- When the need for treatment remains uncertain an observation period can be helpful.

Introduction

In the presence of progressive disease some drugs and medical conditions can cause unexpected but reversible deterioration. Some conditions can give the impression that a patient is dying when, in reality, the cause is reversible and the patient has the potential to recover. Examples are hypercalcemia, hypoglycemia, hyperglycemia, severe anemia and infection. Although these conditions may reflect underlying disease, they do not necessarily reflect a terminal event, and may be unrelated to the underlying disease.[1] It is usually clear from the patient or the circumstances whether treatment is appropriate. In general, if a patient was coping well before the emergency, reversal of the problem will result in a return to the previous lifestyle. However, other situations are more complex and decisions about treating an emergency must include consideration of the issues below.

Issues to consider about the treatment of emergencies in palliative care

A clear understanding of:
- the patient's wishes and the views of the partner or family
- the reversibility of the current problem
- any distress the treatment may cause
- the feasibility and availability of the treatment
- any ethical issues
- why estimates of previous quality of life are *not* helpful.

The time after an emergency can be a valuable opportunity to discuss the progress of the disease and the options for treatment in the future.

When comfort is the only aim

In some situations the deterioration is unequivocally irreversible (e.g. massive hemoptysis) or the patient may have already been deteriorating rapidly because of their primary condition. Alternatively, the patient may refuse treatment, or it may be inappropriate based on a consensus agreed with the clinical team on the patient's behalf in discussion with the partner and family. In these situations the treatment is aimed at relieving distress and discomfort. This does not exclude partially reversing the cause of the emergency. For example, a patient with end-stage cardiac disease who is distressed by severe heart failure may still benefit from intravenous or subcutaneous furosemide, even though the patient does not want to be admitted to hospital.

Sudden collapse

Cardiac or respiratory arrest: At the natural end of a terminal illness cardiopulmonary resuscitation (CPR) is not a treatment choice since it will fail. In other situations, however, it can be the correct treatment.[2,3] Although success is much lower in non-witnessed arrests,[4] some patients will choose CPR even if the success is as low as 10%.[5] When a 'Do Not Resuscitate (DNR)' order is in place, this is only helpful if the current arrest is under the same circumstances as that anticipated in the DNR order. For example, after careful discussion a competent man with ALS/MND makes a DNR order that, in the event of respiratory failure (and being unable to communicate), he would agree to intermittent positive pressure (IPP) ventilation, but would refuse continuous ventilation requiring laryngeal intubation. However, if he aspirates on some food and goes into respiratory arrest, this DNR order would not apply.

Hemorrhage: Treatment of hemorrhage may be possible, but this is often impossible in the presence of very advanced disease, especially if the hemorrhage is severe or the source is inaccessible. Hemorrhage is frightening for the patient and those around. It may be necessary to ease the patient's distress with a benzodiazepine given by whichever accessible route will give the fastest absorption.

Major seizure: These are uncommon in advanced cancer, even in patients with cerebral metastases. However, some patients, especially neurologically impaired children, already have a history of seizures. In these patients, a change in seizure type or pattern can herald either a decline in general health or indicate a concurrent problem such as infection, constipation or the onset of puberty. Parents and carers are sensitive to the changes in seizures and a potential cause should be sought. A tonic-clonic seizure usually resolves by itself in less than one minute. If it continues, prepare to give a benzodiazepine so that if the seizure has not resolved within five minutes the drug is ready to administer promptly. In adults, the standard treatment is diazepam IV or PR. In children and adolescents, midazolam is as effective in controlling seizures as diazepam but has a faster recovery time and can be given IV, IM or intranasally, although the buccal route is better tolerated.[6–10] Buccal midazolam is rapidly absorbed in adults,[11] and as effective as rectal diazepam in adolescents,[12] but there is limited experience of the efficacy of the buccal route in adults.[13] In children, rectal paraldehyde is a useful second-line drug following the benzodiazepines and causes little respiratory depression. Any seizure is a prompt to review anticonvulsant medication, but in children some seizure disorders are ultimately drug-resistant, causing significant morbidity and distress for the child and carers. In addition, adverse effects from anticonvulsant medication include behavioral changes, sleep disturbance and drowsiness. Occasionally, status epilepticus may be a terminal event. Control may be gained using subcutaneous infusion of midazolam either on its own or in combination with phenobarbital.

Drugs

Many drugs have the potential to mimic deterioration due to the disease by causing drowsiness, respiratory depression or hypotension. If a serious adverse effect is causing the patient harm or distress then that adverse effect must be treated. The drug dose should be reduced or the patient changed to a different drug. Patients have the right to be as alert and aware as possible if this is their wish. It is not acceptable to view a serious drug adverse event as inevitable.

Severe agitation

Restless patients with anxiety or mild confusion often need only company and comfort. A few patients, however, are sufficiently agitated that they risk injuring themselves or others, especially if they become aggressive. The aims are to reduce the agitation sufficiently for comfort, and to find a treatable cause if possible. Assessment is essential to exclude a reversible cause of the agitation. This cannot be done if the patient is sedated with benzodiazepines or psychotropic drugs. Consequently sedation is not the aim, since this would make it difficult for the patient to understand what is happening and would hinder assessment. Any drug should be titrated to reduce the agitation that is causing distress to the patient. This is done with the intention of enabling them to express their distress and allowing them to respond to company, empathy and other treatments such as massage and relaxation.

Irreversible agitation: The aims of reducing severe agitation do not change if the cause of the agitation is irreversible. The dose is titrated to the minimum dose that reduces the agitation – there is no evidence that such drugs reduce survival.[14,109,110]

Sedation is not a treatment: The drug doses needed to control agitation may result in drowsiness.[15–21] This is an adverse effect which needs to be minimized. If marked sedation is unavoidable, ideally this needs the permission of the patient if the same doses are to continue, but it may not be possible to obtain this permission in severe agitation. If the patient is not competent for this decision it is helpful to have a clear consensus between the clinical team and the partner or relative. In all circumstances it is essential to have a clear plan (*see* Table 1) to avoid decisions being made on anecdotal experiences.[15,22]

Opioids are contraindicated as a treatment of agitation: Opioids may make the agitation worse through the accumulation of active metabolites, and tolerance

to the sedative effect develops rapidly. *See* Managing the adverse effects of analgesics (p. 53).

Severe pain

The most immediate goal is to reduce pain at rest and to allow the patient to settle sufficiently to allow adequate assessment. Colic needs to be differentiated from other causes of pain as the treatment is very different, but for other causes of pain a strong opioid can be used.

Pain on the slightest movement can be managed with positioning, padding and splints, before excluding a fracture or vertebral collapse. Treatment for pathological fractures are best planned, rather than managed as acute emergencies. If surgery is not possible the pain can be controlled with ketamine, local nerve blocks or spinal analgesia.

Peritonitis: This is a rare complication of obstruction, NSAIDs and inflammatory bowel disease. If surgery is not an option, in our experience intraperitoneal steroid and local anesthetic can provide rapid analgesia for the last hours of a patient's life. Intraperitoneal corticosteroids have been used for ascites.[23]

Pleuritic pain: This may be due to a rib metastasis or pleural inflammation due to infection, tumor or embolus. A local intercostal block can help, as can an intrapleural infusion of local anesthetic.[24]

Table 1: Treating severe agitation

Requirements for treatment

- Agitation causing distress to the patient
- Agitation with the risk of harm to the patient or others
- Agitation preventing assessment
- Permission from the patient (or if non-competent for this decision, a clear consensus for treatment that includes information from the partner and family)
- Documentation of treatment reasons, length and review dates
- Understanding of the drugs used to control severe agitation (e.g. avoiding the use of opioids)
- Willingness to ask for help if agitation persists

Aims of treatment

- Reduce distress by more than half
- Enable the patient to express the reasons for their distress
- Reduce the agitation sufficiently to allow assessment
- Keep drowsiness to a minimum

Table 2: Treating severe pain

Requirements for treatment

- Pain causing distress to the patient
- Understanding of the drugs used to control severe pain (e.g. strong opioids do not control all pains)
- Willingness to ask for help if pain persists

Aims of treatment

- Reduce the pain at rest by more than two-thirds
- Reduce the pain on movement sufficiently to allow essential movements such as going to the toilet
- Keep adverse effects to a minimum
- Plan for medium and long-term analgesia

Persistent agitation or pain: The advice of palliative care, pain and oncology colleagues is essential. Although the agitation or pain may settle, low mood, anxiety and exhaustion may persist (*see* Anxiety (p. 165),

Clinical decision	If YES ⇒ Action
1 Is comfort the only aim?	e.g. rapid deterioration with irreversible cause (e.g. massive hemoptysis, hematemesis or pulmonary embolus), very short prognosis (hour by hour deterioration), or a patient refusing treatment. • Reduce any agitation (*see* cd-4 (p. 207)). • Give analgesia if in pain (*see* Diagnosing and treating pain (p. 39)). • Ensure the patient has company. Keep warm if hypotensive. • Ensure there is support for the patient, partner, family and staff (including you!). • Partial reversal of the cause may still be appropriate for comfort (e.g. furosemide in heart failure).
2 Is this a sudden collapse?	**(a) Cardiac or respiratory arrest:** Cardiopulmonary resuscitation (CPR) should start if: • there is no DNR order *and* successful CPR is possible. Cardiopulmonary resuscitation should not be done if: • this arrest was anticipated *and* a 'Do Not Resuscitate' advance directive exists that has been witnessed and recently reviewed, *or* • the clinical team is as certain as it can be that CPR would fail. For decisions about CPR *see* Issues around resuscitation (p. 193). **(b) Drug toxicity:** *see* cd-3 below. **(c) Hemorrhage:** *If treatment is possible:* obtain IV access, take blood for cross match and start a rapid infusion of 0.9% saline, followed by a plasma substitute while awaiting blood (e.g. Dextran). Consider desmopressin 15–30 microgram IV.[111] Find the bleeding source visually, or using endoscopy or radiology. *If treatment is impossible (or has been refused by patient):* • if the patient is distressed give diazepam 5–20 mg titrated IV (if IV access is not possible, give midazolam 5–15 mg sublingually or IM into deltoid muscle). • if the bleeding is visible (e.g. ulcer, hemoptysis, hematemesis), use dark green or blue towels to make the appearance of blood less frightening to patient, partner and family. • place warm blankets over the patient. • do not leave the patient unattended. **(d) Major seizure (tonic-clonic type):** • Put the patient into the standard recovery position. • Most seizures resolve spontaneously within one minute. If the seizure is not resolving obtain IV diazepam, IV midazolam, or IV lorazepam. • Most seizures resolve spontaneously within 1 minute. If the seizure is not resolving obtain midazolam or diazepam injection. • If the seizure persists, after 5 mins give midazolam 2.5–5 mg bucally (in children give 300 microg/kg), or IM if buccal route not possible. Alternatively, use diazepam 5–10 mg IV, PR (or IM if no other route possible). • If the seizure is persisting, obtain IV access and titrate diazepam 1–10 mg IV over 2 mins until the seizure has stopped. If IV access is not possible consider intramuscular phenobarbital or rectal paraldehyde (for doses in children *see* Drugs in palliative care for children: starting doses (p. 253)). • Review the anticonvulsant medication. **(e) Consider the following as causes:** fall (simple faint, postural hypotension, vertigo, incoordination), hypoglycemia, cardiac arrhythmia, pulmonary embolus, septicemia, or a pericardial effusion (cold, pale, raised pulse rate, BP is maintained initially, poor pulse volume which reduces on inspiration – an exaggeration of normal).
3 Are drugs the cause?	**(a) Reduce the dose or change to an alternative drug.** **(b) If ventilation has been seriously compromised (< 5 respirations/min):** *Opioids:* start 60% oxygen. Dilute naloxone 0.4 mg in 10 ml and titrate IV at 0.04 mg/minute until respiration improves, followed by naloxone infusion (full opioid reversal is not the aim). *Spinal local anesthetics:* ventilation may be needed for 1–2 hours. *Benzodiazepine:* start 60% oxygen. Flumazenil IV 200 microgram over 15 seconds followed by 100 microgram/minute up to 1000 microgram (1 mg). **(c) If severe hypotension is present (systolic < 60 mmHg):** *Spinal local anesthetics:* IV 0.9% saline 500 ml infused rapidly. If the response is brief or insufficient give ephedrine 3–9 mg IV.

Table continued on p. 207

Anger (p. 161) and Withdrawal and depression (p. 177)). This persistence of psychological problems will delay the resolution of the agitation or pain and to avoid disappointment this delay needs to be explained to the patient, partner and staff. In situations when a pain-relieving procedure has to be delayed benzodiazepines can reduce anxiety and distress.

The breathless patient

Severe breathlessness is frightening and simple measures are important first steps. If severe hypoxia is present, the patient may be too agitated to tolerate oxygen and the agitation will need to be reduced to a level where oxygen can be tried.

Air hunger: Fast respiratory rates are distressing and exhausting. It occurs in ketoacidosis due to diabetes mellitus and is usually reversible. It can also occur in the presence of fear or persistent hypoxia at the end of life, requiring support for the patient and family.[29] Gasping is seen in some patients in the last minutes of life, but these patients are deeply unconscious and there is no evidence that it is distressing to the patient. An opioid may help, but may also increase agitation and if there is no improvement the agitation should be treated as in cd-4 opposite.

Chest pain: This may indicate acute problems such as myocardial infarction, pneumothorax, pulmonary embolism or an acute chest infection. Cardiac ischemic pain is more likely if the pain is caused by exertion and radiates to the arms or shoulders.[30] Vertebral metastases or rib metastases can cause chest pain through nerve root compression.

Heart failure: This is common in older patients, especially if they are nursed flat at the end of their illness. Initial treatment is with intravenous furosemide, but longer-term control may be needed with ACE inhibitors, beta-blockers or spironolactone, according to established guidelines.[31]

Acute severe asthma may be related to pre-existing asthma, chronic obstructive pulmonary disease (COPD), or due to an allergic drug reaction. Most bronchospasm will respond to inhaled bronchodilators, but a nebulized bronchodilator and intravenous hydrocortisone may be needed in severe cases.[32]

Pleural effusion: Severe breathlessness due to an effusion requires rapid drainage of the effusion for comfort.

Stridor is due to obstruction of the upper trachea. In cancer, and in the absence of an inhaled foreign body, airway compression by tumor is the commonest cause. A 4:1 helium/oxygen mixture has less viscosity than air and can be breathed more comfortably through an obstruction.[33–35] Dexamethasone will help reduce any edema around the tumor, reducing the obstruction. A cough that lacks its normal force and suddenness suggests a 'bovine' cough that is caused by bilateral vocal cord paralysis with a risk of complete laryngeal obstruction by the paralyzed vocal cords.[36] Urgent referral to the ENT specialists is necessary for Teflon injection of one cord.[37]

Metabolic problems

Adrenocortical insufficiency: Causes include adrenal damage (metastases, infection or infarction), hypothalamic damage (brain metastases, cranial irradiation) or abrupt withdrawal of systemic corticosteroids. It may also occur during physical stress whilst on steroids, or soon after weaning off corticosteroids. All patients on corticosteroids should be given a steroid information card that warns against suddenly stopping corticosteroids.

Hypercalcemia: This is common in some cancers (50% of myeloma, 25% of bronchial carcinomas and 20% of breast carcinomas).[38,39] In 80% of cases the cause is the production of a parathyroid hormone-like protein by the tumor,[39–41] a process which is unrelated to the presence of bone metastases. Symptoms are insidious and mimic the symptoms seen in a dying patient, so that hypercalcemia is often missed or undertreated.[42] Drowsiness, nausea, vomiting, confusion, constipation or thirst may occur, but drowsiness alone is common. Polyuria is also usual, but is very difficult to detect from history alone. Patients who were well 1–2 weeks previously and have deteriorated unexpectedly may be hypercalcemic. Such patients should have blood taken for biochemistry. The corrected total serum calcium may be a better test than ionized calcium and may better correlate with symptoms.[43–47] Values of corrected serum calcium > 2.8 mmol/l are abnormal.[48] (But check local laboratory reference values.) Serum chloride levels are usually unaffected, but if they are raised and combined with low bicarbonate, this suggests primary hyperparathyroidism as a cause of the hypercalcemia.[49]

In hypercalcemia due to malignancy, steroids are only effective in myeloma and lymphoma.[39] For other tumors the bisphosphonates are now the most effective treatment available.[51] Because of polyuria caused by the hypercalcemia some patients will need 48 hours of IV hydration, but those who are drinking normally and not dehydrated will not need IV fluids. Hydration by itself will not achieve useful control of the hypercalcemia.[39,52–55] Pamidronate is given as a

Steroid withdrawal: give hydrocortisone 100 mg IM or slow IV. Restart oral corticosteroid.

Antimuscarinic hypotension (e.g. amitriptyline): usually postural so elevate legs and stop drug. Fit support stockings until the drug effect has reduced.

(d) **If anaphylaxis has occurred (edema, stridor, hypotension):**

Give 1:1000 adrenaline IM every 15 mins until the blood pressure is stable. For adults give 0.5–1 ml. For a child < 1 year = 0.05 ml; 1–2 yrs = 0.1–0.2 ml; 3–5 yrs = 0.3–0.5 ml.

Give antihistamine (e.g. diphenhydramine 25 mg slow IV) and continue PO for 24 hours. Give hydrocortisone 100 mg IM or IV.

If bronchospasm persists give salbutamol 2.5 mg nebulized or 250 microgram slow IV.

(e) **If drowsiness or confusion is present:**

See Fatigue, drowsiness, lethargy and weakness (p. 101) and Confusional states (delirium and dementia) (p. 171).

---

4 Is severe agitation present?

- **If urgent control of the agitation is essential** (e.g. irreversible hemorrhage, severe breathlessness, prevention of injury to patient):
  - do not use opioids to treat the agitation (*see* notes).
  - give midazolam 2–10 mg titrated IV, **or** 2.5–5 mg IM or buccal/sublingual. If necessary, repeat the dose up to three times (for IV repeat at 2 min intervals, for IM/sublingual repeat at 10 min intervals). If the agitation worsens on midazolam, use methotrimeprazine 12.5–25 mg IM or SC.
  - sedation is not the aim unless the distress is overwhelming. Using titration it is possible to settle a patient without causing respiratory depression.
  - ensure the environment is safe (e.g. placing mattress on floor).
  - do not leave patient unattended since staying with the patient is comforting and makes it clear to them that they will not be abandoned.
- **If abnormal experiences are present** (e.g. paranoia, hallucinations): add an antipsychotic (*see* cd-7 in Confusional states (delirium and dementia) (p. 173)).
- **Consider the following as causes:** anger, confusional state, fear, hypoglycemia, hypoxia and pain.
- **If the agitation is persistent and the patient is terminal:** consider phenobarbital SC 600–2400 mg/24hours infusion,[25] or propofol 0.5 mg/kg by slow IV followed by a propofol IV infusion of 2 mg/kg/hour.[26–28]

---

5 Is severe pain present?

(a) **Periodic pain suggesting colic** (i.e. coming and going every few minutes): give hyoscine butylbromide 20 mg IV, SC or IM as single injection, followed if necessary by 60 mg/24 hr, either SC infusion or 10–15 mg q6h. In US use hyoscyamine 0.25–0.5 mg/IV/SC q4h PRN, 0.125–0.25 mg SL q4h PRN, max 1.5 mg/day.

(b) **Provide immediate analgesia:** give hydromorphone as a titrated IV injection (or IM if IV access is not possible) followed by SC infusion. Give 2 mg if not on opioid, otherwise use equivalent of usual 4-hourly dose.

(c) **Pain worsened by the slightest passive movement:**
  - find a comfortable position. Use padding or splints to reduce painful movements.
  - if two breakthrough doses of opioid have been ineffective, give ketamine 5 mg buccal/sublingual, or fentanyl 50 μg (may need to progress to sufentanil 25 μg) 10 mins before moving.

  If this is back pain: check for spinal cord compression (*see* cd-9a on p. 213).

  If a pathological fracture is suspected:
  - too unwell to travel: ensure the patient is on a pressure-relieving mattress, give analgesia before turning or moving (usual breakthrough opioid 30 mins, ketamine 5–10 mg buccal/sublingual or fentanyl 50 μg 10 mins before moving).
  - well enough to travel: plan for an X-ray and orthopedic advice (best done electively, rather than as an emergency). Give analgesia as above prior to travel.

(d) **Peritonitis** (constant abdominal pain, pain on light percussion of abdomen, abdominal wall rigidity):
  - well enough for surgery and agrees to this option: refer urgently for a surgical opinion. Give metronidazole 400 mg as IV infusion over 20 mins.
  - too ill for surgery (or refuses this option): at the site of least pain inject 20 ml 0.25% bupivacaine plus 8 mg dexamethasone intraperitoneally. If the pain is no better after 15 mins, repeat at another abdominal site.
  - for nausea or vomiting give methotrimeprazine 5 mg SC.

Table continued on p. 209

single 2–4 hour infusion, but zoledronic acid is more convenient as it can be given as a 30 minute infusion and is more effective than pamidronate.[56,57,112] Zoledronic acid is as safe as pamidronate, is well tolerated, and renal impairment is an uncommon adverse event.[53,58] Fever is the commonest adverse effect of zoledronic acid, occurring in one third of patients.[59] Hypocalcemia has been noted in some patients 2–3 days after zoledronic acid. There is a delay of 24–48 hours before the bisphosphonate begins to act and therefore it is our practice to give the bisphosphonate at the outset of treatment, particularly as effective rehydration (oral or parenteral) will help to reduce the calcium in the first 48 hours. Calcitonin can be used for rapid reduction of hypercalcemia, but the effects last only a few days and it needs to be combined with pamidronate or zoledronic acid.[60] Following IV bisphosphonate, retreatment may be needed in 2–4 weeks,[61] but the patient is now alert to the symptoms and treatment can begin before the calcium level is high. A 30 minute infusion of zoledronic acid is particularly convenient at home. Home treatment of hypercalcemia is straightforward, especially when treating a second episode that has been identified early. Intravenous bisphosphonates are better tolerated and more effective than oral.[113] Most patients return to their pre-hypercalcemic state with a good quality of life. However, hypercalcemia is an indicator of disease progression, and cancer patients may require a change in their anticancer treatment.

Severe hypoglycemia: It is common for existing diabetics with advanced disease to require less insulin or oral hypoglycemics as their oral intake and activity reduce. Consequently these patients are at a risk of hypoglycemia. Symptoms will normally occur at glucose levels of less than 2 mmol/l, although some patients with diabetes-induced autonomic failure may show few symptoms before they collapse.[62] Treatment should be immediate with glucose replacement. If the patient is drowsy, 50% glucose should be given intravenously. If intravenous access is not possible, then 1 mg glucagon can be given intramuscularly. In a diabetic with advanced disease it is safer to plan for a blood glucose range of 6–15 mmol/l, although for some patients this may be a difficult change to contemplate after a lifetime of tightly controlling their blood glucose.

Severe hyperglycemia: Drowsiness, confusion or coma require urgent treatment. The main goals are to rehydrate, restore a normal blood pressure, treat hypoxia and reduce blood glucose while maintaining potassium levels. Both ketotic and non-ketotic hyperglycemia can be treated in this way. Ketotic patients will be acidotic, and it is appropriate to treat this with sodium bicarbonate if they are hyperventilating, but this is best done where blood gases and pH can be easily monitored. Glucose ranges of 6–15 mmol/l are acceptable as long as patients are asymptomatic. It is more important to avoid hypoglycemia and the aim is to minimize symptoms, not the tight control of blood glucose.[63,64] Patients who have a history of hyperglycemia may tolerate blood glucose levels of 20 mmol/l.

Inappropriate ADH secretion: The syndrome of inappropriate antidiuretic hormone secretion (SIADH) can be caused by malignancy (especially small cell lung cancer and head and neck cancers), brain damage (e.g. meningitis, tumor, injury), respiratory conditions (e.g. pneumonia, tuberculosis, empyema) and drugs (e.g. antidepressants, carbamazepine, cytotoxics, methotrimeprazine, NSAIDs, thiazide diuretics).[65–68] Demeclocycline blocks the action of ADH on the kidney.

Magnesium deficiency: Because magnesium is not routinely checked, a deficiency is often missed despite occurring in up to 17% of patients with end-stage cancer.[69,70] It can be caused by cytotoxics (especially cisplatin), reduced nutrition and alcoholism.[71,72] Magnesium supplementation is effective and can be given intravenously or orally, although nausea or diarrhea can occur with the oral route.[73]

Tumor lysis syndrome: This is seen after chemotherapy in very sensitive tumors such as acute leukemia and high-grade non-Hodgkin's lymphoma.[65,74,75] Treatment requires admission to hospital and is usually appropriate in patients who have agreed to pursue treatment for their malignancy.

Children with inborn errors of metabolism: Children who are known to have inborn errors of metabolism are vulnerable to 'metabolic crises'. They may become acutely unwell with concurrent infection, especially if they have been unable to tolerate their normal feeds. The child will look unwell and may be cardiovascularly compromised with cool peripheries and an increased respiratory rate due to acidosis. It is important to recognize this problem and treat it without delay because irreversible neurological damage can occur over a matter of hours. The basis of treatment is to give high-energy feeds or infusion to provide a substrate for metabolism to try to prevent metabolic decompensation. Usually the individual will have an emergency feeding regime available which would involve rehydration with a high-energy feed such as 'Resource 2'. If no such regime is obtainable, dextrose 10% should be administered either via the gastrostomy tube, nasogastric tube or intravenously. Specialist advice is often needed.

(e) **Pleuritic pain:**
- if two breakthrough doses of opioid have been given, ask a pain or palliative care specialist to consider an intercostal nerve block or an intrapleural infusion of bupivacaine.
- treat the underlying cause if possible, e.g. chest infection.

(f) **If severe pain persists** (pain remains at 50% or more of its severity at the start)
- check through clinical decisions 2–12 in Diagnosing and treating pain (p. 39).
- consider anxiety, anger or depression as factors reducing the patient's ability to cope with pain.
- contact a pain or palliative care specialist to consider regular ketamine, nerve block or intraspinal analgesia.
- if further treatment is to be delayed for more than 2 hours, reduce anxiety and fear with lorazepam 0.5–1 mg PO or sublingually as required, or use midazolam 2.5–5.0 mg q2h SC PRN or 20–30 mg/24 hours SC infusion. Sedation is rarely needed.

6 Is the patient breathless?	(a) **First steps:** - sit the patient upright (or at least semi-prone). - ensure there is cool air over the face (fan or window). - stay with the patient. If the patient is agitated *see* cd-4 (p. 207). - if available, check the oxygen saturation with a pulse oximeter. If the S_aO_2 is 90% or less start 24% oxygen. If the S_aO_2 has improved, or the patient is more comfortable, continue the oxygen. (b) **Air hunger** (gasping type of respiration): *Diabetic ketoacidosis: see* cd-7c (p. 211). *Tachypnea:* a respiratory rate of > 20/min. If it is due to fear treat this as agitation (*see* cd-4 (p. 207)). Otherwise, give morphine 5 mg SC and repeat after 20 mins. If after three opioid doses the patient is still distressed by the tachypnea, treat as for agitation. *Terminal gasping in last stages of life:* this is seen in the last minutes of life of a deeply unconscious patient. This is a normal part of dying and needs no treatment, although the partner or relative will need explanation and support. (c) **Chest pain and breathlessness** Consider the following causes: *Myocardial infarction:* give morphine (5 mg if not on opioid, otherwise 50–100% of q4h dose) as a titrated IV injection (or IM if IV access is not possible) possibly followed by SC infusion. Arrange for ECG and take blood for cardiac enzymes. *Massive pulmonary embolism* (chest pain, collapse, breathlessness which is not relieved on sitting up, chest sounds normal, gallop rhythm): in the context of advanced disease, a massive pulmonary embolism is usually a terminal event. Streptokinase is an option,[50] but is rarely indicated in palliative care. *Chest infection* causing pleurisy. *Pneumothorax* (acute breathlessness, chest pain, trachea may be deviated towards lung collapse, hollow chest on percussion but reduced or absent breath sounds): if the collapse is $> 30\%$, consider intercostal drainage with water seal. (d) **Acute heart failure** (acute breathlessness, pink frothy sputum, hypotension, tachycardia, third heart sound, lung crepitations, raised jugular venous pressure, confusion): - give loop diuretic such as furosemide 40 mg IV, repeat after 5 mins if no better. - consider giving morphine as a titrated IV injection (or IM if IV access is not possible), possibly followed by SC infusion. Give 2.5 mg if not on opioid, otherwise use 50–100% of usual q4h dose. - consider an ACE inhibitor for long-term control (start under hospital control if creatinine > 150 mmol/l, sodium < 130 mmol/l, systolic BP < 100 mmHg, or aged > 70 years). - nurse the patient in a sitting or semi-prone position. (e) **Acute severe asthma** (unable to talk, fatigue, exhaustion, low respiratory rate, using accessory muscles of respiration, cyanosis, chest may have no wheeze): - start 60% oxygen (use 28% if there is a history of COPD with CO_2 retention). - check peak flow and give salbutamol inhaler 200 microgram through a spacer device, then recheck peak flow. Repeat inhaled salbutamol up to 10 times over 10 minutes if necessary.

Table continued on p. 211

Hematological problems

Disseminated intravascular coagulation (DIC): This condition is a paradoxical combination of bleeding and clotting that results in damage to vital organs.[78] It occurs in up to 10% of cancer patients and is often fatal.[79] It is caused by the depletion of clotting factors due to microscopic clotting and is seen in metastatic carcinoma (especially in the presence of infection), promyelocytic leukemia and after surgery for prostate cancer. It is diagnosed by the simultaneous presence of prolonged bleeding times and evidence of clotting shown by the presence of D-dimer, a breakdown product of blood clots.[80] Measuring D-dimers is a useful diagnostic test of clotting in both cancer and non-cancer patients.[81] Treatment will depend on the cause, since DIC in the presence of advanced cancer is likely to be a terminal event, whereas DIC due to a treatable infection may be reversible.[82] For those patients where transfer to an acute unit is inappropriate, low molecular weight heparin can help.[83]

Hyperviscosity: This occurs in up to half of IgM myeloma patients and is caused by an excess of immunoglobulin in the blood. Treatment should be under the care of hematologists.[84]

Neutropenia: This is usually seen 4–15 days after chemotherapy (especially with intensive regimes for Hodgkin's disease), but it can also occur after radiotherapy to large areas of bone marrow or in some leukemias. The risk of infection depends on several factors:

High risk factors for infection[85,86]

Neutrophil count $< 1 \times 10^9$/l
High dose corticosteroids
Indwelling venous catheter
Invasive procedure (e.g. urinary catheterization)
Chronic infection (TB, herpes simplex, fungal infection)
Immunodeficiency (e.g. HIV)
Age < 1 year
Fever persisting more than 24 hours after starting antibiotic
Poor home conditions

In the absence of high risk factors, patients are best managed at home.[87] Fever is an indication for a broad-spectrum antibiotic based on local antimicrobial policy, to which an antifungal should be added if the infection persists.[88] However, persisting fever may also be due to viruses or drug-resistant bacteria, and is one of several reasons for admitting a patient to hospital, ideally to an isolation room in an oncology unit:

Indicators for hospital admission

Neutrophil count $< 0.5 \times 10^9$/l
Presence of one risk factor
Symptoms persisting more than 24 hours after starting antibiotic (fever, sore throat, mouth ulcers, diarrhea, cough, breathlessness, dysuria, skin rash, cold sore)
Bruising or bleeding
Hypotension
Sudden onset of confusion or drowsiness

Problems caused by tumor pressure

Spinal cord compression: Patients deserve to be spared the distress of paraplegia if possible and cord compression requires urgent treatment.[89,90] One third of patients survive at least a year after symptoms develop,[91] with a median survival of 4 months.[92] Up to 5% of cancer patients may develop compression, but the proportion is higher in myeloma and prostatic carcinoma.[93] Back pain in a patient with cancer should alert the carer to the risk of compression.[94] Warning signs are radiating pain (unilateral in cervical or lumbar compression, bilateral and encircling in thoracic compression), and unpleasant sensory changes in limbs. Pain on small movements such as coughing or straining suggests the presence of a spinal instability. Sensory and motor loss occurs initially but sphincter disturbance is a late sign. The final stage is rapid cord ischemia. Slow progression of weakness over 14 days or more has a much higher chance of recovery after treatment while deterioration 48 hours before treatment has the lowest chance of recovery.[95,96] Magnetic resonance imaging (MRI) is a key investigation to determine the presence and extent of compression.[97] Bone scans and X-rays localize the area of damage in only 21% of patients.[91] High dose dexamethasone given immediately will reduce cord edema and may temporarily prevent the onset of cord ischemia. The doses of dexamethasone used for SCC are variable, ranging from initial boluses of 100 mg IV[114] to 16 mg IV.[115] Lower doses may be associated with fewer serious adverse effects.[116] Radiotherapy is the definitive treatment. Surgery is worthwhile in suitable patients if radiotherapy is not possible, skeletal instability is

   – if no improvement give salbutamol 5 mg *plus* ipratropium 250 mg nebulized.
   – if still no improvement give hydrocortisone 100 mg IV and admit to hospital. Danger signs are hypoxia ($S_aO_2 < 92\%$), exhaustion, confusion, silent chest, bradycardia, hypotension.

(f) **Pleural effusion** (acute breathlessness, trachea may be deviated away from the effusion, dull chest on percussion with reduced or absent breath sounds):
   – drain 0.5–1 liters if the patient is distressed. *See* Respiratory problems (p. 131) for advice on management.

(g) **Stridor** (rasping sound from upper airway with a sensation of suffocation)
   Immediate treatment: if available, start a 28% helium/oxygen mixture. Exclude a foreign body obstruction (food or inhaled object). Give dexamethasone 16 mg IV as a slow injection over 2 minutes.
   If a bovine cough is present (weak, ineffectual cough): refer urgently to Ear, Nose and Throat specialist for assessment of vocal cord function and consideration for Teflon injection of a vocal cord – tracheostomy is sometimes urgently required.
   If radiotherapy or chemotherapy are an option: refer to the oncologists.
   If no further radiotherapy or chemotherapy possible: refer to the respiratory physicians for consideration of a bronchial stent.
   Continue high dose dexamethasone until after treatment.

(h) **For persistent breathlessness,** *see* cd-9, p. 134.

7 Is there a metabolic cause?	(a) **Adrenocortical insufficiency** (lethargy, nausea, vomiting, abdominal pain, diarrhea, hypotension, low sodium, raised potassium):
	   – if the symptoms are severe and adrenal failure is suspected take blood for cortisol level and give a trial dose of hydrocortisone 100 mg IV. An immediate improvement supports the diagnosis.
	   – maintain on hydrocortisone PO 20 mg on waking and 10 early evening. It is often necessary to add fludrocortisone 50–200 microgram PO once daily.
	(b) **Hypercalcemia** (drowsiness, nausea, confusion, raised corrected serum calcium > 2.8 mmol/l (but check local laboratory reference values)).
	Commonest in myeloma (50%) and carcinomas of the bronchus (25%) and breast (20%).
	Immediate treatment:
	   – calculate the corrected serum calcium from formula [(40-albumin) $\times$ 0.025] + serum calcium.[76]
	   – start bisphosphonate: either 60–90 mg pamidronate as 4-hour IV infusion in 500 ml 0.9% saline or zoledronic acid 2–4 mg IV infusion over 30 mins. (Hypocalcemia has been noted in some patients 2–3 days after zoledronic acid.)
	   – start regular acetaminophen to prevent bisphosphonate pyrexia (common with zoledronic acid).
	Encourage calcium loss: encourage oral fluids, but if dehydrated and unable to drink give at least 1 liter per 24 hours parenteral fluids for 48 hours either IV or by continuous SC infusion.
	Prevent recurrence: recheck corrected serum calcium at first sign of symptoms returning. Review antitumor treatment.
	(c) **Hyperglycemia** (thirst, polyuria, lethargy, glucose > 15 mmol/l):
	Immediate treatment:
	   – start 28% oxygen (20% of these patients have a low O_2 saturation).
	   – check electrolytes, blood glucose and urinary ketones.
	   – start an IV infusion of 0.9% saline at 500 ml/hour. Give 500 ml 0.9% saline hourly until BP and peripheral circulation are normal and signs of dehydration have resolved.
	   – insulin: give short-acting insulin 6 units IV *or* 20 units IM (the SC route cannot be used until peripheral circulation improves).
	   – potassium: 5 mins after first insulin give 13–20 mmol/liter/hour with saline.
	   – if hyperventilating: the patient needs admission to hospital for close monitoring of blood gases and correction of acidosis.
	Keep glucose under control: check blood glucose hourly, repeat electrolytes 1 and 5 hours after starting. Establish 24-hour requirement of insulin.
	Prevent recurrence: maintain glucose to whatever range controls symptoms (usually 8–15 mmol/l). Convert to once daily insulin (e.g. Ultratlente, 'Humulin-U').[77] Exclude drug causes of hyperglycemia (corticosteroids, octreotide, diuretics).

Table continued on p. 213

present, or if the patient deteriorates whilst receiving dexamethasone and radiotherapy.[98] In sensitive tumors, chemotherapy can be effective.[99] Dexamethasone alone is suitable for patients for whom radiotherapy, chemotherapy or surgery is not possible.[100] Any patients with partial or complete motor loss will require assessment by the physiotherapist and occupational therapist.

Raised intracranial pressure: In palliative care this is usually due to intracranial tumor or metastases. Dexamethasone followed by radiotherapy is the treatment of choice, but chemotherapy has a role in sensitive tumors.[101,102] Occasionally a tumor causes hydrocephalus which may need an intracranial shunt.

Vena caval obstruction: The superior vena cava (SVC) drains the upper half of the body, while the inferior vena cava (IVC) drains the lower half and the symptoms of vena caval obstruction reflect which half of the body is affected (*see* clinical decision table). Obstruction of the SVC is often caused by tumor in the mediastinum (usually due to lung cancer). IVC obstruction can be caused by abdominal tumor, but also may be caused by thrombosis. Vena caval obstruction usually occurs slowly over weeks or months, allowing alternative (collateral) drainage to develop. Occasionally the obstruction occurs rapidly over days and needs urgent treatment. In SVCO, dexamethasone is still useful first-line treatment if the symptoms are severe. Radiotherapy relieves symptoms in 50–95% within the first two weeks of treatment, but chemotherapy is useful in SVCO due to small cell lung cancer.[103,104] In IVCO, a thrombus needs to be excluded with ultrasound or CT scan. If tumor obstruction is the cause then dexamethasone may be helpful. If radiotherapy is ineffective or cannot be used, a stent can be inserted into the SVC or IVC as an interventional radiology technique.[104–106] In acute SVCO the symptoms can include distressing headache and anxiety, which will need treatment.

Is the need for treatment uncertain?

Even after taking all the details into consideration, including amicable discussions with the patient and partner or family, on occasion it can still be difficult to know how appropriate it is to treat the cause of the deterioration. Waiting a short time will often resolve the situation since the new circumstances will make the situation clearer.[107] Continuing deterioration or the onset of coma suggests that treatment should be for comfort only. Partners and family find that such changes make them much less likely to request treatment interventions other than for comfort.[107,108] If the situation remains unchanged this suggests that the patient has sufficient reserves to undergo treatment of the primary cause of the deterioration.

An opportunity for discussion

After an emergency is over, there is an important opportunity for discussing the current progression of the illness with the patient and with the partner and family (if the patient agrees). If the emergency reflects disease progression, some will not want to discuss the situation and this needs to be respected, while others will find this an opportunity for open sharing of information and feelings (*see* Breaking difficult news (p. 25)). Because these discussions can involve difficult news, the individual may become distressed, although many have already suspected progression of the disease and are not surprised by the news (*see* Helping the person with the effects of difficult news (p. 29)).

(d) **Hypoglycemia** (pale, sweaty, drowsiness, coma, glucose < 2.5 mmol/l):
Immediate treatment: give sugar in water orally, but if too sleepy give 20 ml 50% glucose IV (flush needle with 0.9% saline to clear all glucose from the vein and prevent local thrombosis). If IV access is not available give glucagon 1 mg IM.
Maintain glucose levels: ensure glucose is being maintained above 5 mmol/l. Repeat IV 20 ml 50% glucose if necessary. Glucagon 1 mg is an alternative but will be less effective in cachectic patients or with repeated doses. Monitor glucose q4h until 3 normal levels obtained.
Prevent recurrence: reduce the dose of insulin or hypoglycemics. Exclude other causes of hypoglycemia (adrenocortical insufficiency, insulinomas, non-selective β-blockers, pentamidine, post gastrectomy dumping, raised IGF2 paraneoplastic hypoglycemia).

(e) **Inappropriate ADH secretion (SIADH)** (lethargy, drowsiness, confusion, headache, sodium < 120 mmol/l, concentrated urine with osmolality > 300 mosmol/kg).
  – treat causes of SIADH such as drugs (reduce drug dose or change to alternative) or chest infection.
  – avoid using hypertonic saline to correct the low sodium unless the patient is in a hospital high dependency unit.
  – fluid restriction to 500 ml/day can help but is unpleasant for patients.
  – demeclocycline 300–600 mg q12h is simple, effective and convenient for many patients.

(f) **Magnesium deficiency** (lethargy, fatigue, low serum magnesium): if severe, 20 mmol magnesium needs to be given daily by IV infusion over 4 hours. Maintenance is with magnesium 10–20 mmol PO daily (approximately equivalent to 150 mg magnesium oxide).

(g) **Tumor lysis syndrome** (weakness, vomiting, muscle cramps, confusion, high blood levels of potassium, calcium, phosphate and uric acid resulting in renal and heart failure).
  – admit urgently to inpatient unit for IV fluids and correction of biochemical disturbances.

(h) **Crisis in children with inborn errors of metabolism**: if this is felt to be a metabolic crisis (*see* notes) start urgent rehydration and high energy feed, e.g. 'Resource 2'. Ask for specialist help.

8 **Is there a hematological cause?**	(a) **Disseminated intravascular coagulation (DIC)** (bruising, mucosal bleeding, prolonged prothrombin time, low platelets, low fibrinogen <1 g/l, presence of fibrinogen products).
	  – *if the symptoms are mild* (bruising, occasional bleeds): start low dose molecular weight heparin 100–150 units/kg SC once daily and aminocaproic or tranexamic acid PO 1 g q8h. Dose of aminocaproic acid – start at 1 g PO q6h, max up to 30 g PO/24 h. IV – 1 g/h.
	  – *if the symptoms are severe* (hemorrhage, thrombosis): consider urgent admission to an inpatient unit with facilities for close hematological control, but if this is inappropriate *see* cd-2c in Emergencies (p. 205).
	(b) **Hyperviscosity in myeloma** (headache, drowsiness, visual disturbances, retinal hemorrhage, tortuous retinal veins, mucosal bleeding, low platelets, cardiac failure).
	  – refer urgently to the hematologists for treatment.
	(c) **Neutropenia** (4–15 days post chemotherapy, fever, low neutrophils $< 1 \times 10^9$/l)
	If no fever and no risk factors (*see* notes): observe, checking neutrophils daily.
	If a fever is present, but no risk factor: start a broad-spectrum antibiotic according to local antimicrobial policy.
	If the fever persists > 24 hours despite antibiotics or one risk factor is present: consider admission to hospital.

9 **Is a tumor causing local pressure problems?**	(a) **Cord compression** (early signs: mild weakness or sensory change with vertebral pain, especially on coughing or lying; late signs: clear sensory or motor changes; very late signs: sphincter disturbance. Sensory changes are usually one or two dermatomes below site of compression, except in cauda equina lesions where changes are often asymmetrical). – give dexamethasone 16 mg IV as slow injection over 2 minutes, then 16 mg PO once daily. Some protocols use higher initial doses (*see* p. 210). In US, give either

Table continued overleaf

100 mg IV loading dose, then 24 mg PO q6h and taper[114], or 24 mg IV × 1 then 6 mg PO q6h × 2 days then gradually taper down.

If the prognosis allows, arrange an urgent MRI and refer for radiotherapy.

Consider referral for surgical decompression if the patient has late signs, the symptoms are worsening despite radiotherapy, further radiotherapy is not possible, or investigations have shown an unstable spine.

If permanent cord damage has occurred: See Constipation (p. 75), Urinary and sexual problems (p. 151) and Skin problems (p. 139). Arrange for physiotherapy and occupational therapy. Contact rehabilitation medical team for help and advice. Reduce and stop dexamethasone unless this is required for pain control.

(b) **Raised intracranial pressure** (headache, vomiting, drowsiness, papilledema).
 – arrange for a CT or MRI scan to assess the cause.

If cerebral metastases are the cause: start dexamethasone 16 mg PO on waking, reducing to the lowest dose that controls symptoms, and refer for cerebral irradiation.

If hydrocephalus is the cause: refer for neurosurgery.

(c) **Stridor:** *see* cd-6g (p. 211).

(d) **Vena caval obstruction**: SVCO (edema of face or arms, stridor, distended neck veins, chest and arm veins, headache, dusky color to skin in chest, arms and face); IVCO (edema of genitals and legs, distended abdominal and leg veins, dusky color to legs).

If this is IVCO: exclude a vena caval thrombosis.

If tumor is the cause: give dexamethasone 15 mg IV as a slow injection over 2 minutes and start dexamethasone 16 mg PO once daily, reducing to the lowest dose that controls symptoms. If the prognosis allows, refer to the oncologists for urgent investigation and radiotherapy or chemotherapy. Consider referral for vena caval stent.

10 Is the need for treatment uncertain?	• Consult with the partner or relatives as they may offer useful information (e.g. previously stated refusal of a specific treatment in specific circumstances). – any stated refusals of treatment only apply to the circumstances anticipated by the patient (or agreed with the clinical team in the case of a non-competent patient). – partners or relatives of adults do not have the right to demand or refuse treatment, but they can give helpful information on the patient's previously stated preferences. • Consult with the clinical team taking into account the history, rate of deterioration, and the availability of treatment. *See* also Making ethical choices (p. 185) and Decisions around competency (p. 189). • **If the need is still unclear agree an observation period using the rule of 3:** Hour by hour deterioration: review in 3 hours. Day by day deterioration: review in 3 days. *If further deterioration has occurred:* treat for comfort. *If no further deterioration:* consider treating or set another review time or date.
11 Has the situation been explained?	• Explain the circumstances to the patient, if they want to discuss the emergency. • If the patient agrees, explain the situation to the partner or family.

cd = clinical decision

References

B = book; C = comment; Ch = chapter; CS-n = case study-number of cases; CT-n = controlled trial-number of cases; E = editorial; G = guideline; GC = group consensus; I = interviews; Let = letter; LS = laboratory study; MC = multi-center; OS-n = open study-number of cases; R = review; RCT-n = randomized controlled trial-number of cases; RS-n = retrospective survey-number of cases; SA = systematic or meta analysis.

1 Taube AW, Jenkins C, Bruera E (1997) Is a 'palliative' patient always a palliative patient? Two case studies. *Journal of Pain and Symptom Management.* **13**(6): 347–51. (R)

2 Zoch TW, Desbiens NA, DeStefano F, Stueland DT, Layde PM (2000) Short- and long-term survival after cardiopulmonary resuscitation. *Archives of Internal Medicine.* **160**(13): 1969–73. (RS-948)

3 Dumot JA, Burval DJ, Sprung J, Waters JH, Mraovic B, Karafa MT, Mascha EJ, Bourke DL (2001) Outcome of adult cardiopulmonary resuscitations at a tertiary referral center including results of 'limited' resuscitations. *Archives of Internal Medicine.* **161**(14): 1751–8. (RS-445)

4 Brindley PG, Markland DM, Mayers I, Kutsogiannis DJ (2002) Predictors of survival following in-hospital adult cardiopulmonary resuscitation. *CMAJ (Canadian Medical Association Journal).* **167**(4): 343–8. (RS-247)

5 Murphy DJ, Burrows D, Santilli S, Kemp AW, Tenner S, Kreling B, Teno J (1994) The influence of the probability of survival on patients' preferences regarding cardiopulmonary resuscitation. *New England Journal of Medicine.* **330**(8): 545–9. (I-287)

6 Vilke GM, Sharieff GQ, Marino A, Gerhart AE, Chan TC (2002) Midazolam for the treatment of out-of-hospital pediatric seizures. *Prehospital Emergency Care.* **6**(2): 215–17. (OS-86)

7 Chamberlain JM, Altieri MA, Futterman C, Young GM, Ochsenschlager DW, Waisman Y (1997) A prospective, randomized study comparing intramuscular midazolam with intravenous diazepam for the treatment of seizures in children. *Pediatric Emergency Care.* **13**(2): 92–4. (RCT-24)

8 McGlone R, Smith M (2001) Intranasal midazolam. An alternative in childhood seizures. *Emergency Medicine Journal.* **18**(3): 234. (Let)

9 Fisgin T, Gurer Y, Senbil N, Tezic T, Zorlu P, Okuyaz C, Akgun D (2000) Nasal midazolam effects on childhood acute seizures. *Journal of Child Neurology.* **15**(12): 833–5. (OS-16)

10 Geldner G, Hubmann M, Knoll R, Jacobi K (1997) Comparison between three transmucosal routes of administration of midazolam in children. *Paediatric Anaesthesia.* **7**(2): 103–9. (RCT-47)

11 Scott RC, Besag FM, Boyd SG, Berry D, Neville BG (1998) Buccal absorption of midazolam: pharmacokinetics and EEG pharmacodynamics. *Epilepsia.* **39**(3): 290–4. (CT-10)

12 Scott RC, Besag FM, Neville BG (1999) Buccal midazolam and rectal diazepam for treatment of prolonged seizures in childhood and adolescence: a randomised trial. *Lancet.* **353**(9153): 623–6. (RCT-42)

13 Scheepers M, Scheepers B (1998) Midazolam via the intranasal route: an effective rescue medication for severe epilepsy in adults with a learning disability. *Seizure.* **7**: 509–12. (CS-2)

14 Morita T, Tsunoda J, Inoue S, Chihara S (2001) Effects of high dose opioids and sedatives on survival in terminally ill cancer patients. *Journal of Pain and Symptom Management.* **21**(4): 282–9. (OS-209)

15 Morita T, Tsuneto S, Shima Y (2002) Definition of sedation for symptom relief: a systematic literature review and a proposal of operational criteria. *Journal of Pain and Symptom Management.* **24**(4): 447–53. (SA, 32 refs)

16 Beel A, McClement SE, Harlos M (2002) Palliative sedation therapy: a review of definitions and usage. *International Journal of Palliative Nursing.* **8**(4): 190–9. (R, 43 refs)

17 Cowan JD, Palmer TW (2002) Practical guide to palliative sedation. *Current Oncology Reports.* **4**(3): 242–9. (R, 65 refs)

18 Cowan JD, Walsh D (2001) Terminal sedation in palliative medicine – definition and review of the literature. *Supportive Care in Cancer.* **9**(6): 403–7. (SA, 41 refs)

19 Quill TE, Byock IR (2000) Responding to intractable terminal suffering: the role of terminal sedation and voluntary refusal of food and fluids. ACP-ASIM End-of-Life Care Consensus Panel. American College of Physicians-American Society of Internal Medicine. *Annals of Internal Medicine.* **132**(5): 408–14. (GC, 65 refs)

20 Chater S, Viola R, Paterson J, Jarvis V (1998) Sedation for intractable distress in the dying–a survey of experts. *Palliative Medicine.* **12**(4): 255–69. (Q-61)

21 Fainsinger RL, Waller A, Bercovici M, Bengston K, Landman W, Hosking M, Nunez-Olarte JM, deMoissac D (2000) A multicentre international study of sedation for uncontrolled symptoms in terminally ill patients. *Palliative Medicine.* **14**: 257–65. (OS-287)

22 Morita T, Akechi T, Sugawara Y, Chihara S, Uchitomi Y (2002) Practices and attitudes of Japanese oncologists and palliative care physicians concerning terminal sedation: a nationwide survey. *Journal of Clinical Oncology.* **20**(3): 758–64. (I-697)

23 Mackey JR, Wood L, Nabholtz J, Jensen J, Venner P (2000) A phase II trial of triamcinolone hexacetanide for symptomatic recurrent malignant ascites. *Journal of Pain and Symptom Management.* **19**(3): 193–9. (OS-15)

24 Paniagua P, Catala E, Villar Landeira JM (2000) Successful management of pleuritic pain with thoracic paravertebral block. *Regional Anesthesia & Pain Medicine.* **25**(6): 651–3. (CS-1)

25 Stirling LC, Kurowska A, Tookman A (1999) The use of phenobarbitone in the management of agitation and seizures at the end of life. *Journal of Pain and Symptom Management.* **17**(5): 363–8. (OS-60)

26 Mercadante S, De Conno F, Ripamonti C (1995) Propofol in terminal care. *Journal of Pain and Symptom Management.* **10**(8): 639–42. (CS-1)

27 Moyle J (1995) The use of propofol in palliative medicine. *Journal of Pain and Symptom Management.* **10**(8): 643–6. (CS-1)

28 Cheng C, Roemer-Becuwe C, Pereira J (2002) When midazolam fails. *Journal of Pain and Symptom Management.* **23**(3): 256–65. (CS-2)

29 Tarzian AJ (2000) Caring for dying patients who have air hunger. *Journal of Nursing Scholarship.* **32**(2): 137–43. (I-12)

30 Goodacre S, Locker T, Morris F, Campbell S (2002) How useful are clinical features in the diagnosis of acute, undifferentiated chest pain? *Academic Emergency Medicine.* **9**(3): 203–8. (OS-893)

31 Prodigy Guidance: Heart failure (2002) www.prodigy.nhs.uk/guidance.asp?gt=Heart Failure. April. (G)

32 SIGN (Scottish Intercollegiate Guidelines Network): Emergency Management of Acute Asthma (1999) Edinburgh: SIGN (available on www.sign.ac.uk/pdf/sign38.pdf). (G)

33 Hansen JJ, Jepsen SB, Lund J (2000) Symptomatic helium treatment of upper and lower airway obstruction. *Ugeskrift for Laeger.* **162**(49): 6669–72. (R, 22 refs)

34 Curtis JL, Mahlmeister M, Fink JB, Lampe G, Matthay MA, Stulbarg MS (1986) Helium-oxygen gas therapy. Use and availability for the emergency treatment of inoperable airway obstruction. *Chest.* **90**(3): 455–7. (CS-1)

35 McGee DL, Wald DA, Hinchliffe S (1997) Helium-oxygen therapy in the emergency department. *Journal of Emergency Medicine.* **15**(3): 291–6. (R, 37 refs)

36 Hillel AD, Benninger M, Blitzer A, Crumley R, Flint P, Kashima HK, Sanders I, Schaefer S (1999) Evaluation and management of bilateral vocal cord immobility. *Otolaryngology – Head & Neck Surgery.* **121**(6): 760–5. (R, 34 refs)

37 Harries ML, Morrison M (1998) Management of unilateral vocal cord paralysis by injection medialization with teflon paste. Quantitative results. *Annals of Otology, Rhinology & Laryngology.* **107**(4): 332–6. (CS-8)

38 Heath DA (1989) Hypercalcemia of malignancy. *Palliative Medicine.* **3**: 1–11. (R)

39 Bower M, Brazil L, Coombes RC (1997) Endocrine and metabolic complications of advanced cancer. In: D Doyle, GWC Hanks, N MacDonald (eds) *The Oxford Textbook of Palliative Medicine* (2e). Oxford Medical Publications, Oxford. pp. 709–25. (Ch)

40 Kovacs CS, MacDonald SM, Chik CL, Bruera E (1995) Hypercalcemia of malignancy in the palliative care patient: a treatment strategy. *Journal of Pain and Symptom Management.* **10**: 224–32. (R, 51 refs)

41 Rabbani SA (2000) Molecular mechanism of action of parathyroid hormone related peptide in hypercalcemia of malignancy: therapeutic strategies (review). *International Journal of Oncology.* **16**(1): 197–206. (R, 54 refs)

42 Lamy O, Jenzer-Closuit A, Burckhardt P (2001) Hypercalcemia of malignancy: an undiagnosed and undertreated disease. *Journal of Internal Medicine.* **250**(1): 73–9. (OS-71)

43 Riancho JA, Arjona R, Sanz J, Olmos JM, Valle R, Barcelo JR, Gonzalez-Macias J (1991) Is the routine measurement of ionized calcium worthwhile in patients with cancer? *Postgraduate Medical Journal.* **67**(786): 350–3. (OS-188)

44 Nussbaum SR, Younger J, Vandepol CJ, Gagel RF, Zubler MA, Chapman R, Henderson IC, Mallette LE (1993) Single-dose intravenous therapy with pamidronate for the treatment of hypercalcemia of malignancy: comparison of 30-, 60-, and 90-mg dosages. *American Journal of Medicine.* **95**(3): 297–304. (RCT-50)

45 Nussbaum SR, Warrell RP Jr, Rude R, Glusman J, Bilezikian JP, Stewart AF, Stepanavage M, Sacco JF, Averbuch SD, Gertz BJ (1993) Dose-response study of alendronate sodium for the treatment of cancer-associated hypercalcemia. *Journal of Clinical Oncology.* **11**(8): 1618–23. (RCT-59)

46 Thode J, Juul-Jorgensen B, Bhatia HM, Kjaerulf-Nielsen M, Bartels PD, Fogh-Andersen N, Siggaard-Andersen O (1989) Comparison of serum total calcium, albumin-corrected total calcium, and ionized calcium in 1213 patients with suspected calcium disorders. *Scandinavian Journal of Clinical & Laboratory Investigation.* **49**(3): 217–23. (OS-1213)

47 Payne RB, Carver ME, Morgan DB (1979) Interpretation of serum total calcium: effects of adjustment for albumin concentration on frequency of abnormal values and on detection of change in the individual. *Journal of Clinical Pathology.* **32**(1): 56–60. (OS-1693)

48 Lum G (1996) Evaluation of a laboratory critical limit (alert value) policy for hypercalcemia. *Archives of Pathology & Laboratory Medicine.* **120**(7): 633–6. (OS-191)

49 Lind L, Ljunghall S (1991) Serum chloride in the differential diagnosis of hypercalcemia. *Experimental & Clinical Endocrinology.* **98**(3): 179–84. (OS-221)

50 Jerjes-Sanchez C, Ramirez-Rivera A, Arriaga-Nava R, Iglesias-Gonzalez S, Gutierrez P, Ibarra-Perez C, Martinez A, Valencia S, Rosado-Buzzo A, Pierzo JA, Rosas E (2001) High dose and short-term streptokinase infusion in patients with pulmonary embolism: prospective with seven-year follow-up trial. *Journal of Thrombosis & Thrombolysis.* **12**(3): 237–47. (CT-40)

51 Body JJ (2000) Current and future directions in medical therapy: hypercalcemia. *Cancer.* **88**(12 Suppl): 3054–8. (SA, 23 refs)

52 Berenson JR (2001) Zoledronic acid in cancer patients with bone metastases: results of Phase I and II trials. *Seminars in Oncology.* **28**(2 Suppl 6): 25–34. (R, 33 refs)

53 Berenson JR, Rosen LS, Howell A, Porter L, Coleman RE, Morley W, Dreicer R, Kuross SA, Lipton A, Seaman JJ (2001) Zoledronic acid reduces skeletal-related events in patients with osteolytic metastases. *Cancer.* **91**(7): 1191–200. (RCT-280)

54 Cheer SM, Noble S (2001) Zoledronic acid. *Drugs.* **61**(6): 799–805. (R, 14 refs)

55 Gucalp R, Theirault R (1994) Treatment of cancer-associated hypercalcemia. *Archives of Internal Medicine.* **154**: 1935–44. (RCT-46)

56 Major P, Lortholary A, Hon J, Abdi E, Mills G, Menssen HD, Yunus F, Bell R, Body J, Quebe-Fehling E, Seaman J (2001) Zoledronic acid is superior to pamidronate in the treatment of hypercalcemia of malignancy: a pooled analysis of two randomized, controlled clinical trials. *Journal of Clinical Oncology.* **19**(2): 558–67. (RCT-287)

57 Major PP, Coleman RE (2001) Zoledronic acid in the treatment of hypercalcemia of malignancy: results of the international clinical development program. *Seminars in Oncology.* **28**(2 Suppl 6): 17–24. (R, 30 refs)

58 Ali SM, Esteva FJ, Hortobagyi G, Harvey H, Seaman J, Knight R, Costa L, Lipton A (2001) Safety and efficacy of bisphosphonates beyond 24 months in cancer patients. *Journal of Clinical Oncology.* **19**(14): 3434–7. (CT-22)

59 Body JJ, Lortholary A, Romieu G, Vigneron AM, Ford J (1999) A dose-finding study of zoledronate in hypercalcemic cancer patients. *Journal of Bone & Mineral Research.* **14**(9): 1557–61. (MC, CT-33)

60 Zojer N, Keck AV, Pecherstorfer M (1999) Comparative tolerability of drug therapies for hypercalcemia of malignancy. *Drug Safety.* **21**(5): 389–406. (R, 109 refs)

61 Wimalawansa SJ (1994) Optimal frequency of administration of pamidronate in patients with hypercalcemia of malignancy. *Clinical Endocrinology.* **41**: 591–5. (RCT-34)

62 Cryer PE (2001) Hypoglycemia risk reduction in type 1 diabetes. *Experimental & Clinical Endocrinology & Diabetes.* **109** (Suppl 2): S412–23. (R, 67)

63 Poulson J (1997) The management of diabetes in patients with advanced cancer. *Journal of Pain and Symptom Management.* **13**: 339–46. (R, 26 refs)

64 Bower M, Brazil L, Coombes RC (1997) Endocrine and metabolic complications of advanced cancer. In: D Doyle, GWC Hanks, N MacDonald (eds) *The Oxford Textbook of Palliative Medicine* (2e). Oxford Medical Publications, Oxford. pp. 709–25. (Ch)

65 Flombaum CD (2000) Metabolic emergencies in the cancer patient. *Seminars in Oncology.* **27**(3): 322–34. (R, 110 refs)

66 Ferlito A, Rinaldo A, Devaney KO (1997) Syndrome of inappropriate antidiuretic hormone secretion associated with head neck cancers: review of the literature. *Annals of Otology, Rhinology & Laryngology.* **106**(10 Pt 1): 878–83. (R, 30 refs)

67 Woo MH, Smythe MA (1997) Association of SIADH with selective serotonin reuptake inhibitors. *Annals of Pharmacotherapy.* **31**(1): 108–10. (R, 32 refs)

68 Chan TY (1997) Drug-induced syndrome of inappropriate antidiuretic hormone secretion. Causes, diagnosis and management. *Drugs & Aging.* **11**(1): 27–44. (R, 211 refs)

69 Crosby V, Wilcock A, Lawson N, Corcoran R (2000) The importance of low magnesium in palliative care. *Palliative Medicine.* **14**(6): 544. (Let, C)

70 D'Erasmo E, Celi FS, Acca M, Minisola S, Aliberti G, Mazzuoli GF (1991) Hypocalcemia and hypomagnesemia in cancer patients. *Biomedicine & Pharmacotherapy*. **45**(7): 315–17. (OS-61)

71 Lajer H, Daugaard G (1999) Cisplatin and hypomagnesemia. *Cancer Treatment Reviews*. **25**(1): 47–58. (R, 74 refs)

72 Rivlin RS (1994) Magnesium deficiency and alcohol intake: mechanisms, clinical significance and possible relation to cancer development (a review). *Journal of the American College of Nutrition*. **13**(5): 416–23. (R, 48 refs)

73 Martin M, Diaz-Rubio E, Casado A, Lopez Vega JM, Sastre J, Almenarez J (1992) Intravenous and oral magnesium supplementations in the prophylaxis of cisplatin-induced hypomagnesemia. Results of a controlled trial. *American Journal of Clinical Oncology*. **15**(4): 348–51. (RCT-41)

74 Kaplow R (2002) Pathophysiology, signs, and symptoms of acute tumor lysis syndrome. *Seminars in Oncology Nursing*. **18**(3 Suppl 3): 6–11. (R, 7 refs)

75 Doane L (2002) Overview of tumor lysis syndrome. *Seminars in Oncology Nursing*. **18**(3 Suppl 3): 2–5. (R, 19 refs)

76 Iqbal SJ, Giles M, Ledger S, Nanji N, Howl T (1988) Need for albumin adjustments of urgent total serum calcium. *Lancet*. **ii**: 1477. (OS)

77 Bower M, Brazil L, Coombes RC (1997) Endocrine and metabolic complications of advanced cancer. In: D Doyle, GWC Hanks, N MacDonald (eds) *The Oxford Textbook of Palliative Medicine* (2e). Oxford Medical Publications, Oxford. pp. 709–25. (Ch)

78 Stewart C (2001) Disseminated intravascular coagulation (DIC). *Australian Critical Care*. **14**(2): 71–5. (R, 14 refs)

79 Maxson JH (2000) Management of disseminated intravascular coagulation. *Critical Care Nursing Clinics of North America*. **12**(3): 341–52. (R, 14 refs)

80 Horan JT, Francis CW (2001) Fibrin degradation products, fibrin monomer and soluble fibrin in disseminated intravascular coagulation. *Seminars in Thrombosis & Hemostasis*. **27**(6): 657–66. (R, 58 refs)

81 ten Wolde M, Kraaijenhagen RA, Prins MH, Buller HR (2002) The clinical usefulness of D-dimer testing in cancer patients with suspected deep venous thrombosis. *Archives of Internal Medicine*. **162**(16): 1880–4. (OS-1739)

82 Bick RL, Arun B, Frenkel EP (1999) Disseminated intravascular coagulation. Clinical and pathophysiological mechanisms and manifestations. *Haemostasis*. **29**(2–3): 111–34. (R, 179 refs)

83 Hofmann M, Rest A, Hafner G, Tanner B, Brockerhoff P, Weilemann LS (1997) D-dimer, thrombin-antithrombin III-complex (TAT) and prothrombin fragment 1+2 (PTF). Parameters for monitoring therapy with low molecular-weight heparin in coagulation disorders. *Anaesthesist*. **46**(8): 689–96. (RCT-30)

84 Reinhart WH, Lutolf O, Nydegger UR, Mahler F, Straub PW (1992) Plasmapheresis for hyperviscosity syndrome in macroglobulinemia Waldenstrom and multiple myeloma: influence on blood rheology and the microcirculation. *Journal of Laboratory & Clinical Medicine*. **119**(1): 69–76. (OS-22)

85 Price CGA, Price P (1995) Acute emergencies in oncology. In: *Oxford Textbook of Oncology on CD-ROM*. Oxford University Press and Optimedia Ltd, Oxford. (Ch)

86 Castagnola E, Paola D, Giacchino R, Viscoli C (2000) Clinical and laboratory features predicting a favorable outcome and allowing early discharge in cancer patients with low-risk febrile neutropenia: a literature review. *Journal of Hematotherapy & Stem Cell Research*. **9**(5): 645–9. (R, 35 refs)

87 Orudjev E, Lange BJ (2002) Evolving concepts of management of febrile neutropenia in children with cancer. *Medical & Pediatric Oncology*. **39**(2): 77–85. (SA, 51 refs)

88 Bodey GP, Rolston KV (2001) Management of fever in neutropenic patients. *Journal of Infection & Chemotherapy*. **7**(1): 1–9. (R, 77 refs)

89 Husband DJ (1998) Malignant spinal cord compression: prospective study of delays in referral and treatment. *BMJ*. **317**(7150): 18–21. (OS-301)

90 Ingham J, Beveridge A, Cooney NJ (1993) The management of spinal cord compression in patients with advanced malignancy. *Journal of Pain and Symptom Management*. **8**(1): 1–6. (RS-17)

91 Jameson RM (1974) Prolonged survival in paraplegia due to metastatic spinal tumours. *Lancet*. **i**: 1209–11.

92 Solberg A, Bremnes RM (1999) Metastatic spinal cord compression: diagnostic delay, treatment, and outcome. *Anticancer Research*. **19**(1B): 677–84. (OS-86)

93 Kramer JA (1992) Spinal cord compression in malignancy. *Palliative Medicine*. **6**: 202–11.

94 Levack P, Graham J, Collie D, Grant R, Kidd J, Kinler I, Gibson A, Hurman D, McMillan N, Rampling R, Slider L, Statham P, Summers D (2002) The Scottish Cord Compression Study Group. Don't wait for a sensory level – listen to the symptoms: a prospective audit of the delays in diagnosis of malignant cord compression. *Clinical Oncology*. **14**: 472–80. (OS-319)

95 Rades D, Heidenreich F, Karstens JH (2002) Final results of a prospective study of the prognostic value of the time to develop motor deficits before irradiation in metastatic spinal cord compression. *International Journal of Radiation Oncology, Biology, Physics.* **53**(4): 975–9. (CT-98)

96 Rades D, Blach M, Nerreter V, Bremer M, Karstens JH (1999) Metastatic spinal cord compression. Influence of time between onset of motoric deficits and start of irradiation on therapeutic effect. *Strahlentherapie und Onkologie.* **175**(8): 378–81. (OS-96)

97 Rankine JJ, Gill KP, Hutchinson CE, Ross ER, Williamson JB (1998) The therapeutic impact of lumbar spine MRI on patients with low back and leg pain. *Clinical Radiology.* **53**(9): 688–93. (CT-72)

98 Loblaw DA, Laperriere NJ (1998) Emergency treatment of malignant extradural spinal cord compression: an evidence-based guideline. *Journal of Clinical Oncology.* **16**(4): 1613–24. (SA, 52 refs)

99 Friedman HM, Sheetz S, Levine HL, Everett JR, Hong WK (1986) Combination chemotherapy and radiation therapy. The medical management of epidural spinal cord compression from testicular cancer. *Archives of Internal Medicine.* **146**(3): 509–12. (CS-2)

100 Falk S, Fallon M (1997) ABC of palliative care. Emergencies. *BMJ.* **315**(7121): 1525–8. (R)

101 Davey P (2002) Brain metastases: treatment options to improve outcomes. *CNS Drugs.* **16**(5): 325–38. (R, 102 refs)

102 Grossi F, Scolaro T, Tixi L, Loprevite M, Ardizzoni A (2001) The role of systemic chemotherapy in the treatment of brain metastases from small-cell lung cancer. *Critical Reviews in Oncology-Hematology.* **37**(1): 61–7. (R, 44 refs)

103 Donato V, Bonfili P, Bulzonetti N, Santarelli M, Osti MF, Tombolini V, Banelli E, Enrici RM (2001) Radiation therapy for oncological emergencies. *Anticancer Research.* **21**(3C): 2219–24. (OS-43)

104 Rowell NP, Gleeson FV (2001) Steroids, radiotherapy, chemotherapy and stents for superior vena caval obstruction in carcinoma of the bronchus. *Cochrane Database of Systematic Reviews.* **4**: CD001316. (SA, 99 refs)

105 Fletcher WS, Lakin PC, Pommier RF, Wilmarth T (1998) Results of treatment of inferior vena cava syndrome with expandable metallic stents. *Archives of Surgery.* **133**(9): 935–8. (RS-28)

106 Paterson J, Rimmer T, Bowker A, Renwick I (1996) Stenting for inferior caval obstruction. *Palliative Medicine.* **10**(4): 344–5. (Let, CS)

107 De Leeuw R, Cuttini M, Nadai M, Berbik I, Hansen G, Kucinskas A, Lenoir S, Levin A, Persson J, Rebagliato M, Reid M, Schroell M, De Vonderweid U, De Beaufort I, Garel M, Hills M, Kaminski M, Lenard HG, McHaffie HE, Orzalesi M, Saracci R (2000) Treatment choices for extremely preterm infants: An international perspective. *Journal of Pediatrics.* **137**(5): 608–15. (Q-4826)

108 Mezey M, Kluger M, Maislin G, Mittelman M (1996) Life-sustaining treatment decisions by spouses of patients with Alzheimer's disease. *Journal of the American Geriatrics Society.* **44**(2): 144–50. (I-50)

109 Sykes N, Thorns A (2003) Sedative use in the last week of life and the implications for end-of-life decision making. *Archives of Internal Medicine.* **163**: 341–4.

110 Sykes N, Thorns A (2003) The use of opioids and sedatives at the end of life. *Lancet Oncology.* **4**: 312–18.

111 Anwar D, Schaad N, Mazzorato C (2003) Treatment of hemoptysis in palliative care patients. *European Journal of Palliative Care.* **10**(4): 137–9. (R, 26 refs)

112 Neville-Webbe HL, Coleman RE (2003) The use of zoledronic acid in the management of metastatic bone disease and hypercalcemia. *Palliative Medicine.* **17**: 539–53. (R, 61 refs)

113 Mannix K, Ahmedzai SH, Anderson H *et al.* (2000) Using bisphosphonates to control the pain of bone metastases: evidence-based guidelines for palliative care. *Palliative Medicine.* **14**: 456–61.

114 Ettinger AB, Portenoy K (1988) *Pain Symptom Management.* **3**(2): 99–103.

115 Vecht CJ *et al.* (1989) Initial bolus of conventional versus high-dose dexamethasone in metastatic spinal cord compression. *Neurology.* **39**(9): 1255–7.

116 Heimdal K *et al.* (1992) High incidence of serious side effects of high-dose dexamethasone treatment in patients with epidural spinal cord compression. *Journal of Neuro-Oncology.* **12**(2): 141–4.

Drug information

- Drug interactions

- Drugs in palliative care for children: starting doses

- Using drugs off-label

- Alternative routes for drugs

- Problems with syringe pump infusions

Advice on children jointly written with Susie Lapwood

Drug interactions written with advice from Carmel Copeland

Information for enteral feed interactions from
Sarah Charlesworth, *Palliative Care Formulary*

For current drug information *see*
www.palliativedrugs.com for palliative care drugs
and www.bnf.org is a useful site for drug information
but is oriented to the UK

Key points

- Many patients with advanced disease are on multiple medications.
- Potential drug interactions are common.
- Children tolerate some drugs very differently from adults and there is considerable variability between individuals.
- Many drugs can be given by a variety of non-oral routes.
- In the US and Canada, drugs can be prescribed for off-label uses and routes, but basic rules about reducing risk apply.

Important note to readers

While all drugs and formulations listed in this section are available in either Canada or the United States, readers are urged to check their availability in their respective countries.

In the US some medications such as domperidone and methotrimeprazine are not easily available via a regular pharmacy but may be available via compounding pharmacies. To obtain more information regarding compounding pharmacies in the US, including locations, you may contact the Professional Compounding Pharmacy Center of America at 1 800 331 2498.

Drug interactions

- *Interactions are more likely to be a problem:*
  - with the following drug groups: antacids, antibiotics, anticoagulants, antidepressants, antidiabetics, anticonvulsants, antifungals, cardiac drugs, corticosteroids, diuretics, NSAIDs and ulcer healing drugs
  - with the following drugs (in descending order of number of likely interactions): carbamazepine, warfarin, diltiazem, verapamil, furosemide, cimetidine, methotrimeprazine, itraconazole, ketoconazole, amiodarone, dexamethasone, prednisolone and erythromycin
  - in drugs with a narrow margin between therapeutic and toxic doses, e.g. digoxin
  - when an interacting drug is started or stopped.
- *If drugs have to be used together that could interact, the risk of an adverse reaction can be minimized by:*
  - keeping doses low (many interactions are dose-related)
  - monitoring more closely for the potential interaction, e.g. more frequent serum potassium checks for furosemide-dexamethasone interaction
  - taking action to prevent the adverse effect, e.g. using a proton pump inhibitor to prevent gastrointestinal mucosal damage caused by an NSAID-steroid interaction.
- *In the US, MedWatch is the FDA (Food and Drug Administration) safety information and adverse effect program.* Any suspected drug interactions can be reported by telephone to 1-800-FDA-1088, or via www.fda.gov/medwatch/.
- *In Canada, any suspected drug interactions can be reported to Health Canada* (by telephone (toll free 866 234 2345); by fax (toll free 866 678 6789); or by e-mail (cadrmp@hc-sc.gc.ca)).

Instructions for use of drug interaction tables

1 Drugs are listed alphabetically in 20 classes:

2 Find the interacting drug.

Continued overleaf

3 Check the likely importance of the interaction (based on the UK eBNF (www.bnf.org)):
   ▲ = interaction potentially hazardous. Combination should be avoided (or only undertaken with caution and appropriate monitoring).
   ⓘ = interaction possible, but not usually serious. Caution needed.
4 Read the effect of the interaction.
5 Read the necessary action.

Important note: This is a list that is restricted to drugs that may be used in palliative care. If any interacting drugs are not on this list they must be checked in a complete list of interactions.

A useful and ready source for up-to-date interaction information on many drugs is the *British National Formulary* website at www.bnf.org. (Not all drugs listed are available in Canada and the US, and some available in Canada and the US may not be listed.)

Drug	Interacting drug and importance of interaction	Effect of interaction	Action
ACE inhibitors			
All	ⓘ antidiabetics	↓ blood glucose	Monitor blood glucose more frequently
	ⓘ antacids	↓ absorption of ACE inhibitor	Take at least 2 hours apart
	ⓘ benzodiazepines ⓘ baclofen ⓘ β-blockers ⓘ calcium channel blockers ⓘ clonidine ⓘ nitrates ⓘ phenothiazines	Enhanced hypotensive effect with any of these interacting drugs	Monitor BP more frequently
	▲ cyclosporin ▲ diuretics – K⁺ sparing ▲ ketorolac ▲ potassium salts, ▲ high K⁺ foods	Risk of hyperkalemia with any of these interacting drugs	Avoid combination
	ⓘ corticosteroids, NSAIDs	Antagonism of hypotensive effect	Monitor BP more frequently
	ⓘ NSAIDs	Increased risk of renal impairment	Monitor renal function more frequently
	▲ diuretics – any	Risk of severe hypotension on first starting	Use only under specialist advice
	ⓘ erythropoietin	Antagonism of hypotension and risk of hyperkalemia	Monitor BP and electrolytes more frequently
	ⓘ heparins	Risk of hyperkalemia	Monitor electrolytes more frequently
Analgesics			
acetaminophen	ⓘ cholestyramine	↓ acetaminophen effect (↓ absorption)	Take at least 2 hours apart
	ⓘ domperidone (available in US from a compounding pharmacy) ⓘ metoclopramide	↑ acetaminophen effect with either of these interacting drugs	Take at least 2 hours apart

Table continued overleaf

Drug	Interacting drug and importance of interaction	Effect of interaction	Action
acetaminophen – cont.	ⓘ warfarin	Possible ↑ warfarin effect	Monitor INR more frequently
alfentanil	ⓘ erythromycin ⓘ ketoconazole	↑ alfentanil plasma level	Observe for opioid side effects
aspirin	ⓘ antacids	↓ plasma aspirin level (↑ excretion)	Take at least 2 hours apart
	ⓘ corticosteroids	Increased risk of GI ulceration and bleeding ↓ plasma aspirin level may also occur	Avoid or use PPI to protect stomach
	▲ heparin, warfarin ⓘ SSRI antidepressants	↑ risk of bleeding	Avoid combination
	▲ hypoglycemic drugs	↓ blood glucose levels	Avoid or monitor blood glucose more frequently
	▲ NSAIDs	Increased side effects especially risk of bronchospasm in asthmatics	Avoid combination
	ⓘ phenytoin	↑ phenytoin effect	Monitor for side effects and phenytoin levels
	ⓘ spironolactone	↓ diuretic effect	Increase spironolactone if necessary
	ⓘ valproate	↑ valproate effect	Monitor for valproate side effects
celecoxib	ⓘ fluconazole	↑ plasma level of celecoxib	Halve celecoxib dose
dextropropoxyphene	▲ carbamazepine	↑ carbamazepine effect	Avoid combination – use valproate instead
	▲ warfarin	↑ warfarin effect	Avoid combination – use other opioids
ketamine	ⓘ theophylline	Increased risk of convulsions	Avoid combination

Drug	Interacting drug and importance of interaction	Effect of interaction	Action
meperidine	ⓘ cimetidine	↑ meperidine plasma level	Observe for opioid side effects
methadone	ⓘ carbamazepine ⓘ ciprofloxacin ⓘ phenytoin	↓ methadone effect	Observe for increased pain
	ⓘ desipramine	↑ plasma level of desipramine	Observe for desipramine adverse effects
	ⓘ fluvoxamine ⓘ sertraline	May ↑ plasma level of methadone	Observe for opioid adverse effects
morphine	ⓘ esmolol	↑ plasma level of esmolol	Observe for beta-blocker adverse effects
	ⓘ amitriptyline ⓘ chlorpromazine ⓘ doxepin ⓘ haloperidol	↑ risk of myoclonus	Observe for myoclonic jerks. Consider switching to alternative opioid
NSAIDs	ⓘ ACE inhibitors	Increased risk of renal damage	Monitor electrolytes and blood pressure more frequently
	▲ aspirin	Increased side effects	Avoid combination
	ⓘ baclofen	Possible ↑ plasma level of baclofen	Observe for baclofen adverse effects
	▲ digoxin	↑ plasma level of digoxin, risk of renal impairment	Avoid combination
	ⓘ corticosteroids	Increased risk of GI ulceration and bleeding	Avoid or use PPI to protect stomach
	ⓘ diuretics – loop and thiazide	↓ diuretic effect, risk of renal damage	Monitor electrolytes more frequently
	ⓘ diuretics – potassium sparing	Increased risk of hyperkalemia	Monitor electrolytes more frequently
	▲ heparin, warfarin	Possible ↑ risk of bleeding	Monitor INR more frequently
	ⓘ lithium	↑ lithium serum levels	Increase monitoring of lithium levels
	▲ phenytoin	↑ phenytoin effect	Monitor for side effects and phenytoin levels
	▲ sulphonylureas	↓ blood glucose	Avoid combination

Table continued overleaf

Drug	Interacting drug and importance of interaction	Effect of interaction	Action
Opioids – all	ⓘ cimetidine	↑ plasma level of some opioids	Use ranitidine instead of cimetidine
	ⓘ domperidone ⓘ metoclopramide	Reduced effect of interacting drug on GI motility	Consider using higher domperidone or metoclopramide dose
tramadol (not currently available in Canada)	▲ anticonvulsants	Increased risk of seizures	Avoid combination
	▲ antidepressants – all	Increased risk of CNS toxicity	Avoid – use alternative weak opioid
	ⓘ antipsychotics	Increased risk of convulsions	Change to alternative weak opioid
	ⓘ carbamazepine	↓ tramadol effect	Observe for increased pain
	ⓘ digoxin	Reports of digoxin toxicity	Check digoxin levels
	▲ warfarin	May increase warfarin effect	Check INR more frequently
Antacids			
All	ⓘ ACE inhibitors ⓘ bisphosphonates ⓘ cefaclor ⓘ cefpodoxime ⓘ ciprofloxacin ⓘ digoxin ⓘ gabapentin ⓘ itraconazole ⓘ iron ⓘ ketoconazole ⓘ lansoprazole ⓘ methotrimeprazine ⓘ olanzapine ⓘ phenytoin ⓘ tetracycline	↓ absorption of any of these drugs	Take at least 2 hours apart
	ⓘ enteral feeds	Coagulate with feeds	Dilute with 60 ml water and flush well
	ⓘ aspirin	↓ effect of aspirin (↑ excretion)	Take at least 2 hours apart
	ⓘ sucralfate	↓ effectiveness of sucralfate	Take at least 2 hours apart

Anti-arrhythmics

All	▲ other anti-arrhythmics	Risk of myocardial depression	Avoid combination
	▲ antipsychotics	Risk of ventricular arrhythmias	Avoid combination
	ⓘ bupivacaine	Increased myocardial depression	Avoid combination
amiodarone *NB: very long half-life – interactions may occur weeks or months after stopping*	▲ TC antidepressants ▲ haloperidol ▲ erythromycin (IV, IM) ▲ methotrimeprazine ▲ trimethoprim	Risk of ventricular arrhythmias with any of these interacting drugs	Avoid combination
	▲ β-blockers ▲ verapamil	Risk of bradycardia, AV block and myocardial depression	Avoid combination
	ⓘ cimetidine	↑ plasma level of amiodarone	Monitor for amiodarone adverse effects
	ⓘ lithium	May cause hypothyroidism	Monitor thyroid function
	▲ digoxin ▲ phenytoin ▲ warfarin	↑ plasma level of these interacting drugs	Avoid combination
disopyramide	▲ antidepressants ▲ TC antidepressants ▲ methotrimeprazine ▲ ritonavir ▲ sotalol ▲ verapamil	Risk of ventricular arrhythmias with any of these interacting drugs	Avoid combination
	ⓘ antimuscarinics	Increased antimuscarinic effects	Observe for drowsiness, dry mouth, confusion, blurred vision. Avoid combination or reduce doses
	▲ clarithromycin ▲ erythromycin	↑ plasma level of disopyramide	Avoid combination
	▲ diuretics	Cardiac toxicity if hypokalemia occurs	Avoid combination
	ⓘ phenytoin ⓘ phenobarbital	↓ plasma level of disopyramide	Reduce disopyramide dose or change to valproate

Table continued overleaf

Drug	Interacting drug and importance of interaction	Effect of interaction	Action
flecainide	▲ TC antidepressants	Risk of ventricular arrhythmias	Avoid combination
	▲ β-blockers	Risk of bradycardia and myocardial depression	Avoid combination
	ⓘ cimetidine ⓘ fluoxetine	↑ plasma level of flecainide with either of these interacting drugs	Avoid combination or change to ranitidine or alternative SSRI
	▲ diuretics	Cardiac toxicity if hypokalemia occurs	Avoid combination
	▲ verapamil	Risk of asystole	Avoid combination
mexiletine	▲ diuretics	Cardiac toxicity if hypokalemia occurs	Avoid combination
	ⓘ phenytoin	↓ plasma level of mexiletine	May need to increase mexiletine dose
propanolol	▲ bupivacaine	Increased risk of bupivacaine toxicity	Avoid combination
	ⓘ cimetidine	↑ plasma level of propranolol	Use ranitidine instead of cimetidine
	ⓘ muscle relaxants	Increased muscle relaxation	Observe mobility and tone
Antibiotics			
amoxicillin	ⓘ allopurinol	↑ risk of rash	Change to cephalosporin if rash occurs
	▲ warfarin	May alter effect of warfarin	Monitor INR more frequently
cephalosporins	ⓘ bumetanide ⓘ furosemide	↑ risk of renal damage with either of these interacting drugs	Avoid combination in presence of renal impairment
	▲ warfarin	Possible ↑ warfarin effect with some cephalosporins	Monitor INR more frequently
cefaclor	ⓘ antacids	↓ absorption of cefaclor	Take at least 2 hours apart

Drug	Interacting drug and importance of interaction	Effect of interaction	Action
cefpodoxime	ⓘ antacids	↓ absorption of cefpodoxime	Take at least 2 hours apart
	ⓘ cimetidine ⓘ ranitidine	↓ absorption of cefaclor	Avoid or increase cefpodoxime dose
ciprofloxacin	ⓘ antacids ⓘ enteral feeds ⓘ oral iron ⓘ sucralfate	↓ absorption of ciprofloxacin	Take at least 2 hours apart
	ⓘ methadone	↑ plasma level of methadone	Observe for opioid adverse effects
	▲ warfarin	Possible ↑ warfarin effect	Monitor INR more frequently
clarithromycin	▲ carbamazepine ⓘ digoxin ⓘ itraconazole ⓘ methylprednisolone ▲ midazolam ⓘ omeprazole ▲ phenytoin ▲ warfarin	↑ plasma level of any of these interacting drugs	ⓘ Observe for adverse effects of interacting drug ▲ Avoid combination
co-trimoxazole	▲ amiodarone	Risk of ventricular arrhythmia	Avoid combination
	ⓘ thiazides ⓘ loop diuretics	Risk of severe hyponatremia	Check serum electrolytes more frequently
	▲ phenytoin ▲ warfarin	↑ plasma level of either of these interacting drugs	Avoid combination
doxycycline	ⓘ carbamazepine ⓘ phenytoin	↓ doxycycline plasma level with either of these interacting drugs	Use alternative tetracycline or increase doxycycline dose
erythromycin	▲ amiodarone	Risk of ventricular arrhythmia with parenteral erythromycin	Avoid combination

Table continued overleaf

Drug	Interacting drug and importance of interaction	Effect of interaction	Action
erythromycin – cont.	(i) alfentanil/fentanyl (i) buspirone ▲ carbamazepine (i) corticosteroids (i) digoxin ▲ disopyramide (i) felodipine ▲ midazolam (i) omeprazole (i) valproate ▲ warfarin (i) zopiclone (Canada only)	↑ plasma level of any of these interacting drugs	(i) Observe for adverse effects of interacting drug ▲ Avoid combination
	(i) cimetidine	↑ erythromycin plasma level	Observe for erythromycin toxicity, e.g. deafness
flucloxacillin (Canada) **oxacillin** (US)	(i) enteral feeds	↓ absorption of flucloxacillin	Stop feed for 1 hour before to 2 hours after drug
metronidazole	▲ phenytoin ▲ warfarin	↑ plasma level of any of these interacting drugs	(i) Observe for adverse effects of interacting drug ▲ Avoid combination
	(i) cimetidine	↑ plasma level of metronidazole	Observe for metronidazole adverse effects
	▲ phenytoin	antifolate effect	Avoid combination
tetracycline	(i) antacids (i) enteral feeds	↓ absorption of tetracycline	Stop feed for 1 hour before to 2 hours after drug
	▲ warfarin	Possible increased anticoagulation	Monitor INR more frequently
trimethoprim	(i) digoxin (i) sulphonylureas (i) warfarin	Possible ↑ plasma level of any of these interacting drugs	Observe for adverse effects of interacting drug
	▲ amiodarone	Risk of ventricular arrhythmia	Avoid combination
	▲ phenytoin	Antifolate effect	Avoid combination
Anticoagulants			
All	▲ allopurinol	Unpredictable risk of hypothrombinemia and bleeding	Monitor INR and platelets more frequently

Drug	Interacting drug and importance of interaction	Effect of interaction	Action
All – cont.	(i) aspirin	↑ anticoagulant effect	Check clotting more frequently
heparin	(i) ACE inhibitors	↑ risk of hyperkalemia	Check electrolytes more frequently
	▲ ketorolac	↑ risk of bleeding	Avoid combination
	(i) NSAIDs	Possible risk of bleeding	Cover with PPI
warfarin	▲ barbiturates ▲ carbamazepine ▲ St John's Wort ▲ sucralfate	↓ warfarin effect with any of these interacting drugs	Avoid combination
	▲ enteral feeds	↓ absorption of warfarin	Monitor INR more frequently
	▲ amiodarone ▲ celecoxib ▲ cephalosporins ▲ cimetidine ▲ ciprofloxacin ▲ clarithromycin ▲ co-trimoxazole ▲ cranberry juice ▲ erythromycin ▲ fluconazole ▲ ketoconazole ▲ metronidazole ▲ miconazole ▲ tetracyclines	↑ warfarin effect with any of these interacting drugs	Avoid combination or monitor INR frequently
	▲ acetaminophen (i) ampicillin (i) antidepressants ▲ corticosteroids ▲ dextropropoxyphene ▲ diclofenac ▲ flurbiprofen ▲ ibuprofen ▲ methylphenidate ▲ omeprazole (i) trimethoprim (i) valproate ▲ venlafaxine	Possible ↑ warfarin effect with any of these interacting drugs	Monitor INR more frequently

Table continued overleaf

Drug	Interacting drug and importance of interaction	Effect of interaction	Action
warfarin – cont.	▲ phenytoin	Altered coagulation	Monitor INR more frequently
	▲ sulphonylureas	↓ glucose and altered coagulation	Avoid combination
Anticonvulsants			
All	▲ antidepressants ▲ antipsychotics	Increased risk of seizure	Avoid combination if seizures are a risk
carbamazepine	ⓘ tramadol (not currently available in Canada) ⓘ alcohol	Possible increased carbamazepine adverse effects	Avoid combination or use valproate
	ⓘ clonazepam ▲ corticosteroids ⓘ doxycycline ⓘ haloperidol ▲ lamotrigine ▲ methadone ⓘ olanzapine ⓘ paroxetine ⓘ phenytoin ⓘ risperidone ▲ TC antidepressants ⓘ valproate ▲ warfarin	↓ plasma level of any of these interacting drugs	ⓘ Observe for loss of effectiveness of interacting drug ▲ Avoid combination and use valproate
	▲ cimetidine ▲ clarithromycin ▲ dextroprop-oxyphene ▲ diltiazem ▲ erythromycin ⓘ fluconazole ⓘ ketoconazole ▲ fluoxetine ▲ fluvoxamine ⓘ haloperidol ⓘ lamotrigine ▲ verapamil	Increased effect of carbamazepine with any of these interacting drugs	ⓘ Observe for carbamazepine adverse effects ▲ Avoid combination – use valproate
	▲ St John's Wort ⓘ phenobarbital ⓘ phenytoin	↓ plasma level of carbamazepine with any of these interacting drugs	Observe for loss of effectiveness of carbamazepine or avoid combination – use valproate
	ⓘ diuretics	Risk of hyponatremia	Monitor electrolytes more frequently

Drug	Interacting drug and importance of interaction	Effect of interaction	Action
gabapentin	ⓘ antacids	↓ absorption of gabapentin	Take at least 2 hours apart
phenobarbital	ⓘ carbamazepine ⓘ clonazepam ⓘ ethosuximide ⓘ haloperidol ⓘ lamotrigine ⓘ paroxetine ⓘ phenytoin ⓘ valproate	↓ plasma level of any of these interacting drugs	Observe for loss of effect of interacting drug
	▲ St John's Wort	↓ plasma level of phenobarbital with this interacting drug	ⓘ Observe for loss of phenobarbital effect ▲ Avoid combination
	ⓘ methylphenidate ⓘ phenytoin ⓘ valproate	↑ plasma level of phenobarbital with these interacting drugs	Observe for phenobarbital adverse effects
phenytoin	▲ amiodarone ⓘ antacids ⓘ carbamazepine ⓘ clonazepam ▲ corticosteroids ⓘ digoxin ⓘ haloperidol ▲ itraconazole ▲ ketoconazole ⓘ lamotrigine ⓘ methadone ▲ nifedipine ⓘ paroxetine ▲ TC antidepressants ⓘ valproate ⓘ verapamil ▲ warfarin	↓ plasma level of interacting drug	ⓘ Observe for loss of effect of interacting drug ▲ Avoid combination
	ⓘ carbamazepine ▲ St John's Wort ▲ sucralfate	↓ plasma level of phenytoin	ⓘ Observe for loss of phenytoin effect ▲ Avoid combination

Table continued overleaf

Drug	Interacting drug and importance of interaction	Effect of interaction	Action
phenytoin – cont.	▲ amiodarone ⓘ aspirin ▲ cimetidine ⓘ clarithromycin ▲ esomeprazole ▲ fluconazole ▲ fluoxetine ▲ metronidazole ▲ miconazole ▲ nifedipine ▲ NSAIDs ⓘ omeprazole ⓘ sulphonamides ⓘ tolbutamide ⓘ valproate	↑ plasma level of phenytoin	ⓘ Observe for phenytoin toxicity ▲ Avoid combination
	ⓘ lithium	Risk of neurotoxicity	Observe for neurotoxicity
primidone	ⓘ phenytoin ▲ St John's Wort ⓘ tiagabine	↓ plasma level of any of these interacting drugs	Observe for loss of effect of interacting drug
valproate	▲ antipsychotics	Increased risk of seizures	Avoid combination if seizures are a risk
	ⓘ cholestyramine	↓ absorption of valproate	Take at least 2 hours apart
	ⓘ amitriptyline ⓘ diazepam ⓘ lorazepam	Altered plasma level of interacting drug	Observe for altered effect of interacting drug
	ⓘ aspirin ▲ cimetidine ⓘ erythromycin	↑ plasma level of valproate with any of these interacting drugs	Observe for valproate side effects
	▲ olanzapine	Increased risk of neutropenia	Avoid combination
	ⓘ warfarin	↑ anticoagulation	Monitor INR more frequently
Antidepressants			
Any tricyclic	▲ antiarrhythmics ▲ antipsychotics	Increased risk of ventricular arrhythmia with either of these interacting drugs	Avoid combination

Drug	Interacting drug and importance of interaction	Effect of interaction	Action
Any tricyclic – cont.	▲ anticonvulsants	Increased risk of seizure	Avoid combination
	▲ anticonvulsants ▲ antipsychotics ⓘ cimetidine ⓘ methylphenidate ▲ SSRI antidepressants	↑ plasma level of TC antidepressants with any of these interacting drugs	ⓘ Observe for TC antidepressants adverse effects ▲ Avoid combination
	▲ carbamazepine	↓ plasma level of TC antidepressant	▲ Avoid combination
	ⓘ baclofen	↑ muscle relaxant effect	Observe for hypotonicity
	ⓘ hyoscine ⓘ methotrimeprazine	↑ muscarinic side effects with any of these interacting drugs	Observe for dyskinesia, drowsiness, dry mouth, confusion, blurred vision
	ⓘ diuretics	Hypotension	Observe for dizziness on standing, check BP
	ⓘ high dietary fiber	↓ absorption of TC antidepressants	Observe for loss of antidepressant effect
	ⓘ tramadol	Risk of CNS toxicity	Avoid combination
amitriptyline	ⓘ morphine	↑ risk of myoclonus	Observe for myoclonic jerks. Consider changing to alternative opioid
	ⓘ cimetidine	↑ plasma level of amitriptyline	Observe for amitriptyline adverse effects
Any SSRI	ⓘ anticonvulsants	Increased risk of seizures	Avoid combination
	ⓘ methylphenidate	Possible ↑ plasma level of SSRI	Observe for SSRI adverse effects
	▲ St John's Wort	Increased serotonergic symptoms	Avoid combination

Table continued overleaf

Drug	Interacting drug and importance of interaction	Effect of interaction	Action
Any SSRI – cont.	ⓘ TC antidepressants	↑ plasma level of TC antidepressants	Observe for adverse effects of TC antidepressants
	ⓘ tramadol	Risk of CNS toxicity	Avoid, combination
	▲ warfarin	Possible increased effect of warfarin	Avoid, or check INR more frequently
fluoxetine *NB: very long half-life means that fluoxetine effects may last for weeks*	▲ carbamazepine ▲ haloperidol ⓘ nifedipine ▲ phenytoin ⓘ verapamil	↑ plasma level of any of these interacting drugs	▲ Avoid combination ⓘ Observe for adverse effects of interacting drug
sertraline	ⓘ cimetidine	↑ plasma level of sertraline	Reduce sertraline dose or use ranitidine
	▲ methadone	↑ plasma level of methadone	Avoid combination
venlafaxine	ⓘ haloperidol	↑ plasma level of haloperidol	Observe for haloperidol adverse effects
Antidiabetics			
Any antidiabetic	ⓘ ACE inhibitors ⓘ alcohol ⓘ octreotide ⓘ salicylates	↓ glucose level with any of these interacting drugs	Monitor blood glucose more frequently
	ⓘ corticosteroids ⓘ diuretics	↑ glucose level with any of these interacting drugs	Monitor blood glucose more frequently
chlorpropramide (also see sulphonylureas)	ⓘ alcohol	Flushing	No action unless distressing
	ⓘ thiazide with spironolactone	Risk of hyponatremia	Check electrolytes more frequently
glibenclamide (also see sulphonylureas)	ⓘ ciprofloxacin ⓘ miconazole	↓ glucose level	Monitor blood glucose more frequently. Reduce antidiabetic dose if necessary
gliclazide (Canada) **glipizide** (US)	▲ miconazole (topical)	↓ glucose level	Use alternative antifungal
metformin	ⓘ ACE inhibitors	Possible ↓ glucose level	Monitor blood glucose more frequently

Drug	Interacting drug and importance of interaction	Effect of interaction	Action
metformin – cont.	ⓘ alcohol	Increased risk of lactic acidosis	Monitor blood glucose more frequently
	ⓘ cimetidine	↓ glucose level due to reduced excretion of metformin	Use ranitidine instead of cimetidine
	ⓘ octreotide	Possible ↑ metformin effect	Monitor blood glucose more frequently
sulphonylureas (these include: – chlorpropamide – glibenclamide – gliclazide – glipizide – tolbutamide)	ⓘ methotrimeprazine	↑ glucose level	Monitor blood glucose more frequently. Increase antidiabetic dose if necessary
	ⓘ cimetidine	↓ glucose level	Use ranitidine instead
	ⓘ co-trimoxazole	↓ glucose level (rare)	Monitor blood glucose more frequently
	▲ fluconazole ▲ miconazole	↓ glucose level due to ↑ plasma level of sulphonylurea	Use single dose fluconazole, or use ketoconazole or use itraconazole
	▲ NSAIDs	↓ glucose level	Avoid combination – use another antidiabetic
	ⓘ octreotide	Possible ↓ glucose level	Monitor blood glucose more frequently
	▲ warfarin	↓ glucose level and altered warfarin effect	Avoid combination
tolbutamide	ⓘ phenytoin	↑ plasma level of phenytoin	Reduce phenytoin or use sodium valproate
Antiemetics			
dimenhydrinate	ⓘ TC antidepressants ⓘ antimuscarinics	Increased risk of anti-muscarinic adverse effects with these interacting drugs	Observe for drowsiness, dry mouth, confusion, blurred vision, hypotension. May need to reduce doses

Table continued overleaf

Drug	Interacting drug and importance of interaction	Effect of interaction	Action
domperidone (in US available from a compounding pharmacy)	(i) TC antidepressants (i) antimuscarinics (i) opioids	↓ effect of domperidone on GI motility with these interacting drugs	Avoid combination or change domperidone to metoclopramide
haloperidol	▲ amiodarone	Increased risk of ventricular arrhythmias	Avoid combination
	(i) buspirone ▲ fluoxetine, fluvoxamine ▲ venlafaxine	↑ plasma level of haloperidol with these interacting drugs	Observe for drowsiness or extrapyramidal side effects
	(i) indomethacin	May cause profound drowsiness	Use alternative NSAID
	(i) carbamazepine (i) phenobarbital	↓ plasma level of haloperidol with either of these interacting drugs	Observe for loss of haloperidol dose – if necessary increase haloperidol dose
	(i) morphine	Increased risk of myoclonus	Observe for myoclonic jerks. Consider switching to alternative opioid
methotrimeprazine	(i) ACE inhibitors (i) beta-blockers (i) clonidine (i) diuretics (i) nitrates	Increased risk of hypotension with any of these interacting drugs	Monitor BP more frequently
	▲ amiodarone ▲ disopyramide ▲ pimozide ▲ procainamide ▲ sotalol	Increased risk of ventricular arrhythmias with any of these interacting drugs	Avoid combination
	(i) antacids	↓ absorption of methotrimeprazine	Take at least 2 hours apart
	(i) TC antidepressants (i) antimuscarinics	Increased antimuscarinic side effects with these interacting drugs	Observe for drowsiness, dry mouth, confusion, blurred vision. Avoid combination or reduce doses

Drug	Interacting drug and importance of interaction	Effect of interaction	Action
methotrimeprazine – cont.	ⓘ sulphonylureas	Possible ↑ blood glucose level	Monitor blood glucose more frequently
metoclopramide	ⓘ TC antidepressants ⓘ antimuscarinics ⓘ opioids	↓ effect of metoclopramide on GI motility with these interacting drugs	Avoid combination or increase metoclopramide dose

Antifungals

Drug	Interacting drug and importance of interaction	Effect of interaction	Action
fluconazole	ⓘ celecoxib ▲ midazolam ▲ phenytoin ▲ sulphonylureas ▲ warfarin	↑ plasma level of any of these interacting drugs	ⓘ Observe for adverse effects ▲ Avoid combination
itraconazole	ⓘ buspirone ⓘ dexamethasone ▲ digoxin ▲ warfarin ▲ midazolam	↑ plasma level of any of these interacting drugs	Reduce dose of interacting drug or use topical antifungal
	ⓘ antacids ⓘ cimetidine ⓘ ranitidine ⓘ omeprazole ⓘ lansoprazole ▲ phenytoin	↓ plasma level of itraconazole with any of these interacting drugs	ⓘ Increase itraconazole dose or use fluconazole ▲ Avoid combination – use fluconazole
	ⓘ clarithromycin	↑ plasma level of itraconazole	Observe for itraconazole adverse effects
	▲ simvastatin	Risk of myopathy	Avoid combination – use fluconazole
ketoconazole	ⓘ buspirone ⓘ carbamazepine ⓘ corticosteroids ▲ midazolam ▲ warfarin	↑ plasma level of any of these interacting drugs	Reduce dose of interacting drug or use topical antifungal
	ⓘ antacids ⓘ ranitidine ⓘ omeprazole ⓘ lansoprazole ▲ phenytoin ⓘ sucralfate	↓ plasma level of ketoconazole with any of these interacting drugs	ⓘ Use fluconazole ▲ Avoid combination

Table continued overleaf

Drug	Interacting drug and importance of interaction	Effect of interaction	Action
ketoconazole – cont.	ⓘ enteral feeds	↓ absorption of ketoconazole	Stop feed for 1 hour before to 2 hours after drug
	▲ simvastatin	Risk of myopathy	Avoid combination – use fluconazole
miconazole	▲ gliclazide (Canada) ▲ glipizide (US) ▲ phenytoin ▲ sulphonylureas ▲ warfarin	↑ plasma level of any of these interacting drugs	Avoid combination
	▲ simvastatin	Risk of myopathy	Avoid combination – use fluconazole
nystatin	ⓘ chlorhexidine	Reduced effectiveness of nystatin	Take at least 2 hours apart or use systemic antifungal
Antimuscarinics			
All	ⓘ dimenhydrinate ⓘ hyoscine ⓘ oxybutynin ⓘ TC antidepressants	Increased risk of muscarinic effects with any of these interacting drugs	Observe for drowsiness, dry mouth, confusion, blurred vision. Avoid combination or reduce doses
	ⓘ haloperidol ⓘ metoclopramide	Increased risk of movement disorders with any of these interacting drugs	Observe for tremor, Parkinsonian features or restlessness. Avoid combination or reduce doses
Antipsychotics			
haloperidol	See antiemetics (p. 239)		
methotrimeprazine	See antiemetics (p. 239)		
olanzapine	▲ carbamazepine	↓ plasma level of olanzapine	Observe for loss of olanzapine effect
	ⓘ fluvoxamine	↑ plasma level of olanzapine	Observe for olanzapine adverse effects
	▲ valproate	Increased risk of neutropenia	Avoid combination

Drug	Interacting drug and importance of interaction	Effect of interaction	Action
risperidone	▲ carbamazepine	↓ plasma level of risperidone	Avoid combination
Anxiolytics			
benzodiazepines	▲ phenytoin	↑ plasma level of phenytoin	Avoid combination – use sodium valproate
buspirone	ⓘ haloperidol	↑ plasma level of haloperidol	Observe for haloperidol adverse effects
	ⓘ diltiazem ⓘ erythromycin ⓘ itraconazole ⓘ ketoconazole ⓘ verapamil	↑ plasma level of buspirone	Observe for buspirone adverse effects
clonazepam	ⓘ carbamazepine ⓘ phenytoin	↓ plasma level of clonazepam with either of these interacting drugs	Avoid combination – use sodium valproate
	▲ lithium	↑ plasma level of lithium	Check lithium levels
diazepam	ⓘ enteral feeds	Reduced absorption of diazepam	Dilute drug with 30–60 ml water and flush well
	ⓘ esomeprazole ⓘ fluvoxamine ⓘ omeprazole ⓘ sodium valproate	↑ plasma level of diazepam with any of these interacting drugs	Observe for diazepam adverse effects
	ⓘ phenytoin	Altered plasma level of phenytoin and ↓ plasma level of diazepam	Monitor phenytoin levels and observe for loss of effect of diazepam
lorazepam	ⓘ sodium valproate	↑ plasma level of lorazepam	Observe for lorazepam adverse effects

Table continued overleaf

Drug	Interacting drug and importance of interaction	Effect of interaction	Action
midazolam	▲ clarithromycin ⓘ diltiazem ▲ erythromycin ▲ fluconazole ▲ indinavir ▲ itraconazole ▲ ketoconazole ▲ ritonavir ⓘ verapamil	↑ plasma level of midazolam due to ↓ metabolism caused by any of these interacting drugs	ⓘ Observe for midazolam adverse effects ▲ Avoid combination
	ⓘ carbamazepine ⓘ rifampicin	↓ plasma level of interacting drug	Observe for loss of effect of midazolam and consider increasing midazolam dose
zopiclone	ⓘ erythromycin	↑ plasma level of zopiclone	Observe for zopiclone adverse effects
Beta-blockers			
All	ⓘ ACE inhibitors ⓘ anxiolytics ⓘ baclofen ⓘ calcium channel blockers ⓘ diuretics ⓘ methotrimeprazine ⓘ phenothiazines	Risk of hypotension with any of these interacting drugs	Monitor BP more frequently
	▲ adrenaline	Severe hypertension with any of these interacting drugs	Avoid combination
	▲ verapamil	Risk of asystole, severe hypotension and heart failure	Avoid combination
	▲ amiodarone	Risk of bradycardia and AV block	Avoid combination
	▲ anti-arrhythmics	Increased risk of myocardial depression	Avoid combination
	ⓘ antidiabetics	Masking of hypoglycemic symptoms	Monitor blood glucose more frequently
	▲ clonidine	Increased risk of hypertension on stopping clonidine	Withdraw beta-blocker several days before stopping clonidine
	ⓘ pilocarpine	Increased risk of arrhythmias	Avoid combination
esmolol	ⓘ morphine	Possible ↑ plasma level of morphine	Observe for adverse effects of morphine

Drug	Interacting drug and importance of interaction	Effect of interaction	Action
labetolol	ⓘ cimetidine	↑ plasma level of labetolol	Observe for adverse effects of labetolol
metoprolol	ⓘ cimetidine	↑ plasma level of metoprolol	Observe for adverse effects of metoprolol
sotolol	▲ amiodarone ▲ disopyramide ▲ diuretics ▲ phenothiazines ▲ TC antidepressants	Increased risk of ventricular arrhythmia with any of these interacting drugs	Avoid combination
Bisphosphonates			
clodronate	ⓘ antacids ⓘ oral iron	↓ absorption of clodronate with any of these interacting drugs	Use IV route instead of oral
pamidronate zoledronate	ⓘ aminoglycosides	Risk of hypocalcemia	Avoid combination
Calcium channel blockers (CCB)			
All	ⓘ ACE inhibitors ⓘ alcohol ⓘ antipsychotics ⓘ anxiolytics ⓘ baclofen ⓘ beta-blockers ⓘ clonidine ⓘ diuretics	Increased hypotensive effect with any of these interacting drugs	Monitor BP more frequently
	ⓘ cimetidine ⓘ grapefruit juice	↑ plasma level of CCB with either of these interacting substances	Change to ranitidine. Use alternative fruit juice
	ⓘ itraconazole	Increased negative inotropic effect	Change to fluconazole
amlodipine, felodipine	ⓘ itraconazole ⓘ ketoconazole	↑ plasma level of amlodipine with either of these interacting drugs	Change to fluconazole
	ⓘ carbamazepine ⓘ phenytoin	Possible ↓ effect of amlodipine with either of these interacting drugs	Use alternative anticonvulsant

Table continued overleaf

Drug	Interacting drug and importance of interaction	Effect of interaction	Action
diltiazem, verapamil	▲ anti-arrhythmics ▲ beta-blockers	Risk of bradycardia, AV block and severe myocardial depression with either of these interacting drugs	Avoid combination
	(i) buspirone ▲ carbamazepine ▲ digoxin (i) midazolam ▲ phenytoin ▲ TC antidepressants	↑ plasma level of any of these interacting drugs	(i) Observe for adverse effects of interacting drug ▲ Avoid combination
	(i) IV dantrolene	Risk of arrhythmias	Avoid IV administration of dantrolene
	▲ phenytoin	↓ effect of diltiazem and verapamil	Use alternative CCB
felodipine, isradipine (US), **nicardipine** (US), **nifedipine**	(i) carbamazepine (i) phenytoin	↓ plasma level of CCB with either of these interacting drugs	Use alternative anticonvulsant
felodipine	(i) erythromycin	↑ plasma level of CCB	Use alternative antibiotic or CCB
nicardipine nifedipine	▲ digoxin	↑ plasma level of digoxin	Avoid combination
verapamil	(i) alcohol	↑ plasma level of alcohol	Use alternative CCB
CNS stimulants			
methylphenidate	(i) antidepressants (all)	↑ plasma level of antidepressant	Observe for loss of antidepressant effect
	▲ phenobarbital (i) phenytoin ▲ warfarin	↑ plasma level of any of these interacting drugs	(i) Observe for adverse effects of interacting drug ▲ Avoid combination
Corticosteroids			
All (systemic)	(i) antidiabetics	↑ glucose level	Monitor blood glucose more frequently. Increase antidiabetic dose if necessary
	▲ carbamazepine (i) phenobarbital ▲ phenytoin	↓ plasma level of corticosteroid with these interacting drugs	Corticosteroid dose may have to be increased

Drug	Interacting drug and importance of interaction	Effect of interaction	Action
All (systemic) – cont.	ⓘ erythromycin ⓘ itraconazole ⓘ ketoconazole	↑ plasma level of corticosteroid with any of these interacting drugs	Observe for corticosteroid adverse effects – dose may have to be decreased
	ⓘ loop or thiazide diuretics	Increased risk of hypokalemia	Check electrolytes more frequently
	ⓘ NSAIDs	×15 risk of upper GI bleed	Avoid or protect with proton pump inhibitor
	▲ warfarin	Possible changed warfarin effect	Check INR more frequently
Diuretics			
All	▲ ACE inhibitors ⓘ alcohol ⓘ anxiolytics ⓘ baclofen ⓘ beta-blockers ⓘ calcium channel blockers ⓘ phenothiazines ⓘ antidepressants (TC)	Risk of hypotension with any of these interacting drugs	Monitor blood pressure more frequently. Enquire about postural hypotension
	ⓘ carbamazepine	Risk of hyponatremia	Monitor electrolytes more frequently
	ⓘ corticosteroids ⓘ NSAIDs	Antagonism of diuretic effect with either of these interacting drugs	Observe for loss of diuretic effect
	ⓘ NSAIDs	Increased risk of renal damage	Avoid in renal impairment
loop diuretics	▲ aminoglycosides ▲ vancomycin	Increased risk of ototoxicity with either of these interacting drugs	Avoid combination
	▲ antiarrhythmics ▲ digoxin	Cardiac toxicity occurs with either of these interacting drugs if K^+ low	Check electrolytes more frequently
	ⓘ antidiabetics	↑ blood glucose	Monitor blood glucose more frequently
	ⓘ cephalosporins	Risk of renal damage	Avoid in presence of renal impairment

Table continued overleaf

Drug	Interacting drug and importance of interaction	Effect of interaction	Action
loop diuretics – cont.	(i) cholestyramine	↓ diuretic effect (↓ absorption)	Take at least 2 hours apart
	(i) corticosteroids	Increased risk of hypokalemia	Monitor electrolytes more frequently
thiazide diuretics	▲ anti-arrhythmics ▲ digoxin	Cardiac toxicity occurs with either of these interacting drugs if K⁺ low	Monitor electrolytes more frequently
	(i) antidiabetics	↑ blood glucose	Monitor blood glucose more frequently
	(i) calcium salts (i) vitamin D	Risk of hypercalcemia with either of these interacting drugs	Avoid combination
	(i) chlorpropamide (i) trimethoprim	Risk of hyponatremia	Monitor electrolytes more frequently
	(i) corticosteroids	Increased risk of hypokalemia	Monitor electrolytes more frequently
potassium sparing diuretics	▲ ACE inhibitors	Risk of severe hyperkalemia	Avoid combination
	(i) chlorpropamide	Risk of hyponatremia with thiazide and potassium diuretic combination	Monitor electrolytes more frequently
	(i) NSAIDs (i) indomethacin	Possible risk of hyperkalemia	Check electrolytes more frequently
	▲ lithium	↑ lithium toxicity (reduced excretion)	Monitor lithium levels more frequently
	▲ potassium salts (i) high potassium foods	Risk of hyperkalemia with any of these interacting substances	(i) Check electrolytes more frequently ▲ Avoid combination
Muscle relaxant drugs			
baclofen	(i) antidepressants (TC)	↑ muscle relaxant effect	Observe for drowsiness or hypotonicity
	(i) NSAIDs	↑ effect of baclofen due to ↓ excretion	Observe for drowsiness or hypotonicity

Drug	Interacting drug and importance of interaction	Effect of interaction	Action
baclofen, tizanidine	ⓘ ACE inhibitors ⓘ beta-blockers ⓘ calcium channel blockers ⓘ diuretics ⓘ nitrates	Risk of hypotension with any of these interacting drugs	Monitor blood pressure more frequently. Enquire about postural hypotension
dantrolene (IV)	ⓘ diltiazem	Risk of arrhythmias	Avoid IV use of dantrolene in patients on diltiazem
	ⓘ verapamil	Hypotension, hyperkalemia, myocardial depression	Avoid IV use of dantrolene in patients on verapamil
Nutrition			
Enteral feeds	ⓘ antacids	Coagulate with feed	Dilute with 60 ml water and flush well
	ⓘ carbamazepine	Binds to tubes	Dilute drug with 30–60 ml water and flush well. Stop feed for 1 hour before to 2 hours after drug
	ⓘ ciprofloxacin	↓ absorption of ciprofloxacin	Stop feed for 1 hour before to 2 hours after drug
	ⓘ diazepam	Binds to tubes	Dilute drug with 30–60 ml water and flush well
	ⓘ flucloxacillin (Canada) and oxacillin (US)	↓ absorption of flucloxacillin/ oxacillin	Stop feed for 1 hour before to 2 hours after drug
	ⓘ ketoconazole	↓ absorption of ketoconazole	Stop feed for 1 hour before to 2 hours after drug
	ⓘ penicillin V	↓ absorption of penicillin	Stop feed for 1 hour before to 2 hours after drug
	▲ phenytoin	Binds to tubes	Dilute drug with 30–60 ml water and flush well

Table continued overleaf

Drug	Interacting drug and importance of interaction	Effect of interaction	Action
Enteral feeds – cont.	ⓘ tetracyline	↓ absorption of tetracycline	Stop feed for 1 hour before to 2 hours after drug
	▲ warfarin	↓ warfarin effect ↓ absorption of warfarin	Monitor INR more frequently. Stop feed for 1 hour before to 2 hours after drug
Iron	ⓘ bisphosphonates ⓘ ciprofloxacin ⓘ levodopa ⓘ tetracyclines	↓ absorption of interacting drug with any of these interacting drugs	Take at least 2 hours apart
	ⓘ tetracyclines	↓ absorption of iron	Take at least 2 hours apart
Ulcer healing drugs			
cimetidine	ⓘ anti-arrhythmics ⓘ antipsychotics ⓘ benzodiazepines ⓘ beta-blockers ▲ carbamazepine ⓘ calcium channel blockers ⓘ erythromycin ▲ lidocaine ⓘ metformin ⓘ metronidazole ⓘ opioids ⓘ paroxetine ▲ phenytoin ⓘ sulphonylureas ⓘ TC antidepressants ▲ valproate ▲ warfarin	↑ plasma level of any of these interacting drugs	ⓘ Observe for adverse effects of interacting drug ▲ Avoid combination
cimetidine **famotidine** **nizatidine** **ranitidine**	ⓘ cefpodoxime ⓘ itraconazole ⓘ ketoconazole	↓ plasma level of any of these interacting drugs	Use cimetidine
proton pump inhibitors (PPI)	ⓘ digoxin	↑ plasma level of digoxin	Check digoxin levels
	ⓘ ketoconazole ⓘ itraconazole	↓ plasma level of antifungal with either of these interacting drugs	Change to fluconazole

Drug	Interacting drug and importance of interaction	Effect of interaction	Action
esomeprazole, omeprazole	ⓘ diazepam ⓘ phenytoin ▲ warfarin	↑plasma level of any of these interacting drugs	ⓘ Observe for adverse effects of interacting drug ▲ Avoid combination
lansoprazole	ⓘ antacids ⓘ sucralfate	↓ absorption of lansoprazole with either of these interacting drugs	Take at least 2 hours apart
sucralfate	ⓘ ciprofloxacin ⓘ digoxin ⓘ ketoconazole ⓘ lansoprazole ⓘ olanzapine ▲ phenytoin ⓘ tetracyclines ▲ warfarin	↓ absorption of any of these interacting drugs	Take at least 2 hours apart

Drugs in palliative care for children: starting doses[1-6]

Drug pharmacokinetics

Children absorb, distribute, metabolize and eliminate drugs differently from adults:

- *Neonates (under 1 month)* have a low renal and hepatic clearance with a higher volume of distribution. This prolongs the half-life of many drugs so that they require smaller doses relative to their size, but they may need a loading dose to avoid a delay in effect. A pediatrician experienced in neonatal medicine should monitor drug and drug dose selection.
- *Infants (1 month–2 years) and children (> 2 years)* have relatively high drug clearances with a normal volume of distribution. This leads to shorter half-lives compared with adults so that they may need comparatively higher doses at shorter intervals. Children older than 12 years have similar pharmacokinetic profiles to adults.

Drug presentation and routes

Care and imagination are needed when selecting appropriate routes and preparations. Contrary to popular belief, children often prefer tablets to sickly sweet syrups. If liquids are used their taste can be improved with fizzy drinks or fruit juice. The rectal and buccal routes provide effective and rapid absorption and some children are willing to self-administer drugs this way. Subcutaneous infusions using portable, battery-driven pumps are a valuable method of administering many drugs with minimum trouble to the child. The intranasal and sublingual or buccal routes are alternatives.[7-9] Some children already have central venous access catheters in place often with several months' experience of their use.

Opioids

Dosing: Infants in the first year of life are particularly sensitive to opiates, hence a smaller starting dose/kg compared to those in older children is recommended (*see* table). Children also metabolize morphine faster, so some may need short-acting preparations q2–3h rather than q4h and long-acting preparations q8h rather than q12h. As in adults, dose requirements can vary greatly between individuals.[10]

Intranasal opioids are less traumatic than injection and can be useful for testing efficacy, for rapid pain control and for breakthrough pain.[7–9]

Rectal opioids: In situations where oral dosing is difficult (e.g. reluctance, dysphagia, vomiting) rectal dosing is often acceptable.

Fentanyl has a place in the management of stable pain, but it should be used with caution. Fentanyl is a potent opioid and the smallest transdermal patch (25 microgram/hour) is approximately equivalent to 75 mg/24 hours of oral morphine. For children, many Canadian pediatricians obtain an approximate 12.5 microgram/hour dose by occluding (*not* cutting – risk of overdose if patch is cut) half the 25 microgram patch. (This is not promoted by the manufacturer.) The pharmacokinetics of transdermal fentanyl are complex, resulting in delays of up to 14 hours in steady state blood levels and up to 30 hours in reducing to low levels.[11,12] The alternative of using a subcutaneous infusion of fentanyl is less suitable in mobile children. Fentanyl intravenously via PCAs (Patient Controlled Analgesia) is commonly used in some pediatric cancer units in the US (e.g. Memorial Sloan-Kettering Cancer Center, New York, NY). Buccal/sublingual fentanyl (use the injection solution) can be used for short-lived breakthrough pain.[13,14] Fentanyl oral transmucosal units are available in the US, but the absorption rate is variable from person to person. It is commonly used in children although not officially FDA approved in this population. It should not be used in opioid-naïve patients.

Starting doses

Doses for children can be complex since (1) calculations based on weight are often needed, (2) doses can vary greatly between different children and (3) information sources can be presented in many different ways:

Different ways of expressing doses in children

micrograms	Total daily dose
milligrams	Dose per hour
microgram/kg body weight	Single dose
mg/kg body weight	24-hour infusion

At Helen House children's hospice in Oxford, England it is common practice to double check complex dose calculations with a second professional.[15]

  The tables that follow contain suggested starting doses (expressed as total daily dose) and suggested frequency of dosing.

Suggested starting doses expressed as total daily dose or single doses (*single doses in italics*)

Drug	Neonates (under 1 month)	Infants (1 month to 2 years)	Children (2–12 years)	Comments
Non-opioid primary analgesics				
acetaminophen[16] **(oral, rectal)** Susp or elixir: 120 mg/5 ml, Infant susp gtts: 80 mg/ml Chew tabs: 80, 160 mg Supps: 120, 325, 650 mg	10 mg/kg/24 hr 6-hrly divided doses	1–3 m = 40 mg/kg/24 hr 3 m–1 yr = 240 mg/24 hr 1–2 yr = 480 mg/24 hr 6-hrly divided doses	2–5 yrs = 500 mg/24 hr 6–12 yrs = 1 g/24 hr > 12 yrs = 2 g/24 hr 4–6 hrly divided doses	Halve doses if jaundice. Increase doses by 10% for rectal route
ibuprofen Susp: 100 mg/5 ml Pediatric gtts: 200 mg/5 ml Caplets: 100 mg Chew tabs: 50, 100 mg	Not recommended	< 7 kg: not recommended > 7 kg = 20 mg/kg/24 hr 6–8 hrly divided doses	2–12 yrs = 20 mg/kg/24 hr > 12 yrs = 600 mg/24 hr 6–8 hrly divided doses	Not for use in children under 7 kg weight
diclofenac Tabs: 25, 50 mg Supps (Canada only): 50, 100 mg	Not recommended	< 1 yr: not recommended 1–2 yrs = 1 mg/kg/24 hr 6–8 hrly divided doses	2–12 yrs = 1 mg/kg/24 hr > 12 yrs = 75 mg/24 hr 6–8 hrly divided doses	Not for use in children under 12 months of age. Controlled release preparations not recommended for children
Weak oral opioid primary analgesics				
codeine (oral) Syrup: 15 mg/ml (US)/5 mg/ml (Canada) Tabs: 15, 30 mg	Under advice of specialist	< 1 yr: under advice of specialist 1–2 yrs = 3 mg/kg/24 hr 4–6 hrly divided doses	2–12 yrs = 3 mg/kg/24 hr > 12 yrs = 120 mg/24 hr 4–6 hrly divided doses	Reduce doses by 50% in renal impairment. Do not use in renal failure
First line strong opioid primary analgesics Please note: 1 These are starting doses for children **not** previously on weak opioids. 2 Recommended starting doses vary widely so these starting doses are purposefully cautious – be prepared to rapidly titrate the dose upwards if the pain remains uncontrolled.				
morphine (oral) (instant release)	500 microgram/kg/24 hr 4-hrly divided doses (under advice of specialist)	< 1 yr = 500 microgram/kg/24 hr > 1 yr = 1 mg/kg/24 hr 3–4 hrly divided doses	2–12 yrs = 1 mg/kg/24 hr > 12 yrs = 30 mg/24 hr 3–4 hrly divided doses	Can be made up in suppository form
(controlled release)	Not recommended	< 1 yr = 500 microgram/kg/24 hr > 1 yr = 1 mg/kg/24 hr 8–12 hrly divided doses	2–12 yrs = 1 mg/kg/24 hr > 12 yrs = 30 mg/24 hr 8–12 hrly divided doses	

Table continued overleaf

Drug	Neonates (under 1 month)	Infants (1 month to 2 years)	Children (2–12 years)	Comments
Second line strong opioid primary analgesics				
fentanyl (24 hr SC infusion or transdermal) hydromorphone (oral) methadone (oral) oxycodone (oral) (in the US fentanyl, hydromorphone and methadone are commonly used via IV PCAs)	• *For children already on strong opioids:* convert to equivalent dose and then retitrate if necessary (*see* Using opioids (p. 49)). • *For children on weak opioids or no opioids:* ask for specialist advice from palliative care specialist with experience of using these opioids in children.			
Other drugs (starting doses)				
amitriptyline (oral) Susp: 10 mg/5 ml Tabs: 10, 25, 50, 75 mg (in the US also available in 100 and 150 mg)	Not recommended	< 1 yr = not recommended > 1 yr = 500 microgram/kg/24hr as single bedtime dose	*2–7 yrs = 500 microgram/kg/24 hr 7–10 yrs = 5 mg 10–12 yrs = 10 mg Single bedtime dose*	Use with caution in children with cardiac dysfunction. Not recommended for depression
antacids Gaviscon	Half dual sachet of oral powder with or after feeds	Full dual sachet of oral powder with or after feeds	2–12 yrs = 5–10 ml of liquid > 12 yrs = 10–20 ml of liquid Give after meals and bedtime	
baclofen (oral) Tabs: 10, 20 mg (scored)	Not recommended	< 1 yr = not recommended 1–2 yrs = 750 microgram/kg/24 hr 6–8 hrly divided doses	15 mg/24 hr 8-hrly divided doses	Divided doses reduce adverse effects. Start with low dose and titrate at 3 day intervals until effective or adverse effects are a problem
bisacodyl (oral, PR) Tabs: 5 mg Supps: 5 mg (Canada only), 10 mg	Not recommended	*5 mg as single daily dose*	*2–12 yrs = 5 mg as single daily dose > 12 yrs = 10 mg as single daily dose*	If colic is a problem try splitting the dose into two daily doses
carbamazepine (oral or rectal) Susp: 100 mg/5 ml Chew tabs: 100, 200 mg Tabs: 200 mg CR tabs: 200, 400 mg	Not recommended	< 1 yr = 5 mg/kg/24 hr 1–2 yrs = 100 mg/24 hr Start once daily, then move to 8–12 hrly divided doses	1–10 yrs = 5 mg/kg/24 hr > 12 yrs = 600 mg/24 hr Start once daily then move to 8–12 hrly divided doses	For rectal route, use approximately 25% more than oral dose. Start low and increase every 3–7 days. Start once daily, then move to 8–12 hrly divided doses
chloral hydrate or triclofos (oral) Syrup: 500 mg/5 ml	Not recommended	*25 mg/kg as single bedtime dose*	*1–5 yrs = 250 mg 6–12 yrs = 500 mg As single bedtime dose*	Chloral betaine 717 mg ≡ 414 mg chloral hydrate. Triclofos is expensive but may cause less gastric irritation

Drug	Neonates (under 1 month)	Infants (1 month to 2 years)	Children (2–12 years)	Comments
dantrolene (oral) Caps: 25, 100 mg	Not recommended	1 mg/kg/24 hr 12-hrly initially, then 6-hrly	2–12 yrs = 1 mg/kg/24 hr 12-hrly divided doses *> 12 yrs = 25 mg as a* *single daily dose*	
desmopressin Nasal spray: 10 microgram/spray Tabs: 100, 200 microgram (oral) (scored)	*2–5 microgram/24 hr* *Once daily*	*5 microgram/24 hr* *Once daily*	*10 microgram/24 hr* *Once daily*	Can be used < 5 yrs for diabetes insipidus
	Not recommended	Diabetes insipidus: 150 microgram/24hr in 8-hrly divided doses	*Enuresis: 100* *microgram/24hr as single* *bedtime dose* Diabetes insipidus: 300 microgram/24hr in 8-hrly divided doses	Can be used < 5 yrs for diabetes insipidus
dexamethasone (oral, SC) Tabs: 0.5 mg, 2 mg Inj: 4 mg/ml, 10 mg/ml In US also available in 0.25, 0.75, 1.5, 4, 6 mg and elixir 0.5 mg/5 ml, 0.5 mg/0.5 ml	*100 microgram/kg/24 hr* *Once daily*	*500 microgram/24 hr* *Once daily* SC same as oral dose	*2 mg/24 hr* *Once daily* SC same as oral dose	Reduce to lowest dose that controls symptoms. Cushingoid features develop rapidly. Higher starting doses often needed for urgent treatment (e.g. raised ICP)
diazepam (oral) *For muscle spasm* Tabs: 2, 5, 10 mg	Not recommended	200 microgram/kg/24 hr 12-hrly divided doses	2–12 yrs = 1 mg/24 hr > 12 yrs = 3–5 mg/24 hr Once daily	*Maximum 10 mg* *as a single dose*
(rectal, IV) *For seizure* Inj: 5 mg/ml Rectal soln: 5 mg/ml	IV: 300 microgram/kg titrated Rectal: 1–2.5 mg	IV: 400 microgram/kg titrated Rectal: 5 mg	IV: 2–12 yrs = 400 microgram/kg titrated > 12 yrs = 5–10 mg titrated Rectal: 5–10 mg	*Maximum 10 mg* *as a single dose* Repeat after 5–10 mins if necessary
dimenhydrinate dimenhydrinate IM: 50 mg/1 ml as a 1 ml ampoule dimenhydrinate IV: 10 mg/ml as a 5 ml vial multidose vial: 50 mg/ml as a 5 ml vial Tabs: 15, 25, 50 mg Cap: 50 mg Chewtab: 15, 50 mg (Canada only) Liquid: 15 mg/5 ml, 12.5 mg/4 ml, 12.5 mg/5 ml Suppos: 25, 50, 100 mg (Canada only) Gelcap: 75 mg (Canada only)	Not recommended	Not recommended	2–6 yrs = 75 mg/24 hr 6–12 yrs = 150 mg/24 hr	May cause local irritation given SC
diphenhydramine PO – 12.5, 25, 50 mg, 6.25 mg/5 ml, 12.5 mg/5 ml IV/IM formulations – available	Not recommended	Use with caution	5 mg/kg/day divided q4–6h IV/PO	Commonly used in hospital pediatric setting in the US for nausea and vomiting

Table continued overleaf

Drug	Neonates (under 1 month)	Infants (1 month to 2 years)	Children (2–12 years)	Comments
docusate (oral) Canada: Liquid: 20 mg/5 ml, 50 mg/5 ml Caps: 100 mg Drops: 10 mg/ml US: Caps: 50, 100, 250 mg Liquid: 10 mg/5 ml, 50 mg/5 ml	Not recommended	< 6 m = not recommended > 6 m = 37.5 mg/24 hr 8-hrly divided doses	2–12 yrs = 37.5 mg/24 hr > 12 yrs = 100 mg/24 hr 8–12 hrly divided doses	Takes 24–48 hours to act
domperidone (oral) (in US available from compounding pharmacies in strengths of 10 mg and 20 mg) Tabs: 10 mg	Not recommended	600 microgram/kg/24 hr 4–8 hrly divided doses	< 12 yrs = 600 microgram/kg/24 hr > 12 yrs = 30 mg/24 hr 8-hrly divided doses	
fluconazole (oral) Susp: 50 mg/5 ml Tabs: 50, 100 mg Caps: 150 mg	*< 2 wks = 3 mg/kg once every 72 hr 2–4 wks = 3 mg/kg once every 48 hr*	*3 mg/kg/24 hr as a single daily dose*	*50 mg/24 hr as a single daily dose*	Reduce dose or frequency in renal impairment
furosemide (oral, IV) Liquid: 10 mg/ml Tabs: 20, 40, 80, 500 mg Inj: 10 mg/ml	500 microgram/kg/24 hr	500 microgram/kg/24 hr Max 20 mg daily	2–12 yrs = 1 mg/kg/24 hr > 12 yrs = 20 mg/24 hr	Maximum for single dose = 6 mg/kg
gabapentin (oral) Caps: 100, 300, 400 mg Tabs: 600, 800 mg	Not recommended	5 mg/kg/24 hr: *Day 1: 5 mg/kg once daily Day 3: 5 mg/kg 12-hrly Day 5: 5 mg/kg 8-hrly*	100 mg/24 hr *Day 1: 100 mg once daily* Day 2: 100 mg 12-hrly Day 3: 100 mg 8-hrly	In older children, doses up to 2.4 g may be needed. Reduce dosing interval in renal impairment in children < 12 yrs
glycopyrrolate (SC) Inj: 200 microgram/ml	Not recommended	*5 microgram/kg as a single dose* 25 microgram/kg/24 hr as continuous SC infusion	*Single dose: 2–12 yrs = 5 microgram/kg > 12 yrs = 100 microgram* 25 microgram/kg/24 hr as continuous SC infusion	Alternative to hyoscine hydrobromide
haloperidol (oral, SC) Tabs: 0.5, 1, 2, 5, 10, 20 mg Liquid: 2 mg/ml Inj: 5 mg/ml	Not recommended	25 microgram/kg/24 hr 12-hrly divided doses	2–12 yrs = 25 microgram/kg/24 hr 12-hrly divided doses *> 12 yrs = 1 mg as single daily dose*	Avoid high doses or prolonged courses if possible. Only the lowest doses required for nausea
hyoscine butylbromide (SC) (Canada only) Inj: 20 mg/ml Tabs: 10 mg	Not recommended	1.5 mg/kg/24 hr 6–8 hrly divided doses or as continuous SC infusion	2–5 yrs = 15 mg/24 hr 6–12 yrs = 30 mg/24 hr 8-hrly divided doses or as continuous SC infusion	Less sedating alternative to glycopyrrolate. Ineffective orally
hyoscine hydrobromide (SC) (Canada) (known as scopolamine in the US) Inj: 400, 600 microgram/ml	Not recommended	60 microgram/kg/24 hr 6-hrly divided doses or as continuous SC infusion	60 microgram/kg/24 hr 6-hrly divided doses or as continuous SC infusion	More sedating than glycopyrrolate
(transdermal) TD patch: 1 mg/72 hr	Not recommended	Not recommended	2–3 yrs = ¼ patch/72 hrs 4–9 yrs = ½ patch/72 hrs > 10 yrs = 1 patch/72 hrs	Found to be useful in pediatric palliative care

Drug	Neonates (under 1 month)	Infants (1 month to 2 years)	Children (2–12 years)	Comments
imipramine (oral)	Not recommended	Not recommended	*200 microgram/kg/24 hr Once at night*	Alternative to amitriptyline for neuropathic pain. Increase by 50% every 2–3 days
itraconazole (oral) Caps: 100 mg Liquid: 50 mg/5 ml	Not recommended	*3 mg/kg as single daily dose*	*3–5 mg/kg as single daily dose*	–
ketamine (SC, oral) *For analgesia:* Inj: 10 mg/ml, 50 mg/ml	Not recommended	*1 mg as single dose 2.5 mg/kg/24 hr as continuous SC infusion*	*1 mg as single dose 2.5 mg/kg/24 hr as continuous SC infusion*	Analgesic doses are approximately 5% of anesthetic doses. Only for use in specialist units
lactulose Liquid	Not recommended	*1 m–1 yr = 2.5 ml/24 hr 1–2 yrs = 5 ml/24 hr 8–12 hrly divided doses*	*2–5 yrs = 5 ml/24 hr 5–12 yrs = 10 ml/24 hr > 12 yrs = 20 ml/24 hrs 12-hrly divided doses*	Takes 36–48 hrs to act. High doses can cause abdominal bloating and dehydration
loperamide (oral) Caps: 2 mg Syrup: 1 mg/5 ml Quick dissolve tabs: 2 mg	Not recommended	Not recommended for acute diarrhea	*Acute diarrhea: 2–12 yrs = 100 microgram/kg > 12 yrs = 2–4 mg once after each loose stool*	Maximum 16 mg daily. In acute infection, 3–5 days use only. In chronic diarrhea regular 6–8 hrly dosing may be necessary
lorazepam (oral) Tabs: 0.5, 1, 2 mg SL tabs: 0.5, 1, 2 mg	*25–50 microgram/kg as single dose*	*50 microgram/kg as single dose*	*2–12 yrs = 50 microgram/kg/24 hr > 12 yrs = 500 microgram As single dose*	Can be repeated up to 3 times daily
methotrime-prazine Inj: 25 mg/ml Liquid: 25 mg/5 ml Oral drops: 40 mg/ml Tabs: 2, 5, 25, 50 mg	Not recommended	*200 microgram/kg/24 hr as single bedtime dose*	*200 microgram/kg/24 hr as single bedtime dose*	Found to be useful in pediatric palliative care
metronidazole (oral) Tabs: 250 mg Caps: 500 mg	–	*15 mg/kg/24 hr 8-hrly divided doses*	*2–12 yrs = 25 mg/kg/24 hr > 12 yrs = 400 mg/24 hr 8-hrly divided doses*	Doses and regimens vary with the diagnosis
miconazole (oral) Oral gel: 24 mg/ml	Not recommended	*5 ml/24 hr 12-hrly divided doses*	*2–6 yrs = 10 ml/24 hr 12-hrly divided doses > 6 yrs = 20 ml/24 hr 6-hrly divided doses*	–
midazolam (SC) Inj: 1, 5 mg/ml	Not recommended	*150 microgram/kg as a single loading dose 1 mg/kg/24 hr as continuous SC infusion*	*150 microgram/kg as a single loading dose 1 mg/kg/24 hr as continuous SC infusion*	Allows finer titration than diazepam
(nasal)	Not recommended	*200 microgram/kg as a single dose*	*200 microgram/kg as a single dose*	Alternative to buccal route
(buccal)	Not recommended	*300 microgram/kg as a single dose*	*300 microgram/kg as a single dose*	Children prefer this route to other routes

Table continued overleaf

Drug	Neonates (under 1 month)	Infants (1 month to 2 years)	Children (2–12 years)	Comments
octreotide (SC) Inj: 50, 100, 500 microgram/ml (in US also available as 200 and 1000 microgram/ml)	Not recommended	25 microgram/kg/24 hr as continuous SC infusion	300 microgram/24 hr as continuous SC infusion	–
ondansetron Tabs: 4, 8, 24 mg Orally disintegrating tablet 4, 8 mg Liquid: 4 mg/5 ml IV, SC	Not recommended	Not recommended	0.15 mg/kg tid PRN	Commonly used in hospital pediatric setting in the US for nausea and vomiting
omeprazole (oral) Tabs: 10, 20 mg	Not recommended	*700 microgram/kg as single morning dose*	*Single morning dose: 2–12 yrs = 700 microgram/kg > 12 yrs = 20–40 mg*	Available as dispersible tablets
paraldehyde (PR) (Canada only) Inj: 5 ml	*Single dose: 0.5 ml*	*Single dose: <3 m = 0.5 ml 3–6 m = 1 ml 6–12 m = 1.5 ml 1–2 yrs = 2 ml*	*Single dose: 3–5 yrs = 3 ml 6–12 yrs = 5 ml*	Given as an enema. Mix 1 part paraldehyde with 9 parts 0.9% saline or 1 part arachis oil (avoid in peanut allergy)
phenobarbital (oral, SC) Tabs: 15, 30, 60, 100 mg Liquid: 5 mg/ml Inj: 20, 30, 120 mg/ml	1 mg/kg/24 hr 12-hrly divided doses	2 mg/kg/24 hr 12-hrly divided doses	*Single daily doses: 2–12 yrs = 5 mg/kg > 12 yrs = 60–180 mg*	Plasma half-life shorter in young children
promethazine Available in Canada only as a 25 mg/ml injection US preparations: PO – 12.5, 25, 50 mg, 25 mg/5ml PR – 12.5, 25 mg IV/IM formulations – available	Not commonly used for children		0.25–1 mg/kg q4h PRN	Available in US but not commonly used in children
ranitidine (oral) Tabs: 150, 300 mg Liquid: 15 mg/ml	2 mg/kg/24 hr 8-hrly divided doses	<6 m = 2 mg/kg/24 hr 8-hrly divided doses 6 m–2 yrs = 4 mg/kg 12-hrly divided doses	2–12 yrs = 8 mg/kg/24 hr 12-hrly divided doses *> 12 yrs = 300 mg as single night-time dose*	Daily doses should not exceed 300 mg
salbutamol (nebulized) Soln: 5 mg/5 ml Nebules: 1.25 mg/2.5 ml, 2.5 mg/2.5 ml, 5 mg/ 2.5 ml	Not recommended	<6 m = Not recommended 6 m–2 yrs = 2.5 mg/24 hr repeated up to 4 times daily at home	2.5 mg/24 hr repeated up to 4 times daily at home	For older children, administration through a mouthpiece is better tolerated and more effective
senna syrup (oral) Syrup: 1.7 mg/ml, 8.8 mg/5 ml Tabs: 8.6 mg Granules: 15 mg/5 ml	Not recommended	0.5 ml/kg/24 hr 12-hrly divided doses	< 6 yrs = 0.5 ml/kg/24 hr 6–12 yrs = 5 ml/24 hr > 12 yrs = 10 ml/24 hr 12-hrly divided doses	Can be given once daily, but there is less chance of colic with divided doses
spironolactone (oral) Tabs: 25, 100 mg	1 mg/kg/24 hr 12-hrly divided doses	1.5 mg/kg/24 hr 12-hrly divided doses	2–12 yrs = 3 mg/kg/24 hr 12-hrly divided doses *> 12 yrs = 100 mg as single morning dose*	
sucralfate (oral, topical) Susp: 1 g/5 ml Tabs: 1 g	Not recommended	1 g/24 hr 4–6 hrly divided doses swallowed or topical	2–12 yrs = 2 g/24 hr > 12 yrs = 4 g/24 hr 4–6 hrly divided doses swallowed or topical	Used as a hemostatic agent or gastric mucosal coating agent
temazepam (oral) Caps: 7.5, 15, 30 mg	*1 mg/kg as single bedtime dose*	*1 mg/kg as single bedtime dose*	*2–5 yrs = 2.5 mg 6–12 yrs = 5 mg > 12 yrs = 10 mg As single bedtime dose*	
tranexamic/ aminocaproic acid (oral) Tabs: 500 mg Injection: 100 mg/ml	Not recommended	75 mg/kg/24 hr given 8-hrly	2–12 yrs = 75 mg/kg/24 hr > 12 yrs = 2 g/24 hr given 6–8 hrly	Can be used topically to stop bleeding. Via compounding pharmacies in the US

Using drugs off-label

In adult and pediatric palliative care many drugs are not licensed for their intended use or routes. It is accepted, however, that this is a legitimate aspect of practice.[17] The following guidelines are slightly modified from the original ones for the UK.[18]

Guidelines for off-label prescribing

- A drug license applies to the activities of the pharmaceutical company, not the doctor's prescribing practice.
- The cost of testing new uses and routes means that they are unlikely to be tested by pharmaceutical companies to gain a license.
- Preparations that are imported or specially prepared can be prescribed for named patients.
- The responsibilities lie with the prescribing doctor.

The key to safe off-label prescribing and administration of drugs is to keep risks to a minimum. Some basic rules will reduce the risks to the prescriber and person administering the preparation.[18]

Basic rules for off-label prescribing

- The drug or preparation should:
  - be licensed for other uses and routes
  - be well known and studied
  - have been used by others previously for the intended route and purpose.
- The reasons for use should not be trivial.
- In the case of new, or little used, uses and routes, the details should be documented and consent obtained from the patient.

Alternative routes for drugs

Oral route

Most patients prefer this route. When available, patients should be given a choice of preparation. This may be a tablet (plain or coated), capsule, liquid (solution or suspension) or a dispersible preparation.

Non-oral routes

The oral route is not always possible. The intravenous route is sometimes needed for a rapid effect in emergencies. It is also commonly used in patients who already have a central or peripheral line in place. The intramuscular route is suitable for single doses when the intravenous route is not available, but is not suitable for repeated use because of discomfort. However, the subcutaneous, rectal and buccal/sublingual routes provide useful alternatives. Experience and investigation have shown that many drugs can be safely and effectively given by the subcutaneous route.[17-20] Some drugs can also be given topically or through a feeding tube.

For fuller and current information see:

- www.palliativedrugs.com for palliative care drugs
- the book *Care Beyond Cure* from the Canadian Society of Hospital Pharmacists (also available in French).

Continuous subcutaneous infusion (CSCI)

It should be noted that subcutaneous use of medications in palliative care is common in Europe, Australia, Canada and other countries.[18,19] The use is limited but growing in the US. Thus, opioids are commonly used IV via Patient Controlled Analgesia (PCA) pumps. Medications mentioned as being delivered via SC, including CSCI, are often used IV in the US.

Basic rules for CSCI

- Use a plastic cannula rather than a metal butterfly.
- Choose a protected site, e.g. upper anterior chest.
- Use a pump that is familiar to you.
- Use a familiar procedure for priming the line.
- Only use drugs that are known to be safe and effective by the subcutaneous route.
- Use 0.9% saline for diluting drugs. If necessary drugs can be diluted with 'water for injection', except ketamine and octreotide which should be diluted with 0.9% saline.
- Limit the number of drugs per syringe to two.
- Check the pump several times in 24 hours (or instruct the patient, partner or relative to do so).
- Know the procedure needed for infusion failures (check cannula, tubing, syringe, battery and pump) (*see* p. 272).

Gastrostomy/jejunostomy route

Many drugs can be given this way with some precautions:

- Do not use enteric-coated tablets or capsules.
- Do not crush extended-release tablets or capsules.
- Some extended-release morphine preparations such as Kadian™ and Avinza™ can be given this way by opening the capsules and dispensing the granules into the tube.
- Do not use preparations intended for buccal use.
- Avoid crushing tablets of antibiotics, cytotoxics and hormones because of the risk of inhalation by staff.
- If an injection solution is used, it should be diluted with 30–60 ml water.

Available routes for drugs

Drug	Tablet (T)/capsule (C) Ir = immediate release sr = sustained release	Liquid (L) Powder/granules (P,G) Chewable/dispersible (Ch, D)	Buccal/sublingual/nasal	Gastrostomy route possible?[18]	IV	IM	SC CSCI = SC infusion Bolus = bolus injection	Rectal	Topical
acetaminophen	Yes – T(ir)	Yes – L	No	Yes – use oral liquid	No	No	No	Yes	No
amitriptyline	Yes – T(ir)	No	No	No	No	No	No	No	No
amoxicillin	Yes – C (ir)	Yes – L, P	No	Yes – oral suspension or injection solution	Yes	Yes, but not usually used	No information	No	No
amoxicillin/clavulanic acid	Yes – T (ir)	Yes – L, D	No	Yes – use oral suspension but dilute to half strength and flush well	No	No	No	No	No
antacids	Yes – T, C (ir)	Yes – L	No	May interact with feeds. Not needed with jejunal tubes	No	No	No	No	No
baclofen	Yes – T (ir)	No	No	Yes	No	No	No	No	No
bulk laxatives	No	Yes – P	No	No. Use feed with high fiber content	No	No	No	No	No
buprenorphine	Yes – T (ir)	No	Yes (SL)	No information	Yes, but not usually used	Yes, but not usually used	No	No	Yes (transdermal)
calcitonin	No	No	Yes – nasal spray	No	No	Yes	Yes. Bolus or CSCI	No	No
carbamazepine	Yes – T (ir/sr)	Yes – L	No	Yes – use oral liquid diluted with 30 ml water (stop feed 1hr before and after). May interact with feeds	No	No	No	Yes, 125 mg PR = 100 mg orally[21-23]	No
ceftriaxone	No	No	No	No information	Yes	Yes	Yes. Bolus (mixed with 1 ml lidocaine)[24]	No	
chloral hydrate	Yes – T (ir) (Canada) Yes – C (ir) (US)	Yes – L	No	Yes – use oral liquid diluted with water	No	No	No	No (Canada) Yes, 325, 650 mg supp. (US)	No

Drug									
ciprofloxacin	Yes – T (ir)	Yes – L	No	Use crushed tablets in *distilled* or *sterile* water. May interact with feeds	Yes	No	No	No	No
clonazepam	Yes – T (ir)	No	No	Yes–crush tablet with 30–60 ml water. May bind to tube	No	No	Yes Bolus or CSCI	Yes[25]	No
codeine	Yes – T (ir/sr)	Yes – L	No	Yes – use oral liquid diluted with water	Yes, but not usually used	Yes, but not usually used	No information	No information	No
corticosteroids	Yes – T (ir)	Dexamethasone disperses in water	Yes (topical)	Yes – disperse tablet in water, or use injection liquid	Yes over 1 min	Yes, but not usually used	Yes Bolus	Yes (local action)	Yes
desmopressin	Yes – T (ir)	No	Yes (nasal)	No information	Yes, but not usually used	Yes, but not usually used	Yes Bolus or CSCI	No	No
diazepam	Yes – T (ir)	Yes – L	No	Oral solution prepared by pharmacist	Yes	Yes	No	Yes	No
diclofenac	Yes – T (ir/sr)	No	No	No	No	No	No	Yes[26]	No
dimenhydrinate	Yes – T (ir) C (sr)	Yes – L	No	Yes – use liquid	Yes	Yes	Yes. Bolus or CSCI. Can cause irritation	Yes (Canada) No (US)	no
docusate	Yes – C (ir)	Yes – L	No	No information	No	No	No	Yes	No
domperidone (in US available from a compounding pharmacy)	Yes – T (ir)	Yes – L	No	Yes – use oral liquid	No	No	No	Yes	No
fentanyl	No	No	Yes (buccal)	No	Yes, titrated, and as IV PCA in US	Yes, but not usually used	Yes Bolus or CSCI	Yes, but unusual	Yes (trans-dermal)
fluconazole	Yes – T, C (ir)	Yes	No	Yes – use oral liquid	Yes	No	No	No	No
gabapentin	Yes – C (ir)	No	No	Yes – oral suspension prepared by pharmacist	No	No	No	No	No (Canada) Yes from a compounding pharmacy in US

Table continued overleaf

Drug	Tablet (T)/capsule (C) ir=immediate release sr=sustained release	Liquid (L)/Powder/granules (P,G) Chewable/dispersible (Ch, D)	Buccal/sublingual/nasal	Gastrostomy route possible?[18]	IV	IM	SC CSCI=SC infusion Bolus=bolus injection	Rectal	Topical
glyco-pyrrolate	No	No	No	No information	Yes, but not usually used	Yes, but not usually used	Yes Bolus or CSCI	No	No
haloperidol	Yes – T (ir)	Yes – L Tablets disperse in water	No	Yes. Oral solution can cause diarrhea	Yes, but not usually used	Yes, but not usually used	Yes Bolus or CSCI	No	No
hydromorphone	Yes – T (ir) C (sr)	Yes (G)	No[27]	No information	Yes, commonly used in the US as IV PCA	Yes, but not usually used	Yes[28] Bolus or CSCI	Yes,[29] but not used	No
hyoscine butylbromide (Canada only)	Yes but poor absorption T (ir)	No	No	No (poor absorption)	Yes, but not usually used	Yes, but not usually used	Yes Bolus or CSCI	No	No
hyoscine hydrobromide/scopolamine	No	No	Yes (SL, buccal)[9,30]	No information	Yes, but not usually used	Yes, but not usually used	Yes Bolus or CSCI	No	Yes (trans-dermal)
ibuprofen	Yes – T (ir) T, C (sr)	Yes – L	No	Yes – use oral liquid	No	No	No	No	Yes
ketamine	No	Yes – L (injection used orally)	Yes (SL, nasal) but experience is limited	No information	Yes, but not usually used	Yes, but not usually used	Yes Bolus or CSCI	No	No
ketoconazole	Yes – T (ir)	No	No	Yes – oral solution/ suspension prepared by pharmacist (stop feed 1 hr before and after). May interact with feeds	No	No	No	No	No
ketorolac	Yes – T (ir)	No	No	Possible (crush tabs or use injection), but not recommended because of gastric mucosa effects	Yes	Yes	Yes CSCI	No	Only for eyes
lansoprazole	Yes – C (sr)	No	No	Yes – with 40 ml apple juice	No	No	No	No	No

Drug									
loperamide	Yes – C (ir)	Yes – T (quick-dissolve)	Yes – use quick-dissolve tablet	Yes – disperse capsule contents in water. Oral solution can cause diarrhea	No	No	No	No	No
lorazepam	Yes – T (ir)	No	Yes (SL, tab), but absorption may be oral[31,32]	Yes – dissolve SL tablet in water (if can't be given sublingually)	Yes	Yes	Yes	No	No
methadone	Yes – T (ir)	Yes – L	Yes[33]	No information	No (Canada) Yes, used in US as IV PCA	No	No	Yes[34,35]	No
metoclopramide	Yes – T (ir)	Yes – L	No	Yes – crush tablets and disperse in water (takes 5 mins). Oral liquid can cause diarrhea	Yes, but not usually used	Yes, but not usually used	Yes[36] Bolus or CSCI	Yes,[37] but not usually used	No
metronidazole	Yes – T (ir)	No	No	No	Yes	No	No	Yes	Yes
methotrimeprazine (Canada only)	Yes – T (ir)	No	No	Yes – crush tablet with water	Yes, but not usually used	Yes, but not usually used	Yes Bolus or CSCI	No	No
methylphenidate	Yes – T (ir/sr)	No	No information	No information	No	No	No	No	No
midazolam	No	No	Yes (buccal or nasal)[7,38]	Yes – use diluted injection solution	Yes, but not usually used	Yes, but not usually used	Yes[39] Bolus or CSCI	Yes, but not usually used	No
morphine	Yes – T (ir) T, C (sr)	Yes – L, SR cap with granules	SL – no[40] Nasal – yes[41]	Yes – use oral liquid or mix SR granules and flush with 30 ml water	Yes, commonly used in US as IV PCA	Yes, but not usually used	Yes	Yes[42]	Yes[43–45]
ondansetron	Yes – T (ir)	Yes – L	No	Yes – use oral liquid or diluted injection solution	Yes	No	Yes Bolus or CSCI	No	No
octreotide	No	No	No	No information	Yes, but not usually used	No	Yes Bolus or CSCI	No	No

Table continued overleaf

Drug	Tablet (T)/capsule (C) ir=immediate release sr=sustained release	Liquid (L) Powder/granules (P,G) Chewable/dispersible (Ch, D)	Buccal/sublingual/nasal	Gastrostomy route possible?[18]	IV	IM	SC CSCI=SC infusion Bolus=bolus injection	Rectal	Topical
omeprazole	Yes – T (sr)	No	No	Crush the tablet and mix with 10 ml Na bicarb solution (1.6 g NaHCO₃ mixed with water to 120 ml). Administer 50 ml sod bicarb solution via tube, then add omeprazole suspension, then follow with 50 ml sod bicarb solution	No	No	No	No	No
oxycodone	Yes – T (ir) C (sr)	No	No[27]	Yes – crush tablets with water	No	No	No	Yes[46,47]	No
pamidronate	No	No	No	No	Yes, with 500 ml 0.9% saline over 4 hours	No	Yes, diluted in 500 ml 0.9% saline over at least 4 hours[48]	No	No
pantoprazole	Yes – T (sr)	No	No	No	Yes	No	No	No	No
phenobarbital	Yes – T (ir)	Yes – L	No	Yes – use oral liquid	Yes, but not usually used (injection not currently available in Canada)	Yes, but not usually used (injection not currently available in Canada)	Yes Bolus or CSCI	Yes[49]	No
phenytoin	Yes – T (ir), C (sr)	Yes – L, Ch	No	Yes – dilute oral liquid by half with water, flush well. May bind to tube. May interact with feeds	Yes	Yes	No	No	No
ranitidine	Yes – T (ir)	Yes – L	No	Yes – crush tablets in water (takes 5 mins)	Yes	Yes, but not usually used	Yes[50]	No	No
scopolamine/hyoscine hydrobromide	No	No	Yes (SL, buccal)[9,30]	No information	Yes, but not usually used	Yes, but not usually used	Yes Bolus or CSCI	No	Yes (transdermal)

senna	Yes – T (ir)	Yes – L	No	No information	No	No	No	No	No
spironolactone	Yes – T (ir)	No	No	Yes	No	No	No	No	No
sucralfate	Yes – T (ir)	Yes – L	No	Yes – use oral liquid diluted with equal amount of water (stop feed 1hr before and after). Binds to feeds	No	No	No	Yes (local action)	Yes[51,52]
temazepam	Yes – C (ir)	No	No	No information	No	No	No	No	No
tramadol (not currently available in Canada)	Yes	No	No	Yes	No	No	No	No	No
tranexamic acid/ aminocaproic acid	Yes – T (ir)	No	No	Yes – crush tablet with water	Yes, but not usually used	No	No	No	Yes[53,54]
valproic acid	Yes – C (ir)	Yes – L	No	Yes – use liquid	Yes, over 3–5 mins	No	No	Yes[55]	No
warfarin	Yes – T (ir)	No	No	Yes – disperse tablets in water. May interact with feeds	No	No	No	No	No

Drugs suitable for CSCI

Drug	Local irritation*	Diluent	May be incompatible with**	Alternative to CSCI
Commonly used by CSCI				
glycopyrrolate	uncommon	N. saline	dexamethasone	sublingual hyoscine hydrobromide
haloperidol	uncommon	N. saline	dexamethasone hyoscine butylbromide ketorolac	haloperidol as single SC bedtime dose
hydromorphone	uncommon	N. saline		SC dose q4h
hyoscine butylbromide (Canada only)	uncommon	N. saline	haloperidol	hyoscine as SC dose 4–6 hourly
hyoscine hydrobromide/ scopolamine	uncommon	N. saline		sublingual hyoscine hydrobromide/scopolamine patch
methotrimeprazine	occasional	N. saline	dexamethasone	methotrimeprazine as single SC bedtime dose
metoclopramide	uncommon	N. saline		SC dose 8-hourly or domperidone PR
midazolam	uncommon	N. saline	ketorolac	diazepam as single PR bedtime dose
morphine	uncommon	N. saline		SC dose q4h
octreotide	uncommon	N. saline	dexamethasone	octreotide as SC dose 8-hourly
scopolamine/ hyoscine hydrobromide	uncommon	N. saline		sublingual hyoscine hydrobromide/scopolamine patch
Limited experience of CSCI				
alfentanil	uncommon	N. saline		Buccal alfentanil/fentanyl/ sufentanil or transdermal fentanyl
clodronate[56]	limited experience	N. saline (1 liter over 24 hrs)	No experience with other drugs – use alone	IV infusion
dexamethasone	uncommon	N. saline	glycopyrrolate haloperidol methotrimeprazine	dexamethasone as single SC morning dose
fentanyl	uncommon	N. saline		transdermal fentanyl
ketamine	uncommon	N. saline	Limited experience with other drugs	ketamine as SC dose 8-hourly
methadone[57,58] (parenteral form not available in Canada)	common	N. saline	Limited experience with other drugs	methadone as rectal or SL dose
ondansetron, granisetron	uncommon	N. saline	methotrimeprazine, metoclopramide	Give as SC injection 8-hourly
pamidronate[48,56]	can be irritant	N. saline (500 ml over 24 hrs)	No experience with other drugs – use alone	IV infusion
ranitidine[51]	uncommon	N. saline	Limited experience[50]	IM or slow IV (2 mins) or SC 50 mg q6h

* Information on local irritation is based only on CSCI. Bolus SC injections are more likely to cause local pain or irritation.
** Only drugs commonly used by CSCI in palliative care are considered.

Problems with syringe pump infusions

Much of the following table is adapted from the UK edition of this guide, where the use of the Graseby syringe drivers (MS16a and MS26) is almost universal. The Graseby drivers are used in Canada, but CADD and CADD-PCA pumps are used a lot more. Although some of the information in the table is specific to the Graseby syringe drivers, other sections would apply to the use of any pump, including PCA pumps, e.g. leaks, wrong infusion site, dead battery, etc.

- Check pump infusions at least 6-hourly.
- If there is a problem, start from the periphery, checking battery, pump type, correct placement of syringe, syringe contents, line, any filters, connections and insertion site.

In the US, intravenous PCA pumps are often used if opioids are given parenterally. The use of Graseby or CADD pumps/drivers is a less common practice in the US. Also see comments on p. 262.

Clinical decision	If YES ⇒ Action
1 **Infusion running through early?**	• *Wrong pump:* using an MS16a (calibrated in mm/hour) instead of an MS26 (calibrated in mm/24 hours) will result in an infusion running 24 times faster than expected. • *Due to priming line at set-up:* this only happens when the rate is set *before* the syringe's contents are used to prime the line and any filters. This is normal and subsequent infusions will run on time. It has the advantage that the rate can be set at the start of the infusion without a subsequent change. • *Is the boost button being used (on MS26)?* Use of the boost facility should be discouraged as experience suggests that symptom control is not improved and may be compromised. • *Has a smaller syringe size been inserted without changing the rate?* Infusions are calibrated in millimeters of plunger travel, not in volume delivered. This means that if a smaller syringe is inserted the infusion will run through early. If a different sized syringe is used the rate must be recalibrated. • *Pump fault:* mechanical or electrical fault – replace pump.

2 **Infusion running through late?**	• *Battery low or exhausted:* replace battery.
	• *Wrong pump:* using an MS26 (calibrated in mm/24 hours) instead of an MS16a (calibrated in mm/hour) will result in an infusion running 24 times slower than expected.
	• *Due to failure to reset the rate:* this only occurs if the rate is set *after* priming the line. Subsequent infusions will run late unless the rate is changed.
	• *Has a larger syringe size been inserted without changing the rate?* Infusions are calibrated in millimeters of plunger travel, not in volume delivered. This means that if a larger syringe is inserted the infusion will run through late. If a different sized syringe is used the rate must be recalibrated.
	• *Syringe out of position:* check the syringe is correctly positioned and locked in place.
	• *Blocked line:* the pump will usually switch off. A blockage may be due to:
	  – kinked line: replace and refill the line
	  – clamp left on the line: remove the clamp
	  – blood in the needle/cannula: re-site the infusion site (*see* cd-7)
	  – drug precipitation: *see* cd-5.
	  NB: A blocked spinal line should only be checked by a pain or palliative care specialist with experience in spinal lines.
	• *Pump fault:* mechanical or electrical fault – replace pump.

3 **Excess drug effects?**	• *Overinfusion:* check through the reasons for an infusion running through early in cd-1 above. • *Incorrect infusion site:* Subcutaneous: aspirate to check that the needle or cannula is not intravenous. Spinal: contact pain or palliative care specialist with experience in spinal lines. • *Administration error* in making up the drug.
4 **Reduced drug effects?**	• *Leak:* check all connections and lines for signs of leakage. If filters are being used their connectors can easily develop fine cracks. Because infusion rates are very low (0.5 ml/hour or less) leaks may not be obvious, so if a leak is suspected it is best to replace and refill all lines and filters. Many teams no longer use filters in subcutaneous infusions, but they are used in spinal infusions.

- *Drug reactions (when two or more drugs used):* it is possible for a soluble, colourless and inactive product to be produced when two drugs are mixed. This risk is minimized by keeping the number of drugs in the same syringe to a minimum (usually no more than two).
- *Drug precipitation:* check through cd-5 below.
- *Underinfusion:* check through the reasons for an infusion running through late in cd-2.
- *Incorrect infusion site:*
  Subcutaneous: check that the needle or cannula is still in place. Inject 1 ml water to exclude a blockage.
  Spinal: contact pain or palliative care specialist with experience in spinal lines.
- *Administration error* in making up the drug.

5 Change in appearance of infusion solution?	• *Dexamethasone:* add dexamethasone last to other drugs. • *Other drugs:* Check www.palliativedrugs.com or www.pallmed.net for current compatibility data. Ensure water is used as the diluting solution. Dilute drugs by using larger syringe or setting up more dilute 12-hourly or 8-hourly infusions. Consider setting up second syringe driver to reduce number of drugs in one syringe.
6 Site reaction?	• *Swelling:* this is common in subcutaneous infusions and mild swellings only need observation. Infusions for hydration can cause uncomfortable swelling if the wrong sites are used such as the thigh or upper chest. The upper back is the best site for large volumes. Observe if mild, otherwise change site. • *Inflammation/pain:* Stop using highly irritant drugs, e.g. chlorpromazine, diazepam, prochlorperazine. Change to small gauge plastic IV cannula inserted subcutaneously. Consider – adding hydrocortisone 50 mg or dexamethasone 1–2 mg to syringe mixture – rotating sites every 3 days – using other routes, e.g. rectal, transdermal, sublingual (*see* Alternative routes for drugs (p. 262)).
7 Infusion site leaking?	• *Leakage of drug from the infusion site:* this can happen with older sites (7 days or more) even in the absence of inflammation. Change to a new site. • *Bleeding from the infusion site:* this can occur on insertion but stops within minutes. If it persists this may be due to a coagulation disorder: – if bleeding stops within minutes of insertion, flush cannula with 1 ml 0.9% saline, then start infusion – if bleeding persists or starts in an established site, exclude a coagulation disorder and consider alternative routes of drug administration (*see* Alternative routes for drugs (p. 262)).

cd = clinical decision

References

B = book; C = comment; Ch = chapter; CS-n = case study-number of cases; CT-n = controlled trial-number of cases; E = editorial; GC = group consensus; I = interviews; Let = letter; LS = laboratory study; MC = multi-center; OS-n = open study-number of cases; PC = personal communication; R = review; RCT-n = randomized controlled trial-number of cases; RS-n = retrospective survey-number of cases; SA = systematic or meta analysis.

1 *British National Formulary* – 45 (March 2003) London: British Medical Association and Royal Pharmaceutical Society of Great Britain.

2 RCPCH (1999) *Medicines for Children*. Royal College of Paediatrics and Child Health, London.

3 King N (2001) *Guidelines on Symptom Control in Palliative/Terminal Care*. Kent Institute of Medicine & Health Sciences (University of Kent at Canterbury), Canterbury.

4 Jassal SS (2002) *Basic Symptom Control in Paediatric Palliative Care: the Rainbow Children's Hospice Guidelines* (4e). Rainbow Children's Hospice, Loughborough.

5 Institute of Child Health (1994) *Paediatric Analgesia and Antiemetics*. www.ich.ucl.ac.uk/clinserv/anaesthetics/professionals/09analgesics.html.

6 Goldman A (1994) In: *Care of the Dying Child*. OUP, Oxford.

7 Anonymous (2003) Intranasal delivery of morphine may offer better effects. *Clinical Journal of Oncology Nursing*. 7(4): 377.

8 Coda BA, Rudy AC, Archer SM, Wermeling DP (2003) Pharmacokinetics and bioavailability of single-dose intranasal hydromorphone hydrochloride in healthy volunteers. *Anesthesia & Analgesia*. 97(1): 117–23.

9 Zhang H, Zhang J, Streisand JB (2002) Oral mucosal drug delivery: clinical pharmacokinetics and therapeutic applications. *Clinical Pharmacokinetics*. 41(9): 661–80. (R, 101 refs)

10 Siden H, Nalewajek G (2003) High dose opioids in paediatric palliative care. *Journal of Pain and Symptom Management*. 25(5): 397–9. (Let, OS-80)

11 Grond S, Radbruch L, Lehmann KA (2000) Clinical pharmacokinetics of transdermal opioids: focus on transdermal fentanyl. *Clinical Pharmacokinetics*. 38(1): 59–89.

12 Regnard C, Pelham A (2003) Severe respiratory depression and sedation with transdermal fentanyl: four case studies. *Palliative Medicine*. 17: 714–16.

13 Chandler S (1999) Oral transmucosal fentanyl citrate: a new treatment for breakthrough pain. *American Journal of Hospice and Palliative Care*. 16(2): 489–91.

14 Hanks G (2001) Oral transmucosal fentanyl citrate for management of breakthrough pain. *European Journal of Palliative Care*. 8(1): 6–9.

15 Lapwood S (2000) Personal communication to C Regnard.

16 Cranswick N, Coghlan D (2000) Paracetamol efficacy and safety in children: the first 40 years. *American Journal of Therapeutics*. 7(2): 135–41.

17 Bennett M, Simpson K (2002) The use of drugs beyond licence in palliative care and pain management. *Palliative Medicine*. 16: 367–8. (E)

18 Twycross R, Wilcock A, Charlesworth S (2003) *PCF2: Palliative Care Formulary*. Radcliffe Medical Press, Oxford.

19 Palliative Drugs website (2001) www.palliativedrugs.com.

20 Back IN (2001) *Palliative Medicine Handbook* (3e). BPM Books, Cardiff. Also available on www.pallmed.net.

21 Arvidsson J, Nilsson HL, Sandstedt P, Steinwall G, Tonnby B, Flesch G (1995) Replacing carbamazepine slow-release tablets with carbamazepine suppositories: a pharmacokinetic and clinical study in children with epilepsy. *Journal of Child Neurology*. 10(2): 114–17. (MC, CT-31)

22 Neuvonen PJ, Tokola O (1987) Bioavailability of rectally administered carbamazepine mixture. *British Journal of Clinical Pharmacology*. 24(6): 839–41. (RCT)

23 Graves NM, Kriel RL, Jones-Saete C, Cloyd JC (1985) Relative bioavailability of rectally administered carbamazepine suspension in humans. *Epilepsia*. 26(5): 429–33. (OS)

24 Bricaire F, Castaing JL, Pocidalo JJ, Vilde JL (1988) Pharmacokinetics and tolerance of ceftriaxone after subcutaneous administration. [French] *Pathologie et Biologie*. 36(5 Pt 2): 702–5. (CS-8)

25 Rylance GW, Poulton J, Cherry RC, Cullen RE (1986) Plasma concentrations of clonazepam after single rectal administration. *Archives of Disease in Childhood*. 61(2): 186–8. (OS-11)

26 Wennstrom B, Reinsfelt B (2002) Rectally administered diclofenac (Voltaren) reduces vomiting compared with opioid (morphine) after strabismus surgery in children. *Acta Anaesthesiologica Scandinavica*. 46(4): 430–4. (RCT-50)

27 Weinberg DS, Inturrisi CE, Reidenberg B, Moulin DE, Nip TJ, Wallenstein S, Houde RW, Foley KM (1988) Sublingual absorption of selected opioid analgesics. *Clinical Pharmacology & Therapeutics*. 44(3): 335–42. (OS)

28 Vanier MC, Labrecque G, Lepage-Savary D, Poulin E, Provencher L, Lamontagne C (1993) Comparison of hydromorphone continuous subcutaneous infusion and basal rate subcutaneous infusion plus PCA in cancer pain: a pilot study. *Pain*. 53(1): 27–32. (RCT-8)

29 Parab PV, Ritschel WA, Coyle DE, Gregg RV, Denson DD (1988) Pharmacokinetics of hydromorphone after intravenous, peroral and rectal administration to human subjects. *Biopharmaceutics & Drug Disposition*. 9(2): 187–99. (RCT)

30 Golding JF, Gosden E, Gerrell J (1991) Scopolamine blood levels following buccal versus ingested tablets. *Aviation Space & Environmental Medicine*. 62(6): 521–6. (CT-18)

31 Yager JY, Seshia SS (1988) Sublingual lorazepam in childhood serial seizures. *American Journal of Diseases of Children.* **142**(9): 931–2.

32 Gram-Hansen P, Schultz A (1988) Plasma concentrations following oral and sublingual administration of lorazepam. *International Journal of Clinical Pharmacology, Therapy & Toxicology.* **26**(6): 323–4.

33 Dean M (2003) Topical methadone. Bulletin board on www.palliativedrugs.com, 6 June. (PC)

34 Ripamonti C, Zecca E, Brunelli C, Rizzio E, Saita L, Lodi F, De Conno F (1995) Rectal methadone in cancer patients with pain. A preliminary clinical and pharmacokinetic study. *Annals of Oncology.* **6**(8): 841–3.

35 Bruera E, Schoeller T, Fainsinger RL, Kastelan C (1992) Custom-made suppositories of methadone for severe cancer pain. *Journal of Pain and Symptom Management.* **7**(6): 372–4.

36 McCallum RW, Valenzuela G, Polepalle S, Spyker D (1991) Subcutaneous metoclopramide in the treatment of symptomatic gastroparesis: clinical efficacy and pharmacokinetics. *Journal of Pharmacology & Experimental Therapeutics.* **258**(1): 136–42. (CT-10)

37 Hardy F, Warrington PS, MacPherson JS, Hudson SA, Jefferson GC, Smyth JF (1990) A pharmacokinetic study of high-dose metoclopramide suppositories. *Journal of Clinical Pharmacy & Therapeutics.* **15**(1): 21–4. (RCT-14)

38 Lim TW, Thomas E, Choo SM (1997) Premedication with midazolam is more effective by the sublingual than oral route. *Canadian Journal of Anaesthesia.* **44**(7): 723–6. (RCT-100)

39 Gremaud G, Zulian GB (1998) Indications and limitations of intravenous and subcutaneous midazolam in a palliative care center. *Journal of Pain and Symptom Management.* **15**(6): 331–3. (Let, CT)

40 Coluzzi PH (1998) Sublingual morphine: efficacy reviewed. *Journal of Pain and Symptom Management.* **16**(3): 184–92. (R, 30 refs)

41 Pavis H, Wilcock A, Edgecombe J, Carr D, Manderson C, Church A (2002) Pilot study of nasal morphine-chitosan for the relief of breakthrough pain in patients with cancer. *Journal of Pain and Symptom Management.* **24**(6): 598–602. (CS-9)

42 Moolenaar F, Meijler WJ, Frijlink HW, Visser J, Proost JH (2000) Clinical efficacy, safety and pharmacokinetics of a newly developed controlled release morphine sulphate suppository in patients with cancer pain. *European Journal of Clinical Pharmacology.* **56**(3): 219–23. (RCT-25)

43 Krajnik M, Zylicz Z, Finlay I, Luczak J, van Sorge AA (1999) Potential uses of topical opioids in palliative care – report of 6 cases. *Pain.* **80**(1–2): 121–5. (OS-14)

44 Twillman RK, Long TD, Cathers TA, Mueller DW (1999) Treatment of painful skin ulcers with topical opioids. *Journal of Pain and Symptom Management.* **17**(4): 288–92. (CS-9)

45 Krajnik M, Zylicz Z (1997) Topical morphine for cutaneous cancer pain. *Palliative Medicine.* **11**: 325–6. (CS-6)

46 Leow KP, Cramond T, Smith MT (1995) Pharmacokinetics and pharmacodynamics of oxycodone when given intravenously and rectally to adult patients with cancer pain. *Anesthesia & Analgesia.* **80**(2): 296–302. (RCT-12)

47 Leow KP, Smith MT, Watt JA, Williams BE, Cramond T (1992) Comparative oxycodone pharmacokinetics in humans after intravenous, oral, and rectal administration. *Therapeutic Drug Monitoring.* **14**(6): 479–84. (RCT-48)

48 Duncan AR (2003) The use of subcutaneous pamidronate. *Journal of Pain and Symptom Management.* **26**: 592–3.

49 Graves NM, Holmes GB, Kriel RL, Jones-Saete C, Ong B, Ehresman DJ (1989) Relative bioavailability of rectally administered phenobarbital sodium parenteral solution. *DICP.* **23**(7–8): 565–8. (OS-7)

50 Dickman A (2003) SC ranitidine or omeprazole. Bulletin board on www.palliativedrugs.com, 11 Feb. (PC)

51 Banati A, Chowdhury SR, Mazumder S (2001) Topical use of sucralfate cream in second and third degree burns. *Burns.* **27**(5): 465–9. (RCT-85)

52 Regnard CFB, Mannix K (1990) Palliation of gastric carcinoma haemorrhage with sucralfate. *Palliative Medicine.* **4**: 329–30. (Let, CS-1)

53 De Bonis M, Cavaliere F, Alessandrini F, Lapenna E, Santarelli F, Moscato U, Schiavello R, Possati GF (2000) Topical use of tranexamic acid in coronary artery bypass operations: a double-blind, prospective, randomized, placebo-controlled study. *Journal of Thoracic & Cardiovascular Surgery.* **119**(3): 575–80. (RCT-40)

54 McElligot E, Quigley C, Hanks GW (1992) Tranexamic acid and rectal bleeding. *Lancet.* **337**: 431. (Let, CS-1)

55 Yoshiyama Y, Nakano S, Ogawa N (1989) Chronopharmacokinetic study of valproic acid in man: comparison of oral and rectal administration. *Journal of Clinical Pharmacology.* **29**(11): 1048–52. (OS-8)

56 Walker P, Watanabe S, Lawlor P, Bruera E (1996) Subcutaneous clodronate (and pamidronate). *Lancet.* **348**: 345–6. (Let, CS-2)

57 Mathew P, Storey P (1999) Subcutaneous methadone in terminally ill patients: manageable local toxicity. *Journal of Pain and Symptom Management.* **18**(1): 49–52. (CS-6)

58 Bohrer H, Schmidt H (1992) Comment on Bruera et al. Local toxicity with subcutaneous methadone. Experience of two centers, *Pain,* **45** (1991) 141–143. *Pain* **50**(3): 373. (Let)

Index